*Changing Hospitals*

*Contributors*


| | |
|---|---|
| ELIZABETH BARNES | Assistant Secretary, King Edward's Hospital Fund for London |
| RUSSELL BARTON | Physician Superintendent, Severalls Hospital, Colchester, Essex |
| W. J. H. BUTTERFIELD | Professor of Medicine, Guy's Hospital Medical School, London |
| N. F. COGHILL | Consultant Physician, West Middlesex Hospital, Isleworth, Middlesex |
| D. J. DEAN | Head of Nursing Services, Napsbury Hospital, St Albans, Hertfordshire |
| HILARY LEIGH | Research Assistant, Guy's Hospital Medical School, London |
| R. W. REVANS | Research Fellow, European Association of Management Training Centres, Brussels, Belgium; and Guy's Hospital Medical School, London |
| GEORGE F. WIELAND | Assistant Professor, Graduate School of Management, Vanderbilt University, Tennessee, USA |

# *Changing Hospitals*

A REPORT ON THE HOSPITAL INTERNAL COMMUNICATIONS PROJECT

Edited by
GEORGE F. WIELAND and HILARY LEIGH

Assisted by ELIZABETH BARNES

Introduction by R. W. REVANS

Foreword by W. J. H. BUTTERFIELD

TAVISTOCK PUBLICATIONS

*First published in 1971*
*By Tavistock Publications Limited*
*11 New Fetter Lane, London EC4*
*Printed in Great Britain*
*In 10 point Times 2 points leaded*
*By Northumberland Press Limited, Gateshead*

SBN 422 73590 6


*Portions of the evaluation report appeared in*
*an earlier version entitled 'A Preliminary*
*Evaluation Report on the Hospital Internal*
*Communications Project'.*

*Distributed in the USA*
*by Barnes & Noble, Inc.*

# Contents

# *Foreword*

It is a great privilege to write the foreword to this book because it reports the efforts of so many people from so many backgrounds who worked together in ten hospitals towards a common aim, namely better understanding of themselves and their institutions.

Although they were involved in the organization of medical care, it is unlikely that many began their careers with any intention of becoming administrators. As a general rule, doctors and nurses start out with an impulse to help, and their professional education is orientated towards the individual patient, and the prime focus of our efforts. This is a very proper professional ethic and one that we must never lose.

It is only later on that, as doctors and nurses, we are likely to get involved with administration and organization, usually through being drawn into serving on committees and so on. And until recently, we have taken part in such decision-making activity with rather bad grace: we were 'not trained to sit around tables talking' and we have tended to despise it as an occupation. Good clinicians have often been heard referring to their 'having to serve on hospital working parties' as their 'penance', indicating again our general displeasure when responsibility is thrust upon us. We feel ill at ease, it seems, when we have to side with the administration – the same administration that makes unpopular hospital rules or fails to provide quickly enough what we think our individual patients should get if we are to give them the best of modern treatment.

However, we doctors and nurses are just beginning to realize that such carping against administration and management is not good enough, for a variety of reasons that are being borne in on us day by day.

For example, we are beginning to grasp the fact that the NHS is taking ten per cent of the National Budget, equal to an estimated five per cent of the Gross National Product, or about £2,000 million each year. It has suddenly become apparent that the NHS is 'big business' in financial terms, but with the important difference that we cannot draw up a balance sheet each year, because our profits in terms of relief of suffering are not tangible. Consequently our management decisions have to be based on a new sort of objective – the most efficient, humane service feasible with the available resources, buildings, equipment, manpower, skills, treatment, and preventive procedures.

A second point is that the NHS has a complex structure. When we look at how the health budget is spent, it is immediately obvious that there are many branches and activities and that there are interactions between them. Reading the NHS budget and the lists of personnel involved, it requires a very egocentric personality to see oneself simply as an individual fighting a personal crusade for the rights of one's own patients. The NHS is not simply and solely an organization backing my, or any other individual's, ambitions to heal the sick.

Furthermore, doctors and nurses do need to remind themselves from time to time that for historical reasons there are three main divisions of NHS effort – the community services of general practitioners and dentists and their supporting staffs, the local authority services controlled by medical officers of health, and the hospital service. In many parts of the country, especially in the big conurbations, these three divisions worked more or less in isolation for the first fifteen or twenty years of the NHS. At the time of writing, two Green Papers have been published, one by the last Minister of Health – Mr Kenneth Robinson – and one by the first Secretary of State for Health and Social Security – Mr Richard Crossman, both aiming to integrate these various divisions and reorganize them on an Area basis. If adopted, the plan would involve working closely with other members of our professions outside hospitals, some of whom we have, until recently, often misunderstood! To accomplish what will be needed, we shall have to discard many conceits, many shibboleths; but this is easier on an Area than on a national basis.

A third point drawing many of us into new views about management responsibilities is that those of us who work in hospitals – over two-thirds of the NHS manpower – are becoming more and more aware that our institutions, also, have a tripartite structure – the administrative, nursing, and medical professions. With financial restrictions, we are becoming conscious that somehow or other we have got to learn to work together to improve our efficiency and our prospects of finding ways and means of establishing the improvements we want to see in our hospitals – whether it be a better out-patient service, or a renal dialysis unit, or an intensive care unit, or quicker letters to general practitioners, or better follow-up arrangements. For we cannot expect bigger hospital budgets without first being able to demonstrate our improved 'productivity' in terms of efficiency. The sooner we realize that this is the demand Government will make of us, the earlier will come the chances of more funds for the NHS. Tripartite organizations may at first appear unwieldy, but we should be used to them by now in the United Kingdom, from our government – Monarchy, Church, State – and from the established religion – the Holy Trinity. The main point is that if they are to succeed, each part needs to understand the other two.

This brings me to the present study. Since scientists helped in decision-making in World War II, managers are becoming more and more interested in using scientific methods of inquiry to get objective information as the basis for the better understanding needed in industrial organizations. Perhaps most important for readers of the present book, interest and active participation in organization and management problems is becoming more and more respectable among young scientifically trained doctors – the men who tend to be the intellectual trend-setters.

At last, then, it is appropriate to bring R. W. Revans onto the scene. In a letter from Lord Platt, I was asked to see if my department could help Revans launch a study of Hospital Internal Communications. Revans came to have lunch with me. By the emphasis he gave to the results of his study of the reasons behind the resignations of student nurses, showing that they were really an indication of the social health of the whole hospital, he had suddenly emerged from Manchester as someone who might be able to help doctors, nurses, and hospital administrations, in their new role of understanding each other, someone who might be able to help us diagnose hospitals' own health, by making us think about group interactions, ask questions about them, set up inquiries, analyse the results and use them. This might lead to our being able to 'treat' the hospitals we work in. Furthermore, he could suggest non-authoritarian ways of doing this, by taking some hospitals and letting them discover for themselves the power of such internal inquiries into their state of social health.

I appreciated that the idea behind Revans's approach assumes that all is not perfect, that we as individuals could be biased in our ideas about our own role or about the importance or the real extent of our influence. Revans's approach implied criticism and was therefore likely to inflame personal passions in much the same way as did Freud's ideas about sex because, for many of us, our personal image of ourselves at work is coming to represent an important facet of our egos. After all, it's us 8-10 out of 24 hours. But Revans's ideas could help us understand ourselves at work, particularly such things as those outbursts of irrational resentment against our colleagues which may or may not be openly expressed. Or, equally serious though widely practised, the habit of attacking (often covertly) some other part of the hospital community – 'those surgeons', 'those research people', 'those nurses', 'those people in the office'.

I realized too that when this idea of internal inquiry was put forward later among hospital people, many of them would say, 'This is not new – we've been using this sort of approach in management, conducting inquiries before making decisions, for years.' However, the fact of the matter is that we usually collect information about medicine or administrative or nursing matters without thinking much of the other two parts of the hospital. Everything we aim to do produces interactions and problems between administrators, doctors, and nurses. We avoid unpleasant interactions and problems in our own departments by discussions; how often do we have discussions between the administrators, nurses, and doctors? Only alas, at Board level.

As our lunch went on, remembering how we used any means of inquiry as a basis for collecting information for decision-making during my service with the Army Operational Research Group, I knew I was committed personally to help Revans, as best I could, with his Hospital Internal Communications Project. The rest is recorded in what follows, except perhaps to say how very much I personally have been helped throughout by my colleague at Guy's, Dr J. A. D. Anderson.

Over the years, there have, of course, been ups and downs with the H.I.C. Project. We had to feel our way forward. It emerged that we were slow to identify the full educational requirements involved in the studies in ten different hospitals, to use the notion of management by objectives, to structure meetings for a specific purpose. But our stumbling progress seems to me to be proof of the original contention that the idea was new. We just have not thought enough, inquired enough, or done enough about internal communications.

In retrospect, the whole Project has been a fascinating, sometimes frustrating, experiment. The first phase is now complete, and two reports have been written, one a detailed account and evaluation of the overall project, and the other reporting what happened in the ten co-operating hospitals, which we hope will provide 'case records' of general interest for those with administrative responsibility in hospitals up and down the country.

We have, of course, confirmed that our hospital internal communications are often, indeed usually, inadequate and that thoughtful people with responsibility in hospitals or other health, or non-profit, organizations should strive to improve them. In fact, if your organization cannot gauge its success each year in a financial statement, the best alternative is to assess the communication impact you have had on people's minds and thinking!

Obviously, there will have to be a pause in this sort of H.I.C. inquiry in the NHS while we all take stock of things and ask ourselves two questions. First, how can we find the time and resources to do a better job personally in communicating in our hospital work?

Secondly, we might ask ourselves whether the sort of self-inquiry and devotion to internal communications reported here for hospitals might not be expanded to an Area basis – that is between the three divisions of the NHS. My personal experiences with the Thamesmead project, which is a sort of prototype Area Health Board, certainly convince me of the potential value of such an inquiry into the communication problems between general practitioner, hospitals, and local authorities. Even if it were undertaken in an informal way between leaders in the different branches of the NHS in an Area, there could be few better ways of preparing for any new NHS legislation about Area Health Boards.

So, I believe, if you read the accounts of what happened with this Project in the various hospitals, you will come to some interesting conclusions not only about yourself, but about your hospital and about your local community as a whole.

To act, one must understand; to understand, one must inquire; before acting, it pays to explain.

*Guy's Hospital Medical School* W. J. H. BUTTERFIELD
*October 1970*

# *Editorial note and acknowledgements*

This book, together with its companion volume (Revans, in press), is the final report on the Hospital Internal Communications Project. It represents the work of many individuals and organizations who were courageous enough to support, and actively involve themselves in, a very unusual action-research project.

Perhaps the greatest debt of gratitude is due to those staff members of the ten hospitals who took part in the Project and who subsequently agreed to the publication of our joint efforts. However, without the initiative and persistence of Miss Janet Craig of the King's Fund Hospital Centre in organizing the initial conferences, it is doubtful whether the Project would have got off the ground. Together with the chairman of the Hospital Centre, Mr Philip Constable, and the (then) director, Mr W. E. Hall, Miss Janet Craig and Professor R. W. Revans successfully interested the secretaries of the four metropolitan regional hospital boards and members of the Department of Health, in particular Mr John Cornish and Miss Marjorie Simpson. It was their joint efforts in organizing, supporting, and actually taking part in the early meetings at the Hospital Centre that led some of the senior staff of ten London hospitals to agree to take part in the Project.

The Department of Health and Social Security financed the major part of the Project for over four years. Mr John Cornish and Miss Marjorie Simpson represented the Department on the Project's advisory committee and, we feel, showed great dedication and courage in supporting the Project, particularly in their intellectual and scientific curiosity (and risk-taking propensity) to promote actions that might improve the hospital service.

The Hospital Centre, which helped in so many ways, also housed the central team and the evaluation team, and provided meeting facilities and secretarial help for most of the Project period. We had a most enjoyable and fruitful stay there and would like to thank all the staff of the Hospital Centre especially the director, Mr Miles Hardie, and the assistant director, Miss Janet Craig, for their generous and willing help.

Together with Mr Constable, Mr Hardie and Miss Craig also served on the advisory committee. In addition to their many other contributions they performed a very important function as committee members. They continually reminded us of the situation of the hospitals and the many conflicting demands made upon their resources, as well as keeping to the fore the idea that Project efforts should eventuate in better patient-care.

Guy's Hospital Medical School played a major role in this Project. Through Professor W. J. H. Butterfield of the Department of Medicine and Dr J. A. D. Anderson of the Department of Community Medicine, the School employed the Project staff and administered the grant. As chairman of the advisory committee Professor Butterfield had a particularly difficult task, for, as the reader will learn, the committee found itself faced with executive as well as advisory functions. His skill and insight in encouraging, interpreting, and integrating the interests of all those involved was much appreciated.

Throughout the Project, Dr J. A. D. Anderson was a source of unfailing support and help in unravelling the complex administrative problems of the Project staff. For his patience and personal concern in carrying out this task we should like to express our very special thanks.

The advisory committee and many others, not least of all the ten participating hospitals, enabled the Project to go forward. Among these we should like to mention particularly the following:

Mr Robert Harcourt, senior lecturer in the School of Social Sciences, Brunel University, who gave advice and assistance with projects at Queen Mary's Hospital, West Middlesex Hospital, and Hillingdon Hospital; Mr Norman Sida, Head of the Faculty of Arts at Enfield College of Technology, and three lecturers, Mr Trevor Holley, Miss Adrienne Mead, and Mr Phil Bourne, who helped with a project at North Middlesex Hospital; Mr A. J. C. Lewis, senior lecturer in the Department of Business Studies, Croydon Technical College, and four of his students, Mr G. D. Braham, Mr A. H. Ellson, Miss B. Nicholson, and Mr B. B. Reid, for their help in a project at Mayday Hospital; the staff of the computer department at Brunel University who assisted Hillingdon Hospital; and the staff of the computer department at Essex University who assisted Severalls Hospital.

The conception of the Project and the vital, successful bringing together of hospitals, central team, and evaluation team, as well as other supporters, was effected by Professor R. W. Revans. It will be clear that his ideas provided the central intellectual and practical action basis of this Project. We hope this report will in some small way fulfil the expectations and beginnings provided by Revans.

The presentation of a full, detailed, and multi-faceted report of the Project was envisaged at an early point by the advisory committee. Throughout the somewhat lengthy gestation, committee members have read and commented on successive drafts. We have also benefited from the comments of others who have read portions of the text, especially Mr Duncan N. Smith, Dr N. F. Coghill, Dr J. S. Stewart, Dr Robert Rapoport, Professor Maurice Kogan, and Mr Brian Moores. Financial support during the writing was provided by the Department of Health and Social Security. Additional thanks for supporting revision and editorial activities by Wieland are due to the Graduate School of Management, Vanderbilt University, who also generously provided hospitality and facilities for part of that period to Leigh.

As acknowledged on the title page, we have been able in part to meet our editorial responsibilities through the advice and help of Miss Elizabeth Barnes, who has commented and made detailed suggestions on the central team's report. Together with Mrs Sheila Hillier, she also helped with earlier versions of the hospital reports.

Acknowledgements are also due to Mrs Sheila Hillier, Miss Moira Jones, and Miss Marilyn Hopkinson for their help in preparing data for Chapters 4 and 6, and to Mr Ewbank of the Hospital Centre who drew the hospital projects chart.

Portions of the manuscript were typed by Mrs Angela Yardy, Miss Angela Jarvis, and Miss Stella Mill. Further thanks are due to a number of individuals who worked on the evaluation study and these are acknowledged in the introduction to the evaluation report. Finally we should like to thank Dr G. J. Leigh for his patience, and unremitting support, and practical help in reading, checking, and commenting on seemingly endless revisions of our manuscripts.

It will become clear to the reader that this Project was intended to be, and did develop into, separate action and evaluation programmes. Consonant with this, we have been careful to see that the separate substantive viewpoints of the project and the evaluation were not altered or affected by each other. Within this rather severe constraint, however, we have attempted to reduce redundancy and unnecessary and distracting stylistic idiosyncracies, and in other ways to integrate editorially all parts of the volume, while preserving the different perspectives and conclusions that emerged from the Project. While acknowledging the help of the many people cited above, we must, both as editors and as authors, accept full responsibility for the decisions made in these roles.

Lest we exhaust the reader before he even begins the text, we close this note with a brief outline of the make-up of the book. Three different vantage points of the Project are represented in Parts 2, 3 and 4 of this volume, while Part 1 provides the prologue to these separate views.

In Part 1, the reader is provided with an introduction and the background of the H.I.C. Project. First (Chapter 1), Revans describes the antecedents, including an analysis of the practical problems facing hospitals, which led him to set up the H.I.C. Project. Leigh (Chapter 2) then provides a chronicle of the life of the Project, giving the reader an overall view and an introduction to some of the terms and issues to be examined subsequently. Next (Chapter 3), Wieland provides a view of the Project from the perspective of research and practice in the new discipline of 'planned organizational change'.

The remainder of the volume provides the details of the Project's operation, of its consequences or outcomes, as well as conclusions and reflections upon its value. However, no single set of conclusions – agreed upon by all participants – is provided, nor do we feel this would be desirable, since the Project can and did mean different things to different people. Thus, the reader will have to turn to each of the three remaining parts of the volume to obtain these conclusions.

In Part 2, the central team describes the recruiting of hospital participants and the organizing of the Project, including the initial training courses (Chapter 4). Chapter 5 describes the assembling and organization of the central team to give assistance to hospitals in carrying out their individual projects (Chapter 6), and to provide a series of meetings to facilitate Project work (Chapter 7).

The hospitals describe their experiences in Part 3. The reports of two hospitals have been chosen to give this perspective; the remainder of the reports appear in the companion volume to this book (Revans, in press). The central emphasis in these reports is the practical meaning of the hospital project work for the functioning of the hospitals and for the top staff who comprised the hospital teams.

Finally, Part 4 comprises an independent evaluation of what was done and what was accomplished by the H.I.C. Project. Acknowledgements and an account of the origins of the evaluation team and the evaluation design are provided (Introduction and Chapter 10). Next (Chapters 12-14) come analyses of the effects of the H.I.C. Project on length of patient stay, on staff turnover and absenteeism, and on communications and problem-solving. Detailed analyses of the apparent antecedents of the results of the Project are recounted in Chapters 15-18, followed by a summary and the conclusions of the evaluation study in Chapter 19, the last chapter of the book.

*Department of Community Medicine* G. F. W.
*Guy's Hospital Medical School* H. E. L.
*April 1970*

# *Participants*

PROJECT DIRECTOR

| | |
|---|---|
| R. W. Revans | Research Fellow, European Association of Management Training Centres, Brussels; and Guy's Hospital Medical School, London |

ADVISORY COMMITTEE

| | |
|---|---|
| J. A. D. Anderson (Secretary) | Head of Department of Community Medicine, Guy's Hospital Medical School |
| W. J. H. Butterfield (Chairman from 1966) | Professor of Medicine, Guy's Hospital Medical School |
| P. H. Constable | Chairman, King's Fund Hospital Centre Committee (until 1968) |
| J. B. Cornish | Statistics and Research Division, Department of Health and Social Security |
| Janet Craig | Assistant Director, King's Fund Hospital Centre |
| R. Gedling (Chairman until 1966) | Under-Secretary, Ministry of Health (until 1966) |
| W. E. Hall | Director, King's Fund Hospital Centre (until 1966) |
| M. C. Hardie | Director, King's Fund Hospital Centre (from 1966) |
| Marjorie Simpson | Nursing Officer (Research), Department of Health and Social Security |

CENTRAL TEAM

| | | |
|---|---|---|
| Elizabeth Barnes | Group discussion organizer | January 1966 – December 1968 |
| | Administrator | July 1967 – December 1968 |
| | (part-time) | April 1968 – December 1968 |
| Barbara Bellaby | Information officer | March 1965 – December 1966 |
| Sheila Hillier | Research assistant | April 1967 – November 1968 |
| Hilary Leigh | Research assistant | October 1965 – December 1969 |
| | Administrator | January 1967 – June 1967 |
| A. C. Ogborne | Research assistant (part-time) | May 1967 – November 1967 |
| Rosalind Pinder | Research assistant | December 1966 – February 1967 |
| D. N. Smith | Director | January 1965 – January 1967 |

*Student Members*

| | | |
|---|---|---|
| P. D. Casson | Brunel University | July 1966 – December 1966 |
| Jennifer Coghill | Enfield College of Technology | June 1967 – September 1967 |
| Leela Damodaran | Brunel University | July 1967 – December 1967 |
| Marion Dries | Sussex University | July 1966 – August 1966 |
| Pauline Earnshaw | Loughborough University | April 1967 – December 1967 |
| K. G. Eason | Brunel University | July 1966 – December 1966 |
| Helen Harrison | Sussex University | July 1966 – August 1966 |
| J. A. Holland | King's Fund College of Hospital Management | November 1965 – January 1966 |
| Marilyn Hopkinson | Loughborough University | April 1968 – September 1968 |
| A. Z. Jankowicz | Brunel University | August 1967 – December 1967 |
| Moira Jones | Brunel University | April 1968 – September 1968 |
| Gillian Lincoln | Brunel University | July 1966 – December 1966 |
| B. Scott | Brunel University | July 1966 – December 1966 |
| C. G. Shelley | Brunel University | July 1967 – December 1967 |
| Elizabeth Stenning | Brunel University | September 1966 – December 1966 |
| H. C. Y. Wagener | Leiden University, Holland | June 1966 – August 1966 |
| R. J. T. Watts | Loughborough University | April 1967 – December 1967 |

*Secretarial Staff*

| | | |
|---|---|---|
| Barbara Beskin | King's Fund Hospital Centre | June 1968 – December 1968 |
| Carol Kippin | Guy's Hospital Medical School | January 1969 – July 1969 |
| Linda Sparrow | Guy's Hospital Medical School | February 1969 – July 1969 |
| Angela Yardy | King's Fund Hospital Centre | January 1965 – June 1968 |

EVALUATION TEAM

| | | |
|---|---|---|
| Patricia Day | Research assistant | September 1967 – January 1969 |
| A. C. Ogborne | Research assistant (part-time) | September 1966 – April 1967<br>May 1967 – November 1967 |
| Elizabeth Stenning | Research assistant | September 1967 – September 1968 |
| R. J. T. Watts | Research assistant | September 1968 – October 1969 |
| G. F. Wieland | Evaluator | May 1966 – October 1969 |

*Secretarial Staff*

| | | |
|---|---|---|
| Angela Archer | Part-time | June 1966 – July 1967 |
| Kathleen Chapman | Part-time | September 1967 – July 1969 |

*Interviewers*

| | | |
|---|---|---|
| Marion Anderson | Part-time | February 1967 – January 1969 |
| Gillian Cowan | Part-time | February 1967 – January 1969 |

While they were working on the Project, D. N. Smith and G. F. Wieland were research associates and all other central and evaluation team members were research assistants in the Department of Medicine, Guy's Hospital Medical School.

HOSPITAL-TEAM MEMBERS

| | | |
|---|---|---|
| W. Alderson | North Middlesex | Assistant group secretary |
| T. H. Arie | The London | Senior lecturer in social medicine |
| W. E. Bardgett | Hillingdon | Group secretary |
| R. Barton | Severalls | Physician superintendent |
| Marjorie Bell | Lewisham | Matron |
| Pamela Birleson | The London | House governor's assistant |
| D. E. Bolt | West Middlesex | Consultant surgeon |
| Vera Boyce | Mayday | Matron |
| June Brett | St Nicholas | Consultant anaesthetist |
| A. J. Brooking | Lewisham | Group secretary |
| J. T. Bryant | Mayday | Deputy hospital secretary |
| G. H. L. Bullmore | St Ebba's | Deputy medical administrator |
| Margaret Bunyan | West Middlesex | Assistant matron |
| R. C. Cains | Lewisham | Administrator |
| J. H. Carter | West Middlesex | Deputy hospital secretary |
| A. Cavendish | Lewisham | Consultant surgeon |
| B. Chant | North Middlesex | Group catering officer |
| Ruth Clarke | Severalls | Matron |
| N. F. Coghill | West Middlesex | Consultant physician |
| L. Collis | St Ebba's | Hospital secretary |
| J. T. Cooper | Mayday | Deputy group secretary |
| J. K. Corbett | Severalls | Director of nursing |
| T. W. Cummings | St Ebba's | Assistant chief male nurse |
| Margaret Cutliffe | The London | Deputy matron |
| D. J. Dean | Severalls | Senior assistant to director of nursing |
| Deborah Donohoe | Edgware | Sister |
| Sandra Dreier | West Middlesex | Sister |

| | | |
|---|---|---|
| G. W. Duncan | Hillingdon | Medical administrator |
| R. Dunkley | Hillingdon | Deputy group secretary |
| S. H. Dunmall | St Nicholas | Hospital secretary |
| C. H. Dunn | West Middlesex | Senior consultant anaesthetist |
| R. W. Durrant | Queen Mary's | Deputy group secretary |
| D. J. P. Ellis | Severalls | Psychiatric registrar |
| A. M. Evans | West Middlesex | Hospital secretary |
| C. A. R. Evans | North Middlesex | Group secretary |
| M. J. Fairey | The London | Deputy house governor |
| D. Findlay | St Nicholas | Superintendent radiographer |
| R. Fox | Severalls | Consultant psychiatrist |
| W. Gamble | St Ebba's | Chief male nurse |
| F. P. Haldane | West Middlesex | Consultant psychiatrist |
| St. J. V. Hall | Severalls | Principal tutor |
| J. L. Hamilton-Paterson | Edgware | Consultant pathologist |
| W. Harman | Edgware | Senior hospital medical officer |
| D. J. Hooton | Severalls | Group secretary |
| I. Joffee | St Nicholas | Consultant surgeon |
| Dilys Jones | Queen Mary's | Matron |
| Isobel King | Edgware | Group medical records officer |
| Kay Kenrick | North Middlesex | Matron |
| G. S. A. Knowles | North Middlesex | Consultant anaesthetist |
| Joanna Laidman | West Middlesex | Matron |
| C. H. Langley | Mayday | Group secretary |
| S. L. Last | The London | Consultant psychiatrist |
| D. N. Lawson | Queen Mary's | Medical administrator |
| B. E. W. Mace | Lewisham | Consultant in physical medicine |
| L. Manners | Severalls | Deputy director of nursing |
| H. S. C. Marsh | Edgware | Deputy group secretary |
| Barbara Merchant | Edgware | Deputy matron |
| C. A. Merrick | Severalls | Group secretary |
| June Monk | St Nicholas | Medical records officer |
| J. A. Monro | Hillingdon | Consultant anaesthetist |
| Winifred Morgan | St Nicholas | Matron |
| Dorothy Murdock | West Middlesex | Theatre superintendent |
| W. Page | St Nicholas | Principal administrative assistant |
| D. J. Parry | West Middlesex | Senior registrar |
| Marie Perkins | Hillingdon | Deputy matron |
| K. G. Perona-Wright | Queen Mary's | Group secretary |
| Doreen Plews | Mayday | Home sister |
| D. R. Preston | St Nicholas | Group secretary |
| Lucy Pulsford | West Middlesex | Assistant matron |
| E. J. Randall | Severalls | Deputy matron |

| | | |
|---|---|---|
| Mary Rea | St Ebba's | Matron |
| Hannah Roberts | St Nicholas | Assistant matron |
| Dorothy Rogers | St Nicholas | Sister |
| Eleanor Roker | Hillingdon | Matron |
| J. L. C. Scarlett | The London | House governor |
| A. Smith | North Middlesex | Deputy hospital secretary |
| C. A. Steel | West Middlesex | Group domestic manager |
| Pamela Steele | North Middlesex | Deputy matron |
| E. M. Steffens | West Middlesex | Hospital secretary |
| J. S. Stewart | West Middlesex | Consultant physician |
| June Swan | The London | Administrative sister |
| Audrey Thomas | West Middlesex | Deputy matron |
| J. W. Thompson | Lewisham | Hospital secretary |
| P. H. Tooley | The London | Senior consultant psychiatrist |
| L. Trotter | Edgware | Group secretary |
| Margaret Ulyatt | Mayday | Consultant anaesthetist |
| Monica Veale | West Middlesex | Acting matron |
| Pauline Vick | Edgware | Matron |
| W. H. Vine | Queen Mary's | Assistant hospital secretary |
| Dorothy de M. Warren | West Middlesex | Acting matron |
| J. P. Watson | Severalls | Hospital secretary |
| Beryl Webster | The London | Assistant matron |
| Grace White | Lewisham | Ward sister |
| J. A. Whitehead | Severalls | Consultant psychiatrist |
| Brenda Whittle | Queen Mary's | Deputy matron |
| Grace Woods | St Ebba's | Medical administrator |
| Elizabeth M. M. Zucker | West Middlesex | Head medical social worker |

PART ONE

# *Background to the Project*

# 1 *Introduction*

## *R. W. REVANS*

### BEFORE: BACKGROUND AND AIMS OF PROJECT

For almost eight years a group of research workers in what was then the department of industrial administration at the Manchester College of Science and Technology studied the sickness and wastage of nurses in a small sample of Lancashire hospitals (Revans 1964b). The results of this work form the starting-point of the Hospital Internal Communications Project, but only as much of the previous research as seems necessary to introduce the later Project is presented here.

### COMMUNICATION AND LEARNING PROCESSES

The communication system of a hospital is normally intended to bring rapid and accurate information about patients, or about services provided for patients, to the attention of those in responsible positions; both the doctor and the matron wish to be aware of emergencies that arise on the ward. If, from time to time, trouble develops that is not effectively dealt with, the management committee or the senior officers may hold an inquiry and, apart from the allocation of blame, any faults revealed in the communication system will be treated at least in a formal way. New instructions may be issued or new forms of report devised. But it is not generally recognized that junior members of the hospital staff, and patients, are (or feel themselves to be) also in need of information. What is more, they feel this need at the moment when the information is important to them, rather than at some time convenient to those who may be able to supply it. A patient uncertain about his condition, or a junior nurse given incomplete or contradictory instructions, may experience anxiety as a result. This anxiety may perhaps be endurable if some explanation intelligible to the patient or the nurse is forthcoming; whether or not this is possible depends upon the relations between the patient and the nurse, or between the nurse and her superior. An explanation that is technically intelligible and convincing to a qualified staff nurse or to a registrar may be incomprehensible to a first-year student or to a patient. This Manchester research suggested, from many incidents reported during the associated attitude surveys, that where the junior nurse is unable readily to approach the ward sister, the patient cannot approach the junior nurse. Moreover, where the sister is not on easy terms with the consultant she cannot be on easy terms with her own ward staff. The social mechanism is simple: if the consultants appreciate the suggestions of the ward sisters, or even seek them, the sisters will be anxious to have ready for those consultants the maximum information about the patients. To get this information, the sisters will encourage their nurses to discuss the patients with them. This, in turn, means that the nurses will tend to communicate more with the patients, and this communication will encourage the patients also to ask questions. If, on the other hand, the consultants do not regard their ward sisters as important sources of information or advice about the patients, the ward sisters in turn will have little cause for encouraging the nurses to discuss and report on patients in detail. The nurses, therefore, will not be motivated to observe patients closely. In these conditions, the junior nurses and the patients will be deprived of those conversations with their superiors that are among the chief media for their learning and for their adjustment.

There is a simple cycle known in engineering terms as the feedback loop; a machine is controlled by a device that monitors its performance, slowing the machine down should it be too fast, speeding it up should it be too slow. *Learning is also a feedback process, and it consists essentially of seeing the effect of one's own behaviour or getting the answer to one's own question.* Unless one receives intelligible responses to, or clarifying information about, what one is trying to do, it is impossible to learn. Somebody in doubt may have his doubt resolved if he receives an answer to his question about his doubt; his doubt is not removed if he is given information, in whatever quantity, but not in response to his own statement or question that expresses the doubt. Sometimes he may even need help in the framing of his question, because the doubt is of so deep an order that he is completely unable to express it, or even identify it. Hence, if his superior is too busy, too impatient, or too authoritarian to help him in the framing of his own questions, he will find it hard to learn. This, essentially, is the situation of many patients and of many nurses in the hospital ward. The institution is seen as alien, impersonal and secretive.

## ANXIETY AS A CHARACTERISTIC QUALITY OF THE HOSPITAL

Hospitals are communities cradled in anxiety. Patients are anxious not only about their own health but about the welfare of their families. Junior nurses are anxious about the difficulties of training, and often tormented by the fear that they may be inadequate in their treatment of the patients. Sisters are often anxious about the good order of their wards and about their relations with the matron and the consultants. Although the task of ward sister, taken day in and day out, must be one of the most satisfying in the whole field of human employment, it is charged with frequent emotional crises that reveal the sister in a flash of revolt against her superiors. Anxious that they may be driving their nurses, the sisters project upon the matron the image of the battle-axe; anxious that they may not be living up to their own standards of patient care, they project upon their junior nurses the image of an irresponsible flightiness. Consultants, for all their marmoreal composure, are often anxious men at heart because they must be constantly taking important decisions on incomplete information. The opposition now manifested by some consultants to studies of their roles, in an attempt to understand better some of the grave problems of hospital administration, can be partly explained as a symptom of indefinable anxiety. Many administrative officers of hospitals are uneasy about their relations with the hospital management committees; and the latter often work off their anxieties by regarding regional boards as arbitrary and dictatorial bureaucrats knowing little of hospital life. Faced with requests from the Department of Health, some group secretaries proceed more cautiously than a tomcat on a barbed wire fence. All this is evidence of an ever present uncertainty. It is a striking fact that on most hospital wards the only persons who seem permanently secure are the domestics; middle-class patients rarely fail to comment about the cheerfulness and equanimity of the cleaners, and frequently turn to them for information or help rather than to the nursing staff. This is not a matter of temperament; it is a freedom from insecurity, since the cleaner knows precisely what she has to do and, in an atmosphere of tension and anxiety, alone may radiate a reassuring calm.

## THE ONSET OF PARATAXIS

A patient must, nevertheless, have confidence in those who treat him. A man with a dependent family, unhinged by pain or even by the fear of death, demands that those who look after him know their business. The junior nurse, too, may wish only for precise instructions in a stressful emergency, when she senses neither need nor opportunity to question. The consultant, therefore, at least by the majority of his patients, is called upon to give an appearance of omniscience. Many respond superbly. But what if the doctor is asked a question by the nurse or by the patient to which he does not know the answer? It would be unprofessional to fabricate some reply that might quieten but mislead the questioner. On the other hand, young ward sisters confess that they often bluff their junior nurses. One simple way of dealing with questions to which one does not know the answer is to discourage such (and so, all) questions, and some hospital staff seem to employ this defence as a matter of course.[1] Such behaviour sets in motion a self-generating and pathological process. Anxiety, always latent, is enhanced by uncertainty. Uncertainty, in turn, is magnified by communication failure. But the difficulties of communicating, and of being communicated with, are in turn heightened by their own very consequences – namely, unrealistic ideas of one's own role, knowledge, status, and other features of the self-image. Those who believe that the way to deal with questions to which they do not know the answer is to discourage such questions are unrealistically defensive. Psychology has a term for such misperception: parataxis.[2] Parataxis inhibits the very communication from which alone patients or nurses may learn. Hence the self-generating process progresses cycle by cycle. Anxiety produces uncertainty; uncertainty blocks communication; blocked communication enhances parataxis; parataxis breeds further uncertainty. The intensity of the process reaches a level that not only the junior nurse, but also the ward sister, can no longer endure, and they may leave the hospital. The Manchester studies also showed these same reactions at work among the matrons, and it would be remarkable if, in different hospitals, according to the richness or transparency of their communication, the consultants did not hold significantly different perceptions of their own dependence upon others and of the dependence of others upon them. Certainly the deep study of managerial attitudes in industry suggests the influence of the particular institution upon levels of satisfaction and of achievement.

### PARATAXIS AND SOCIAL LEARNING

A hospital fraught with anxiety is faced with a problem of understanding itself. Its first need is to obtain a clear picture of its problems. The staff in many hospitals, from the hospital secretary to the porters, are often aware of specific difficulties that may confront them, such as a chronically inefficient records system or a temporary ill-feeling produced by the preparation of the nurses' off-duty rota. Such infelicities may be widely and painfully experienced. But it is one thing to sense such trouble; it is another to be clear about its origins within, or its impact upon, the hospital as a whole, and something else altogether to be clear about one's own responsibility for causing or helping to cause it. What to do about it and how to do it may present still greater challenges. It is one thing for a patient to be aware of pain and discomfort; it is quite another to know specifically what is wrong with him in order to treat it, and something else altogether to effect in him a change of habit or behaviour to bring about a cure.

A general attitude survey conducted by outsiders may produce an emotional map of the hospital that in its entirety would be unrecognizable by the hospital staff as a whole, although particular members might be well aware of its local features. The results of such a survey might then be used for generating inquiry and discussion among those involved in the hospital. Such inquiry and discussion might lead to a demand for the deeper investigation of some part of the system; this, in turn, might lead to the staff asking questions of themselves and their work that had never before been posed. They might gain, in other words, a more realistic view of their own place in the hospital and of the effect of their own behaviour upon others. This would tend to diminish parataxis and, with it, anxiety. Such change would not be easy. We know, at the moment, little about the processes of social learning in circumstances of extreme anxiety, from which participants perceive better both the system to which they belong, and also their own personal influence upon the functioning of that system.[3] It is learning at this emotional depth that is likely to help the hospital. Parataxis is not to be cured by resolutions of management committees nor by memoranda circulated by superior officials. Such action may, if anything, tend to make parataxis worse by reinforcing in those in positions of nominal authority an unrealistic view of their actual power to improve the hospital communication system. The process of social learning, of course, should involve the hospital management no less than it involves the ward sisters or the consultants. If a hospital management's view of what should be its relations with the matron is different from that of the matron herself, and if, as a result, the matron feels she is not supported by her committee, she, in turn, cannot support her sisters. There is evidence that the information about any hospital on which the views of its policy makers must inevitably be formed is often incomplete and, not seldom, biased by the anxieties of the hospital secretary and other senior officers. Indeed, the whole question of what ought to govern the relations of the hospital management to its senior officers and, *a fortiori*, those of a regional board to the local hospital management, is one to which our answers are at present shadowy and incomplete.[4] Yet the evidence is that these relations vitally affect what happens on the wards, and, in particular, help to determine the fate of the individual patient and of the student nurse whose desire it is to care for him.

It was with these beliefs in the chance of promoting insight and commitment to change, based upon former researchers, that, with the encouragement of the King's Fund Hospital Centre, the Hospital Internal Communications Project was conceived.

## EDUCATIONAL ASSUMPTIONS

The assumptions of the Project can be stated simply:

(a) that most people are normally willing to work at whatever they are doing;
(b) that, in this work, they welcome, and may even seek, opportunities for self-expression;
(c) that one important aspect of self-expression is self-development, which demands learning;
(d) that, since the learning process requires one to know the effects of one's own performance, true self-expression must depend upon, among other things, a two-way communication process with others in the work situation.[5]

In a successful learning process, it is not that the subject demands public approval for his efforts; he needs to know when he is falling short of standard just as readily as when he has surpassed it. It may be that he can know this only if others tell him, directly or indirectly. This knowledge must be a constant support; learning from a situation must go with living through that situation. The learning process is not merely a didactic exercise reserved for the classroom or the formal seminar. But if everyday experience is to be our teacher, it must be faced in a way that makes learning possible. Some occupations may be so stereotyped that those following them know as little at the ends of their careers as at the start. Few institutions are designed on the assumption that the first need of those who serve them is to make them into better institutions. Even when, as in a modern hospital, the technology on which the organization relies begins to change more rapidly in a decade than it had done since the dawn of history, one operational responsibility of its staff is still perceived as the application of fixed procedural rules in defence against, and in treatment of, their familiar problems. Thus, to managers everywhere, not only in hospitals, the first object of attention is the immediate trouble, the pressing problem; it is rarely the search below the surface of affairs for first causes. The manager's principal perception is not of objectives nor of resources, not of goals nor of means, but of problems. Perhaps it is only the problem-oriented man, one plentifully charged with aggressiveness, who can tolerate the responsibilities of modern institutional life.

Since the Project was primarily designed to take the study of operational problems back to their organic origins, and by such study to engender the notion and practice of institutional learning or organizational psychotherapy, it might here be appropriate to exhibit one of the earliest manifestos aimed at explaining the Project. It was circulated early in 1966 to the participating hospitals and was thereafter used as a basis for discussion by the central team.

'*Aims and Intentions of the Project*

1. Normally, the demands for order and economy oblige hospital staff to develop procedural rules for overcoming operational problems. If no precise rules exist it is expected that those in authority will use precedent or judgement to settle whatever need may arise. Even if the powers and duties of staff have not been set forth in detail there will exist within every hospital an expectation as to who should handle the emergent problem.

2. In such conditions, staff tend not to examine the origins of problems, only to allocate responsibility for dealing with them, or to attribute blame should they not be dealt with. Thus, there is little true learning, certainly no education, the first objective of which is to encourage the ability to ask those questions most likely to lead to the solution of a problem. Education aims to develop the general capacity to inquire, to show people how to set about finding out. Since it seems that the principal defect of many hospitals is a lack of awareness of their internal problems, education in this sense is of great importance. The Hospital Internal Communications Project aims to provide it.

3. We are, as I see it, primarily trying to help those in charge of hospitals

and of their services at all levels, to use better their own resources in identifying and tackling their working problems. We choose this approach both because we believe that these are the greatest resources that the hospitals have available, and because we also believe the hospitals possess at all levels a considerable fund of latent goodwill and ability. Without exception, all research shows that, given the organized opportunity of working through a problem of concern to them personally, those who serve even in the most stressful conditions and who may have seemed most incapable of coping with them can rise to unexpected heights of insightfulness and resolution.

4. Any first hospital project should on this account be seen as a growth point, as a kindergarten in co-operation. It should involve a few people, say up to ten, quite significantly, in collecting data and in discussing the meaning of the data and the relevance of it to the tasks of those involved with it. Beyond this committed core, there should be a supporting force of partisans, not deeply involved, but willing to give help when asked for it, and thus ready to be involved should the project be extended into their territory. Beyond these, all other employees in the hospital should at least know that the project is going on.

A well designed project should have the following qualities:

(a) It should demand the co-operation at all stages of a group of persons whose tasks are interlocked; a study assigned to one or two individuals, to produce a report for others to implement, is useless. The choice of project, its depth and scope, the methods of study to be used, the forms of co-ordination between individuals, the nature of any report to others outside the group, the methods of putting into effect the findings of the project, and so forth, are all essential subjects for agreement between the team leaders and those whose work will be woven into the study.

(b) It should demand, not only co-operation at all stages within the group, but also an appeal to sources of information or ideas outside the group. These at first may be limited to purely technical affairs, such as asking for help from the H.I.C. central team on methods of interview or data classification. Or it may turn out that the working group, in order to make real progress, will need to share the experiences of another hospital, or even to inquire about the treatment of similar problems in industry. For this reason, the hospital team should, at a fairly early stage, be in touch with any local college of technology or commerce with a department of management or administration.

(c) It must be limited in time; from the outset there should be agreement as to when particular stages of the work should be completed. Once such a project is started the interest aroused can be so great that unnecessary delay in taking action may lead to disillusion and hostility in the very places where enthusiasm and co-operation has once been generated.

(d) It should, when completed, suggest another project, elsewhere in the same hospital but involving largely different persons.

5. In work on the project, the framework of authority should be temporarily thrown away. Those involved in it are faced with a new situation; how to define the need, how to collect information, how to work with others, how to measure progress and, above all, how to employ their own abilities. It is as if, by stripping away the hypothetical framework of authority, we are trying to understand how individuals think and act as the persons they are. They are being given an opportunity, like children whose teacher has suddenly left the class-room, to compare notes among themselves as to how a problem can best be solved.

6. The project should teach each of those who work on it at least all of the following:

(i) To observe how the group responds to the originally unstructured situation.

(ii) To question what behaviour on his part will best help himself or the group.

(iii) To act, whether in words or otherwise, of his own volition; as for example, in collecting data or in trying out an idea that seems to him to contribute to the definition or solution of the problem.

(iv) To sense the effects of his words or actions; he learns how his behaviour has affected others and thus can test the adequacy of his self-understanding.

(v) To generalize from this learning; in the project he will begin to sense the accuracy or otherwise of his own impressions and of those of others; he will see how he and others respond to different attempts to influence and be influenced; how differing goals and desires, if contrasted and evaluated freely, lead to learning and to an improved understanding of communications.

7. It follows that, to be successful, the groups must be highly informal and that the imposition of the traditional framework of authority upon their project must be avoided. I have little fear, now that I begin to know some of the senior staffs of the hospitals personally, that such impositions will deliberately occur, once experience of open discussion has been gained. Nevertheless, its removal must be accomplished by slow degrees; senior staffs must gain confidence in free exchanges before subordinates, and in this I feel both the H.I.C. central team and the hospital teams have a role first to learn and then to enact.'

An important assumption behind this manifesto is that self-development is not only possible, but possible within the framework of these proposed action studies. Training may be the acquisition of particular skills or methods for mastering particular difficulties or situations; education is the development of a general ability to learn, that is, *to make those inquiries, including inquiries about one's own role, of any situation, in order to master it by understanding it.* This ability to see one's place in a given situation, either as an agent helping to bring the situation about in the first place, or as an agent likely to help in resolving it – or even as a double agent, with a hand in both its creation and its resolution – is an essential product of education. It can rarely be engendered by adhering to procedural rules. Moreover, as the world changes and new underlying causes are invisibly called into play, the old procedural rules become a fabric of deception and those who try to live by them pass from surprise, through disappointment, to despair, as they progressively recognize that the ancient magic has lost its power. The more we place our trust in the procedural rules, the more cause we have to regret the passing of the 'good old days'. We may, from time to time, of course, bring in new sets of procedural rules, handed down by some newer Moses; we are then faced with the task of unlearning the old rules and taking up the new. But administrative spring cleaning is a tricky and onerous task, and the broom of high authority is rarely long enough to sweep the procedural cobwebs from the organizational rafters. Institutional reflexes, once acquired, can effectively inhibit, and not seldom oppose, any desire for understanding what is new.

## ORGANIZATIONAL LEARNING

It is, therefore, necessary to experiment with practical exercises in self-teaching. Since it is essential that those in the working situation shall also learn their own part in it, these exercises must involve a responding group. The solitary learner has little opportunity to judge his own performance – unless, like the suburban golfer, he is able to practise his swing before a looking-glass. Secondly, the exercises had better choose reality as their theme. One cannot expect a group of persons striving to master some real problem X to do so by perfecting their solution to some different and imaginary problem. For the mastery of problem X demands first its precise identification. Those who work in the real world must define this for themselves. It may prove the hardest stage of their total task. However helpful may be an understanding of the general properties of all problems belonging to some imaginary series, the hope that reality problem X might belong to the same series may be false and so could perplex and confuse. We all tend to attack the problems we think exist, rather than those that can be more exactly identified with a little extra trouble.

We have no general theory of search that enables us to diagnose by automatic rules what may be the nature of our problem; it is an important educational task that we should learn to define it for ourselves. For this reason, courses of training that rely upon the analysis of highly documented examples (case studies) often fail to remind the student that reality carries no such documentation hanging around its neck. Problem identification is, as academics are not seldom inclined to overlook, itself an initial and unavoidable *practical* problem demanding hard-headed solutions. These, in turn, demand the development of the subject's most powerful weapon, observation, so often left unused during most other so-called methods of education.

Our studies must begin, therefore, not only with some group exercises that, issuing from a familiar reality, offer genuine motivation to those who undertake them, but also with an invitation to the group to examine how each of them responds to the unstructured situation. The responses of the members of the group faced with the unknown problem X (such as aggression, clowning, withdrawal, hostility to the power structure, mutual recrimination, fear, overconfidence, rejection of the problem, or whatever it may be) are parts of the problem itself. It is useless to go ahead until this variety of initial responses has been understood; from it must follow both an appreciation, however dim or inaccurate, by each of his own first responses, and a sight of how the group gradually works from these first responses to some kind of collective definition of what problem X eventually might turn out to be.

### AWARENESS OF ROLES AND OF RESPONSES

At this critical point, the group members should encourage themselves to ask, on the one hand, what kind of behaviour they are displaying, namely, what kind of behaviour others see them as displaying; and, on the other hand, what kind of behaviour on their parts could best help the group to make progress, namely, what behaviour their fellows are beginning to expect of them. This may be more than some convenient reallocation of duties in accordance with old rules. For only when the detailed allocation of personal duties or individual contributions comes to be considered can there be any definition of the essential problem X. Unless the implications of one's own behaviour are made clear in the face of the supposed problem, there is no clarification of the problem itself. One may still be able to make an eloquent speech against it – like professors of political science denouncing their own students for striking against professorial authority – but one gains no more power over reality by so doing, unless one also recognizes the need for change within oneself. It is here that the first members of the hospital teams from different hospitals must offer each other the firmest and most sympathetic support. And it is here that all such professional competence as the central team can summon must be made available to them.

The precise involvement of the individual members of a hospital team cannot be laid down in any general specification. The study of an operating theatre, a casualty department, a records system, or whatever other object of attention is selected, must be so specific in itself, and the individualities of its members so different from those of any other group, that the members must work out a detailed programme on their own. Yet progress must always observe the five stages of the general model of the learning process, namely, to find the answer to the five following questions, either openly, or by implication:

1. What facts (including some view of desirable goals, as well as of our problems and resources) can we observe or be given?
2. What first expectations do these seem to suggest?
3. How can we try these expectations out?
4. What results do we actually get by this try-out?
5. What do we conclude after comparing our first expectations with these subsequent results?[6]

A team may be still feeling its way towards its first practical move, deciding, for example, what aspects of the records system to examine or what sample of nurses' opinion to draw; or it may have become deeply involved in the interpretation of a hundred pages of classified observations; or it may have reached its first goal and, encouraged by a small success, be bracing itself to reach a second and greater. Whatever a team may be doing, it must observe the critical framework of this model. Our educational objective is to learn how this can best be done under hospital conditions. It is incidental (but not unimportant) that some particular sub-system studied in a hospital might, in the course of this learning exercise, also be improved. This constant need for each participant to see the study, whatever may be its official description, as a dialogue between a strengthening of his self-image through interactions with others in the group, on the one hand, and an understanding of the learning process by a comparison of result and expectation, on the other, will make severe demands upon the operational team. Should the hospital service one day embark upon a policy of continual training for its managers, one of the most important assets it would need for its support would be the presence, in every hospital, of a person skilled in conducting free discussion groups. The example set by one or two mental hospitals (Main, 1946; Jones, 1962 and 1968) deserves to be widely followed in other branches of the hospital service. There is much, of course, to be learned from the researches of those who have become known as 'change-agents' in other fields, such as in industry and in banking. But the hospital service is so vast, its needs so great, and its grasp upon traditional ideas so tenacious, that there is a case, existing in its own right, for research into its peculiar problems of change. We need not only to know the outcome of these efforts to study what can be done to excite the constructive curiosity of a few courageous pioneers, but we need also to ask whether it is possible to generalize from this sample of ten different but mutually supporting endeavours. This is a powerful justification for involving the university departments of social science in the detailed progress of the studies.

### ON CULTURAL FLEXIBILITY

We live in a culture dominated by the need for each to be successful. None may dare admit that he is wrong, nor even that he has changed his mind in the face of new evidence. An attitude of eternal cocksureness seems particularly necessary to maintain one's position in public life today. The conscience of a nation must never admit to being mistaken, and thus its guardians must be protected from any opportunity of confession or atonement. Hospitals have more urgent needs. If they are to be learning organizations, those who command them must learn too; they must be open to the questions and criticisms of their juniors and they must be willing to perceive that even the most humble members of their staff may have constructive ideas. It was for this reason that, at each hospital involved in the H.I.C. Project, a team of its most senior staff was formed to ensure that, as far as possible, the subordinate members of all departments would feel encouraged to join freely in the studies. The personal involvement of the chief officers in this way is, of course, no guarantee that the lines of upward communication would eventually open where they might previously have been closed. The learning process of a human institution is not suddenly accelerated by administrative decree nor even by sincere exhibitions of friendliness from on high. The Rock of Ages is not cleft as readily as some might suppose. But all who have watched children burst into a discussion of how to solve a classroom problem the moment their teacher has gone outside must, even if they deplore the collapse of discipline, applaud the explosion of learning. We have, perhaps, a changing morality in these affairs. Children helping each other to learn in this way often used to be punished for cheating; the helper was flogged along with the helped. Our central problem is still to find that relation between differences in levels of authority, between command and obedience, that enables the system to adjust by encouraging it to learn. It is not enough to talk about such an idea, nor even to hear more and more people say that they believe in it; our task is to examine constructively the conditions of success or failure that attend the efforts of those who try to act upon it.

### PREPARATORY MOVES

The King Edward's Hospital Fund for London has a long and respected record of innovation: it has used its substantial income to encourage a wide range of hospital activity, from the production of house journals to the introduction of digital computers. Though generous in its grants to particular hospitals for particular needs, one of its principal aims is to promote new ideas, and the Hospital Centre maintained by the Fund in the West End of London offers useful facilities for doing so. The Centre has four main functions; information and advisory services, exhibitions, investigation and research, and conferences and meetings. The independence and impartiality of the Fund and the Centre's blend of practical demonstration, professional insight, and administrative competence, have given them both a reputation among hospital staff sufficient to guarantee the worthiness of most causes that they may take up. When, therefore, an assistant director of the Centre, Janet Craig, suggested that the Manchester research team might present their findings to an invited audience of persons likely to be interested in following them up, the team felt that the initiative would be seen as non-directive and free from any attempt on their own part to display their findings or to offer their advice, much less their services. It was further decided that the invited audience should be chosen, not only by the staff of the Hospital Centre, but also by the secretaries of the four metropolitan regional hospital boards, who, from their commanding positions in the administration of this complex public service, might know those most likely to accept the invitation. It was cardinal that, at these meetings, each hospital be represented by a team of three; the chairman of the medical committee, the matron, and the chief administrative officer, usually the secretary of the group management committee. If the general aim was to improve hospital communication patterns so that those within the hospital could form a more realistic view of their own roles, nothing would be lost by encouraging co-operation between heads of services from the very outset.

The Project began with no one yet knowing how to improve hospital performance. Hospitals needed to learn to improve themselves; the experts could only learn with them. Learning always needs to start at the top, and those at the top must share this learning with everyone responsible to them. The hospital staffs, on this account, were invited to the meetings to argue and discuss and choose for themselves, from the several methods explained, the methods they considered best suited to their own hospitals.

Speakers at the first meetings, which were held at the Hospital Centre during late autumn of 1964, included, as well as the Manchester research team, Sir Robert Platt, then retiring from the office of president of the Royal College of Physicians, who lent to the proceedings a prestige no less than that of the King's Fund itself, and Dr David Clark, physician superintendent of Fulbourn Hospital, Cambridge, who on the strength of his own writings brought his professional authority to the support of this venture in social analysis (Clark, 1964). The short-term purpose of these meetings was to discover whether a handful of hospitals would each be prepared to give enough members of their staffs the time to study, among themselves, the internal communication systems of their own hospitals. For, in the meantime, the officers of the Ministry of Health concerned with research problems had promised that, should enough interest to launch such efforts be displayed, the necessary financial help would be recommended. And Professor W. J. H. Butterfield, director of the department of medicine, Guy's Hospital Medical School, had agreed that the School would administer the research grant and, more important, had offered the support and advice of his department.

In the event, the senior officers of ten hospitals convinced their management committees that this group effort to examine their own communication systems might prove, at least, marginally instructive. At a further meeting, for the chairmen and other members of committees administratively responsible to the regional boards, some research workers with experience of organizational change attempted to forecast some of the difficulties that participation in the project would inevitably create, and to suggest how they could be met. It was also then made clear that the proposals for analysis and action on which the Project as a whole was based, although specific in principle, were still uncertain in detail.

## THE BEGINNING OF THE LEARNING PROCESS

In retrospect, it is instructive to review the immediate effects of these meetings. The responses of the audience were ambivalent in the extreme, a blend of hot hostility and frigid enthusiasm, of eagerness to be told what to do and of opposition to any advice, simultaneous urges to obedience and to mastery often swelling in the heart of the same person. In matters so close to the self, it is clear that ready-made proposals actively canvassed by 'experts' do not make disciples, and those who believe otherwise must expect to be discouraged. Indeed, even when one's case from the platform is of the starkest logic, namely, 'You say that your hospitals have problems. None but yourselves can solve them. How do you propose to do so?', one must still expect hostility and rejection. If one is at last enticed by the audience to outline a few shadowy proposals for action, one should be encouraged if they are still saluted by a vigorous confusion. Silence can imply withdrawal, perhaps a reinforcement of the very blockages under review, consolidating a second condition even worse than the first. Spontaneous enthusiastic approval may imply misunderstanding, a failure to grasp the need for personal implication, a belief that a crusade to improve *others* is being launched. But a clamorous barrage of dissent means that some in the audience are now seeing problems in the light of their own possible involvement, and that the specific proposals on offer may cut across – or appear to cut across – plans already in their own awakening imaginations. The learning process, implicit in the dialogue between abstract generality (a need to improve communications) and practical action (to find the means of improving them) has begun and may now be left to look after itself for a while. It would, at this point, have been fatal for the team to set forth some prefabricated programme of operations in the hope that it might be accepted as an easy relief from the self-questioning uncertainty. One must simply listen to what is now being said, not only patiently and courteously, which for some of us is hard enough, but also intelligently, constructively, and responsibly, which for most of us is even harder. Apart from answering specifically posed questions, and countering the grosser threats to the progress of the meeting with the question: 'What is your alternative?', there is little need for further input from the platform.

The danger of patronage is too close – and expert knowledge is too likely to be seen as the expression of it – for a prudent man to try impressing, much less coercing, those who carry the real responsibility for running the hospitals. On the contrary, there must be the admission from the platform that nobody yet knows how to tackle the particular problems of the particular hospitals, simply because nobody has tackled them before. In the event, it was enough to remind the meeting that the Hospital Centre exists specifically to encourage people to address themselves to difficult issues previously unexplored. Thus, the willingness of the hospital staffs to make use of the Manchester research findings was significantly advanced, on the one hand, by the emphasis that the responsibility to act was theirs alone and, on the other, by the confidence they held in the staff of the Hospital Centre.

In one sense, these early meetings, held as preparations to the introductory courses to be described in the next chapter, were not a success. The compromise eventually reached upon how much time could be devoted to these preparations was the product of forces far removed from any theory or practice of learning. Nobody at the meetings had any accurate idea of how to prepare busy and experienced adults to study their own problems in a new and objective fashion. Nobody pretended that doctors or nurses could learn in any reasonable period the skills of interviewing and analysing acquired by a social science graduate in three years. Nobody knew what was the absolute minimum of technique that they should have mastered before an inquiry was set in hand on the floor of a hospital. On these very practical issues all were in the dark. Nothing is now to be gained, therefore, by reminding those from the hospitals who attended the conferences of their campaign of attrition, to whittle down the time to be devoted both to preparation before the projects began, and to the projects themselves once they had got going. After successive economies, it was agreed that three days full time would have to be adequate to acquaint the senior team of three from each hospital with their roles in each project; and that one month full time would have to suffice for preparing the operational teams to begin their studies. It was further suggested – and assumed – that the members of these two teams would include, on level terms, a doctor, a nurse, and an administrator.

Subsequent experience suggests that, at least in the orientation of hospital participants, the whole exercise should have taught us a great deal. Firstly, the senior teams should have been much more deeply involved in the design and launching of their study projects; this involvement might have been spread over several months, to include a review of the minor surveys to be made in their own hospitals. More effort should have been made to involve the medical committees. Secondly, the operational teams should have been given more practical field exercises as their training material; they should have gained more insight into the study methods of social science by using them rather than by listening to lectures about them. Perhaps some of the hospitals who eventually joined the Project would be willing to train future operational teams by offering them the opportunity to study some of the problems uncovered, but not yet treated, by their first involvement. Whether or not this is a realistic proposal, these tasks of practical indoctrination will always need to be faced, and they will need to be faced on the floor of the hospital as part of the attack upon a real problem or set of problems. We may take it that, in principle, the self-study of hospital organization must, and can, become part of normal administrative practice, linked with programmes of management education. For all that, a good deal of debate is still needed around the points of practice. We can assert with confidence that, at any future series of evangelizing conferences, the case for the more adequate training of our missionaries could now at least be supported by evidence of previous disappointments.

## AFTER: REFLECTIONS AND RECOMMENDATIONS

It was originally intended that the hospitals choosing to take part in this Project should form a self-governing consortium, calling on the skills of the central team. Instead, they remained ten separate hospitals, held together by the central team.

The disclosure of their inner thoughts and feelings in the presence of colleagues from other hospitals was new for nurses, doctors, and hospital administrators as a group in 1964/65. They needed more time than was allowed, to become used to working upon and talking about their shortcomings, both personal and institutional. More time, too, was required for them to recognize their own strength, to marshal their ability to promote changes of attitude in their own hospitals, and to develop inter-hospital links and advisory panels.

Two influences from outside the consortium of hospitals themselves exacerbated their lack of preparation:

1. In order that the necessary financial support could be given, the hospitals were asked if they would join the Project too soon after the first meeting, which had been designed only to promote discussion about it.
2. The hospital staff needed preparation for project work; in an effort to get started, the training courses organized by the central team took time and effort that should have been invested by the hospitals in uniting and deciding upon their own line of action.

The primary objective of the consortium of ten hospitals was to offer to members of the staff of each of them the structured opportunity to examine some of their problems of organization. These problems, it is argued, create blockages in the free flow of information and questions, lead to inefficient working, and, above all, hamper the hospital community in its ever-present task of adjustment to change. It is thus possible, at a different level, to regard the work of the consortium itself as an exercise in learning, both individual and institutional. How far did those who designed the Project as a whole, and who spent so much effort in exhorting others to reflect upon their places in hospital life, turn inward this light of self-examination? If the process of learning one's own role in a reality situation is encouraged only if one gets information about the effect of one's own actions, then by what criteria is it possible to say whether or not the promoters of the whole enterprise have themselves learned anything? A professional evaluation of this has been made by Dr George Wieland as part of his general review of the Project as a whole, but it may also be of interest to set down what the writer feels to be those aspects of its design and execution that he would strive most to improve should another experiment of this nature be attempted.[7]

## INVOLVEMENT OF SENIOR STAFF

It is now abundantly clear that, from start to finish, the success of any project depends upon the interest shown in it by those holding the senior posts at the hospital.[8] This commanding influence of those in authority is not confined to hospitals alone; in the analogous industrial consortia, it is again clear that the perception of the top management about the importance of the study project is the principal determinant of its progress and of its outcomes.[9] Since it often appears that the senior staff are seen by their subordinates in a highly unfavourable light,[10] and since the evidence to justify these negative views can be so massive as to threaten the senior staff in a highly personal way, it is essential for studies such as these to be so designed as to protect them from ill-informed interpretations of the evidence. There is a limit to the challenge that even the most hardened of bureaucrats can endure or be expected to face. Nevertheless, it is equally true that throughout the institutions of Western Europe as a whole there is, more often than not, a profound dissatisfaction among the middle and technical managers about how these institutions are run; one complaint is that the information vital to doing a good job is frequently missing, and this leads staff members to feel that the system is wasting their time. It is no less true that much of this dissatisfaction becomes projected upon the person or persons in charge. The general effect is usually manifested in hostility towards top management, whoever they may be and whatever their personal qualities. Such hostility can only increase if top management refuses to recognize it, or takes personally what is essentially a characteristic of all complex systems undergoing the stresses of rapid and unforeseeable change. The administrative problem is how to encourage top management to face this hostility and how to interpret it constructively, as evidence that the institution is organizationally sclerotic and unable to adjust rather than that the top management are the innocent victims of some personal vendetta. It is clear that the internal problems of many hospitals will not be ameliorated unless they are, in some degree, brought into the open, and no less clear that they cannot be brought into the open without the top management sometimes feeling themselves the target of vindictive and ill-founded accusations. How effectively to support the senior staff who might feel themselves thus attacked is a major problem in this kind of institutional therapy.[11] Certainly, the stronger the links built by a consortium between those in charge of its separate institutions the greater the hope of helping them individually; only if each sees intellectually and feels emotionally that this hostility may be the common fate of all senior staff, and that it resides in the inevitable inertias of the institution, and not in the defects of the particular person, is there much promise of the support of those at the top for investigations likely to challenge the way things are now done. Even so, the support will hardly be enthusiastic, as it may be too discouraging to hear in specific detail the charges that frustrated human nature can level against its leaders. Thus the later experiments in organizational therapy, built up on experience of this consortium of London hospitals, and carried out in industry, concentrate attention upon the needs and problems of those in charge of the enterprises in which the studies are made.[12] In future, not only should this be done among hospitals, but no hospital should be chosen for study if its senior staff appear to suffer from an insecurity unable to withstand the hostility uncovered, and inadequate to respond to the support of colleagues from other hospitals facing equal challenges. This rigorous condition may mean that the very hospitals most in need of better understanding of their problems of adjustment will most effectively deprive themselves of the means to understand them. But for the present there is no alternative; the notion of institutional learning, of adult persons making a collective study of why they feel that the system in which they work needs to be improved, and thereby effecting the necessary improvements, is still too new, still too much under the shadow of an authoritarian and hierarchichal administrative tradition, to be put to unnecessary risks. We must also welcome other challenges to this tradition and see our auto-therapeutic approach as but one force in a grand alliance. It is, for the present, satisfactory to observe how the more secure senior staffs, called upon to face the stresses that such self-analysis creates, are prepared to work through them. In this, the experimental design of any future programme must promise a more adequate support; something is needed beyond an introductory course of three days.

### TRAINING OF OPERATIONAL TEAMS

The hospital teams were prepared for their tasks by a month's course, mainly of training in practical techniques, such as the conduct of free interviews or the use of survey instruments and other questionnaires. While it is essential somehow to engender an opening balance of operational skills, it would probably be a better use of teaching resources to go more deeply into the nature and use of such skills after the teams have had a little first-hand field experience of trying them out in simple situations. As in all true learning, a new grasp of research methods demands knowledge of what happens when these methods are used, and in something so novel, an interplay of application and feedback is essential if true learning is to be secured. It is true that in the event all hospital teams spent a week during their month's course in trying out their new methods in hospitals other than their own, and that they found this week, and the discussion between the pairs of hospital teams that followed, of great use. Some found it, indeed, the most interesting part of the course; a few thought it the only element at all worth while. Yet an extended opportunity of discussing their operational problems of observation and project design more fully with each other and with their tutors would have been welcomed. In particular, after having chosen the theme for the project on which they were to work in their own hospitals, they should have been able, before actually starting on it, to discuss its implications more fully, with their own seniors, with others, both in their own and in collaborating hospitals, and with the central team. Even this suggested improvement still leaves the cart before the horse. What, more precisely, are the expected goals of the chosen studies? What are the reasons for the hospitals – or for the coalitions within the hospitals that hold the power of decision – choosing the themes they do? Whatever makes them volunteer to join the consortium in the first place? What perceptions do they hold of their administrative problems and what true hope do they have of ameliorating them, either through the administrative therapy here suggested, or by other means? Indeed, while we are on the subject, to what extent are they able to grasp the idea, inherent in the consortium, that it is for them – and almost for them alone – to settle, for good or ill, what kind of hospital, against the background of the hospital service as a whole, they wish their own to be?

This lofty question leads directly to others perhaps more practical. What do those in the hospital team see themselves as doing? What briefing about their new tasks and new roles have they received from the coalition of power? What do they feel as they assemble with a group of strangers to discuss such unusual topics as communications, learning, change, decisions, and so forth? On whose behalf do they see themselves as working? What are the ambiguities in their new (and part-time) roles? Even if they have come in small groups from the same hospital, what can the nurse be thinking as she sits down with the doctor or with the secretary to delve into, say, the problems of questionnaire design? It is, in retrospect, perfectly apparent that to these miscellaneous questions one would receive an even more miscellaneous set of replies. It is equally apparent that the participants must be offered an opportunity, more profound than any they were given during this first experiment, to discuss the experience on which they saw themselves about to embark. A skilful therapist should have spent more sessions with these teams in order that each member might either convince himself or herself of the necessity for what they were doing, or admit, by withdrawing, that he or she had been enticed to join what was still perceived as a chimerical mission. It is quite unrealistic to expect, as the writer at the time expected, a party of doctors, nurses, and administrators, nourished in a hospital tradition of authoritarian directiveness, to accept without discussion or argument the proposition that they would be able to recommend how the hospital system could be improved *if only they could assemble and interpret a first-hand knowledge of where that system needed to be improved*. Some members might believe that any improved operating efficiency is not worth securing – even if it could be secured – at the price, in terms of undermined authority, demanded by the easiest project. Others might say that they are clear enough about their problems already, and that, with better staff, they could be solved. Nor is this all. Even if, in a general way, each member of the team recognized that the internal communications of the hospital were important to its effective functioning – indeed, vital to the stability of its staff and even to the treatment of its patients – it must be a disturbingly novel proposition that they, the team, could be expected to improve these communications by some kind of alchemy passing itself off as social science. Instead, therefore, of having been a show of *ex cathedra* teaching, about the nature of research and the propositions of behavioural science, the course should have offered fuller opportunities of drawing from the participants their perceptions of their new experience. This would also have brought out, for their own benefit no less than that of the central team, their perceptions of how they saw the problems of their own hospitals. It would, moreover, have provided an opportunity for examining those problems afresh, especially in the light of their being treated by those within the system.

Such discussions would have presented the proposed projects in a more realistic setting and would have shown more clearly the opportunities for change they might offer. At appropriate points in the design of each project, the senior teams should have become more deeply involved; this would have been possible if the operational teams had been more confident of their roles and of the objectives of the consortium as a whole. Looking back, it is easy to see that any lack of role definition and any lack of clarity in objectives could alike be traced to insufficient examination, by the teams themselves, of the unusual activity in which they had become caught up. It is not much of an excuse to point out that, on the other hand, the initial courses had to be provided while the enthusiasm of the participating hospitals was still high, and that, in order to get the doctors, nurses, and administrators released for the course at all, it was essential both to cut it down to the barest minimum of time and to load it with (what was thought to be) the greatest content of operationally useful instruction. These were real constraints, it is true; nevertheless, the balance of the time available should have been differently distributed between *ex cathedra* instruction and participative discussion. In this sense, our own introductory courses reflected the very arbitrariness of authority that the whole enterprise was designed to avoid: the experts thought they knew best. This declaration of humility may, however, be some indication that those behind the consortium were able to learn a little from having worked with it; the question is whether any who might replicate the experiment would also be bold enough to organize the preliminary training in the manner now recommended, namely, by encouraging the hospital teams to begin by examining in depth both their personal and their hospital needs and also their project proposals, alike in their own hospitals and in collaboration with the others.

## NOTES

[1] The way of a fool is right in his own eyes, but he that hearkeneth unto counsel is wise' (Prov. 12:15).

[2] In psychology, parataxis is 'the development of skills, attitudes, and ideas without bringing them into relationship with other aspects of one's personality; living in watertight compartments' (English and English, xxxx). As used here, the ambit of its meaning has been extended to include interpersonal and intergroup relationships.

[3] But we are learning. A new social role is being evolved, that of change agent. In an industrial consortium based upon the project here under review, a score of Belgian managers have been exchanged between their enterprises to encourage the process of social learning here proposed. 'Know ye not that a little leaven leaveneth the whole lump?' (I Cor. 5:6).

[4] The second Green Paper on the future structure of the National Health Service has now been published (see Department of Health and Social Security, 1970).

[5] 'The wise in heart will receive commandments, but a prating fool shall fall' (Prov. 10:8).

'The simple believeth every word, but the prudent man looketh well to his going' (Prov. 14:15).

[6] In practice, this model forms the basis of several apparently different learning processes, just as decision theory lies behind all operational research techniques, whether, for example, linear programming or inventory control. The most common learning processes are:

(a) trial and error; or passively finding out what happens without first perceiving that degree of order in Stages 1 and 2 necessary to forecasting the outcomes to be expected at Stage 4;

(b) insight; or securing this order to an extent sufficient to narrow the choice of trials in Stage 3;

(c) mimesis; or copying the actions of others in the expectation of achieving the same results as they do; Stage 1 then becomes the facts of one's own problem coupled with the facts of what one can see others doing about the same problem;

(d) instruction; or the helpful intervention of some other person at any one of the five stages.

In the striving of our hospital teams it is hardly necessary – and would probably be confusing – to go into these distinctions. It is enough to have somebody in the hospital group who can, from time to time, review progress in the light of the five main stages.

[7] The Inter University Programme in Advanced Management, noted (p. 33) by the Mant Report of The British Institute of Management (Mant, 1970) as 'the best example of this trend' (towards involving the enterprise as well as the individual), is based upon the H.I.C. Project.

[8] 'As the judge of the people is so are his officers, and what manner of man the ruler of the city is so are all those that inhabit therein' (Ecclesiasticus 10:1-2).

[9] In an industrial consortium set up three years later among a score of Belgian enterprises this intention was made good. It is the presidents of the firms, not the research team, who are now pressing for the programme to be repeated. Moreover, in a second action consortium successfully completed at the time of writing and staged by the Egyptian Government to involve the staff of its industrial enterprises in the identification, analysis, and resolution of their internal problems, it was made a condition of membership that the chief executives of the participating enterprises became themselves operationally involved. Goodwill or encouragement from on high is no longer considered sufficient; each president must be continuously involved, with his own staff and with other presidents, in the progress of the field studies. It is by now recognized that the principal function of the president, like that of a headmaster, is to provide the conditions in which he and his subordinates best can learn.

[10] There are exceptions; in some organizations junior staff may hold opinions of their superiors markedly more favourable than these can imagine.

[11] Managers of industrial enterprises are paid salaries high enough to enable them to endure attacks of this nature.

[12] For example, all project themes were strategic, namely, concerned primarily with the corporate planning of the enterprises.

# 2 *The H.I.C. Project in outline*

*HILARY LEIGH*

This chapter provides a brief account of a four-year action-research project that can be described as an attempt at organizational development (or change) in hospitals. The Project was initiated by Professor R. W. Revans with the primary aim of trying to help small teams of senior administrators, doctors, and nurses from ten 'self-selected' hospitals in the London area to make better use of their own resources in identifying and tackling their working problems. After an initial period of training, the teams selected and carried out nearly forty projects in their own hospitals, assisted, when requested, by a small central team.

The organization of project staff was unusual in that it consisted of separate 'independent' action and evaluation teams. The Project also had an advisory committee which came to play an important and active role – and to whom the central team was responsible.

Whereas there is general agreement that overall the effects of the Project were relatively modest, demonstrable improvements did occur within participating hospitals, and the evaluation data provide a basis for more effective efforts in similar directions.

The Hospital Internal Communications Project derived in part from Revans's earlier hospital studies which showed that low morale, particularly among nursing staff, tended to be associated with communication problems (Revans, 1964b). For example, where ward sisters felt their relations with matron were inadequate, student nurses tended to feel that ward sisters did little teaching and that it was difficult to ask questions or get satisfactory answers about matters affecting their work. In addition there was a tendency for relations between ward sisters and their consultants to be poor. Such hospitals tended to be characterized by relatively high wastage rates of student nurses, relatively high turnover amongst nursing and other staff, and longer than average patient stay. These findings led Revans to suggest that the effectiveness of a hospital communication system was likely to exert a major influence on both staff stability and length of patient stay.

The Project also reflected Revans's views on management and management education (Revans, 1965 and 1966). He defines management as problem-solving and believes that this can be best learnt through direct practical experience.

'The hospitals themselves, personified by their administrators, their doctors and their nurses . . . , must learn how to conduct surveys, to interpret their findings, to seek the structure of the problems so revealed and to build the programmes of participation by which these problems may be ameliorated' (Revans, 1964b).

It was the expression of this view that led Janet Craig of the King's Fund Hospital Centre to initiate a series of collaborative discussions between Revans and a number of hospitals on how these ideas could be put into practice. These meetings, which were encouraged by members of the (then) Ministry of Health, took place during late 1964 and early 1965, and from them a plan to carry out the H.I.C. Project was evolved. Ten hospitals, comprising seven general hospitals, one teaching hospital, one paediatric hospital, and one mental hospital, agreed to participate.

The ultimate general objective of the H.I.C. Project was to improve hospital functioning through focusing attention on a number of goals, namely improved communications, problem-solving, and changes in the process of problem-solving. In practice, no single goal took any general precedence although better communication (as the Project title implies) was the major theme.

One of the most important and unusual aspects of the Project was the degree to which senior hospital staff became actively involved. Each hospital nominated a two-tier team of representatives from each of three professional groups. The senior or supporting part of the team (consisting of the matron, a group or hospital secretary, and a senior consultant) took part in a three-day residential appreciation course in which they were introduced to the Project and presented with some social science concepts and research findings.

The junior or operational part of the team (consisting of a deputy or assistant matron, a deputy group or hospital secretary, and a senior registrar or another consultant) participated in a one month residential course. Although principles of organizational functioning, of group dynamics, and of communications generally were outlined in the course, the main emphasis lay on introducing survey methods. Lectures, discussions and practical exercises were focused on interview and questionnaire design, statistics, report writing, and so on. One week was devoted entirely to 'learning by doing' through carrying out a practice project. Each team visited a hospital other than their own among the ten and selected a particular staff group for study. Every team designed its own questionnaire, administered interviews, organized a discussion group, analysed the data and produced a report. During the final week the projects were discussed and assessed. The initial training courses were completed in December 1965.

It was intended that supporting and operational teams would jointly select areas for study. The operational teams would then work out the details and execute specific projects, devoting up to one third of their time to the task. In the event the supporting and operational teams did select their own projects, decide on the methods to be used, and attempt to carry out as much of the work themselves as was possible considering the extent of their knowledge and the time available.

To co-ordinate Project activities and assist the hospital teams a small central team was recruited. This consisted of a central-team director with considerable training and administrative experience, a group discussion organizer, a sociology graduate, and a management graduate. Later, when it became evident that most of the operational teams had insufficient time to collect survey data, a number of social psychology students joined the team. Each student spent up to six months working with a particular hospital team on a specific project. The chief function of the central team was to provide assistance to the hospitals on request. Its members were not intended to direct or control the hospital projects.

Another important function of the central team was to organize a series of inter-team meetings, which gave an opportunity for hospital teams to learn from and support each other and share information about their projects. It was hoped these meetings would also help the teams in carrying out feedback activities in their own hospitals. An attempt was also made to encourage groups and individuals to learn from the current situations in which the hospital teams found themselves.

The central team was in turn responsible to an advisory committee consisting of representatives of the (then) Ministry of Health (who financed the major part of the Project, including the evaluation), the King's Fund Hospital Centre (responsible for bringing the hospitals together, housing Project staff, and providing meeting facilities), and Guy's Hospital Medical School (who administered the funds and employed Project staff). Unlike most advisory bodies, this committee became fairly closely involved in the actual running of the Project. In part this arose from the necessity of coping with changes in both the leadership of the Project and the central-team staff and in part from the intense concern of some committee members to protect the interests of the hospitals against undue influence by the central team.

In May 1966, nine months after the project started, an evaluator was appointed to work independently of the central team to assess the effects of the Project. His team (of two to three members) collected a variety of data on the H.I.C. Project. The advisory committee, the central team, the hospital teams, and other hospital participants were interviewed and some also completed postal questionnaires; meetings of these various groups were observed; and, finally data on staff turnover and absenteeism, and on length of patients' stay, were collected from hospital records.

During the three years following the initial courses the ten hospital teams undertook thirty-eight projects, ranging from two in some hospitals to nine in another hospital. Some projects involved several hundred staff; in others only a few key staff participated.

The aims were often broad, for example to learn more about the problems of a cross-section of hospital staff or about those of particular departments or professional groups. In other projects the aims were specific, for example, to study patients' anxieties concerning clinical ward rounds or to analyse the work load of medical social workers.

The pattern of participation varied considerably in different hospitals and in different projects. It was comparatively rare for the whole hospital team to be involved in carrying out a project. Usually one member of the supporting team and two from the operational team, with perhaps one departmental manager, were actively involved. The activities of the teams were often progressive, leading from one project to another, and it was not unusual for different team members or other hospital staff to be involved in subsequent projects. However, this meant it was sometimes difficult to take advantage of accumulated experience from previous projects. Greater benefit might have accrued if the hospital teams had been encouraged to plan and guide an integrated programme of projects aimed at affecting specific aspects of hospital performance.

Most teams embarked on their studies with considerable enthusiasm although later they faced many difficulties. About half the operational-team members found they had insufficient time to undertake all the necessary work on their projects and some felt they lacked adequate support from their senior colleagues. Often the team members were not closely related in their everyday work and they found it difficult to choose projects in which most of them were professionally implicated. There was a tendency to choose topics that members felt were important but which did not directly involve their own work. Often the initial studies aimed at identifying problems, while later projects tended to be concerned with gathering more information about known problems and improving the work of other staff in the hospital.

In the selection and initial planning stages of projects and, later, in discussing the results with staff and taking action on findings, the hospital teams often worked alone. Although the central team was invited to assist in some of the planning of projects, it was chiefly at the data collection stage that help was requested. In over half of the thirty-eight projects central-team members collected the data, analysed them (occasionally with the hospital teams), and wrote a report. In some projects they took part in feedback activities as well. Very few projects were undertaken entirely by the hospital teams. All but one of the hospitals used the central team at some stage in most of their projects.

As a result of the emphasis of the training courses, survey methods were widely adopted during the course of the H.I.C. Project, not only as a means of diagnosing problems but, for those who used them, as a way of enlarging knowledge about hospital functioning. The more difficult task of 'building the programmes of participation' for dealing with problems needed much more help of a different kind, which the central team was insufficiently equipped to provide.

It is perhaps not surprising that sometimes the hospital teams were reluctant to try out problem-solving methods, which could be time-consuming, and could appear likely to disturb existing authority relationships without any guarantee of any improvement over what was being achieved by the use of more traditional methods. The difficulties inherent in trying to integrate a policy of self-direction by the hospitals with the objectives of the Project (general though they were) gave rise to concern among the advisory committee, the central team, and the hospitals.

In mid-1967 the hospital teams met together, alone at first and, towards the end of that year, with the Project advisory committee, to discuss the future of the Project, which was due to terminate at the end of 1967. As a result it was decided to extend the Project for a further year. However, in the spring of 1968 the hospital teams decided to end the third series of centrally organized inter-team meetings, and few further hospital projects were undertaken.

Action was taken on the basis of over half the total number of projects; the rest did not go beyond the report stage. For example, one survey was followed by the setting-up of an appointments system for patients required to reattend the accident and emergency department, the introduction of lectures into a practical course for post-registration nurses in the department, and improvements in nurses' off-duty rotas. Another project contributed to the introduction of a hospital-wide messenger system. No projects appeared to lead to the solution of major problems, and much of the action taken consisted of administrative adjustments in functioning.

In terms of improving communication the overall effects of the Project seemed relatively modest although there was considerable variation both within and between different hospitals. Some team members who played a very active part in their hospital projects felt they had developed relationships established during the training courses which later resulted in beneficial effects on their day-to-day work. These members also learnt more about the functioning of their hospitals and the problems of other staff. Some members, particularly the nurses, said they had learnt to 'listen more' and 'explain things more' to other staff. There were instances of potentially wider improvements, such as better relations between two or three departments and the innovation of regular meetings for departmental managers and senior staff.

The H.I.C. Project has successfully demonstrated that administrators, doctors, and nurses from the same hospital are willing to work together, and with similar staff from other hospitals, to learn different methods of tackling their own management problems. Some action resulted and there were some improvements in communication although these appear to have had little effect on hospital performance as measured by the evaluation study. The methods used by the hospital teams did not become widely diffused throughout the hospitals, and by the end of the Project period (December 1968) most of the hospital teams appeared to have disbanded.

In order to improve the level of achievement so that some measures of hospital performances are affected, it is suggested that the following modifications should be seriously considered – given the context of the H.I.C. Project (namely senior hospital staff selecting and carrying out projects with the assistance of a relatively small, 'low powered' central team exerting little influence). The projects selected need to concern problems recognized (but not necessarily clearly defined) by those whose work is directly affected, including at least one member of top management, who want to improve the situation and take an active part in the process. The links between specific problems and their effects on organizational performance need to be carefully analysed so that priorities can be determined and efforts expended where maximum potential benefit may be obtained. More emphasis needs to be placed on developing effective feedback systems through consultation and discussion with key staff at the very earliest stages. Probably the central team would need to collect any necessary survey data, but, more importantly, its members need to be sufficiently experienced to take a more effective training role in planning, feedback, change, and continuing evaluation activities with the hospital staff.

Finally, there are undoubted advantages of an independent evaluation, particularly to the critical researcher. However, it is the author's belief that evaluation activities should form an integral part of any organizational development project. An action-research project such as H.I.C. needs to contain continual feedback from researchers specifically concerned with evaluation. They should collaborate *both* with the project team and with the hospital staff in defining common goals and differentiating between these and the goals of each participant group. Working through the implications of these goals may help in defining more clearly what can be achieved.

# 3 *The H.I.C. Project and organizational change*

*GEORGE F. WIELAND*

In the view of the evaluation team, the H.I.C. Project was not so much about changing hospitals as about changing organizations. To understand the Project and its outcomes requires that we use the knowledge acquired by scientific study and changing of organizations such as factories, schools, churches, banks, as well as hospitals.

In the preceding chapters, the reader has been provided with the background and an overview of the H.I.C. Project as seen by Revans (Chapter 1), together with a relatively detailed objective description of the activities during the Project (Chapter 2). This chapter introduces some concepts from the academic world in an attempt to place the H.I.C. Project in the context of other efforts of the same generic nature – in the context of organizational change efforts. To evaluate the Project as a whole requires one to compare it with other apparently similar activities – or efforts at changing and improving organizations.

Following a brief discussion of organizational change, there is a presentation of some of the available research findings on the role of communications in hospital functioning. Next, some analytical distinctions are made to characterize efforts at changing different aspects of organizations. The H.I.C. Project is viewed as a technological approach to change emphasizing cognitions and objective orientations. After a discussion of influence relationships and clarity in change programmes, attention is finally focused on some concepts for understanding the sequence of change.

If we are to classify the H.I.C. Project as an effort in organizational change, we must begin by defining what we mean by an organization. A convenient, succinct definition fairly typical of many sociologists is provided by Mouzelis (1967), who

> 'define[s] organization or formal organization as a form of social grouping which is established in a more or less purposive manner for the attainment of a specific goal. Thus purposiveness and goal specificity seem to be the two crucial criteria differentiating organizations from other types of social units. For instance a firm, a political party or a voluntary organization are typical examples of formal organizations. In all these cases men, in a purposive manner coordinate their activities and efforts in order to achieve a specific goal' (p 4).

In organizing to achieve their fairly specific purposes, people 'structure' their activities; they specialize in delineated jobs and roles, which are co-ordinated by making relationships within and between specializing units predictable.

To change such an organization is to alter some of its basic characteristics – to alter the goal of the organization or its purposive grouping or structure. Later on we shall add 'people' and 'technology' to 'structure' as important and more or less interdependent elements of an organization. Because these elements are to some degree interdependent, change in one may have some effect on another or on the goal attainment which is the outcome of the functioning of the organization.

One probably must be somewhat arbitrary in defining change – how much of a difference really constitutes a difference or a 'change'? It seems most useful to view organizational change as a change of one of the basic elements of the organization sufficient to make a difference to another of the elements – to change one or more of them, and especially to change significantly the nature of the goals or their attainment, i.e. the *raison d'être* of the organization as a whole.

In the light of these definitions it is clear that the H.I.C. Project as a whole was an organizational change project, not a project to change a few individuals or a sub-grouping in the hospital. While the immediate focus of the Project was on only six individuals from each hospital (the hospital teams), the ultimate aim was to improve the way the hospitals functioned in the attainment of their major goal, the care of patients. This is clear from the background of the Project in Revans's earlier research findings about the relationship between communication, morale, and length of patients' stay[1] and also clear from some of the avowed aims of the Project (see especially Chapters 1 and 11). Below we shall try to examine some of the possible routes to eventual change in goal attainment by the H.I.C. hospitals. Some of these alternative ways to organizational change involve changing the procedures for obtaining information in the hospitals and then changing other work procedures. Other alternatives entail change in the attitudes of key staff and still others entail changes in the authority structure of key staff members. The ultimate aim of all these alternatives – and all were attempted in one way or another during the H.I.C. Project – was to improve patient-care. Because the Project was an attempt to change some of what we have termed basic characteristics of organizations and because the ultimate aim of these initial changes was improvement in patient-care, it is quite clear that the H.I.C. Project was an exercise in organizational change.

Before looking at the H.I.C. Project in detail it is of some value to examine briefly the origins of work on organizational change, because apparently similar approaches may arise from different assumptions and views of the basic nature of what is to be changed. The effects of a number of disciplines and fields of practice are particularly evident in work on organizational change. Programmes of change built around the sensitivity or training group (e.g. Schein and Bennis, 1965) and an emphasis on emotional, irrational man and his conflicts derive in part from Freud and from psychotherapeutic practice in changing the characteristics of individuals. The organizational sociotherapy of Jaques (1951) also has similar origins.

From another quarter comes the work of practising managers and management consultants who developed notions of the optimal structure or patterning of formal relations in organizations (see, e.g., Urwick, 1956). Later scientific study of informal relations (of, for example, the emotional needs and unplanned relationships of people in organizations) began as a reaction to an apparent overemphasis on the rational, formal aspects of man and his organizations. Both of these approaches have been examined and utilized to some degree in the development of an empirically-based science of organizations and organizational change, starting with the Hawthorne experiments, the 'human relations' movement, and evolving into views of change that incorporate both structural and 'human' considerations (see, e.g., Likert, 1961).[2]

Because most of the studies of (or efforts at) organizational change and improvement have been undertaken by psychologists and sociologists concerned with either 'people' or 'structure', or both, another scientific approach to change has been more or less neglected until recently – namely the technology approach, which assumes a 'rational' man who will freely accept technological changes that are efficient and in his interest. The psychologist or sociologist will frequently argue that man is not rational, that approaches to organizational change based on scientific management, work study, or other views of man as an object and manipulator of objects, can have only negligible effects limited by the meagre extent of man's rationality. Despite these views, the place of technology in organizations has continued to grow, thereby emphasizing the usefulness of viewing man and his organizations in rational terms.

We may now have reached the point where the rational approach and the non-rational approach to man are converging in the study and practice of organizational change. At the present time, there is discussion of collaboration between operational researchers and social scientists (Beckhard, 1969). Similarly, study by social scientists of the 'utilization of technology' may be only a preliminary step to the use by social scientists and others of such a dual approach to changing organizations (Havelock and Benne, 1966; Cherns, 1968).

The H.I.C. Project represents a 'hybrid' effort at organizational change, combining a rational, technological approach with a non-rational, social science approach. This is evident in the staffing of the Project, for example. Revans, the originator of the Project, is himself a practitioner in operational research, while the backgrounds of the remainder of the H.I.C. staff range from management to psychology, and from sociology to psychiatry.

The H.I.C. Project is unusual in that its aims were, in practice, to change the human and the structural characteristics of hospitals, although starting from a technological orientation to change. There are a number of other relatively unusual aspects to this Project. One is that it is a scientific study of organizational change, since relatively few such studies have been done.[3] Furthermore, most of these studies have been based on one or two organizations with a rather limited number of change-agents, (i.e. facilitators of change) involved in the change programmes. Thus the present study has a potential advantage in permitting comparisons of various different approaches to change. Also an advantage, but potentially detrimental in some respects as well, is the independence of the evaluation from the research component (see Wieland, 1968a).

## COMMUNICATION AND THE H.I.C. PROJECT

Before moving to a more detailed examination of the nature of the change programme attempted in the H.I.C. Project, we shall examine the role of communication in the Project. Does 'communication' in the title of the Project really indicate what it was all about? Furthermore, what does the available research evidence tell us about the role of communication in hospitals?

First of all, to what extent was this Project about communication? Revans's (1964b) view of the difficulties in hospitals hinges upon information and communication as a way of alleviating the lack of information. The H.I.C. Project was, as described in Chapters 1 and 2, a way of improving communication by bringing survey methods into hospitals. However, the way in which surveys were brought into the hospital is very important, for the surveys were to be done by hospital people themselves, completely under their own direction. It was up to the hospital people how they would use this instrument for improving communication.

In other words, the H.I.C. Project was concerned with bringing to hospitals the capacity to use surveys themselves. The H.I.C. Project was not a study of communication practices in hospitals, the effects of these practices, or their modification, but, rather, its essence was to introduce survey techniques to hospitals and thereby improve communication (see Chapter 6).

Apparently because the emphasis in the H.I.C. Project was on bringing the capacity to use surveys to hospitals, rather than the study of current communication practices, no systematic diagnosis was made of communications practices in H.I.C. hospitals. In connection with this kind of diagnosis, Georgopoulos and Mann (1962) suggest some of the aspects of communication that one might examine in relation to organizational functioning:

'The consequences of particular communication practices for organizational behavior will depend on such specific considerations as who talks with whom, about what, under what conditions, in what manner, how frequently, and how long. Both the quantitative and the qualitative characteristics of communication are important. Similarly, both the formal and informal channels of communication in the organization, and their relative availability and use are important. How much relevant, and/or irrelevant, information is passing through the various formal and informal channels will affect the detection and solution of problems, decision making, and successful role performance on the part of organizational members. It is clear, however, that not all communication in a hospital, or any other organization, is functional. Too little communication or, less frequently, too much communication, communication of the wrong kind or with the wrong people, may well be dysfunctional for the organization and the performance of its members. It is, therefore, important to ascertain the communication practices and patterns which facilitate or impede performance in the organization' (p. 622).

Of course, some of the surveys within the H.I.C. Project hospitals were used to study some of the aspects of communication practices detailed by Georgopoulos and Mann. Nevertheless, the most common thread running through the activities of the H.I.C. Project was the use of surveys to change hospitals and particularly to change the amount of information available. It was the use by hospitals themselves of surveys to obtain information, not the communications aspect of the information, that was important. In this sense communication was part of the H.I.C. Project.[4]

To the extent the H.I.C. Project did examine communication practices in some of the surveys, it is relevant to ask about the role of communication in hospitals and the relationship of such communication to the task of caring for patients. If the central team or hospital team had studied communication, what kind of model could they have used? The Georgopoulos and Mann study had been done several years earlier, and excerpts from it were used as background reading material for members of the H.I.C. Project. However, the emphasis in the excerpts chosen was on the apparent direct relationship between co-ordination and patient-care, and not on the apparent lack of any direct relationship between communication and patient-care, which Georgopoulos and Mann had also reported.

In their comprehensive examination of factors that seem to affect patient care, Georgopoulos and Mann listed co-ordination, shared expectations, and certain communication and supervisory practices that facilitate co-ordination, as well as staff composition ratios, staff–patient ratios, etc. No communication practices were directly related to patient-care. The closest relevant variables concerned shared expectations. Now shared expectations could well flow from communication practices, but these are probably in the nature of a special kind of communications – *influential* communications (Wieland, 1968b). Thus the comprehensive investigation by Georgopoulos and Mann of organizational characteristics related to the quality of patient-care showed that communication might play a role, but only indirectly as mediated by such factors as shared expectations or co-ordination, which are in turn related to patient-care. According to Georgopoulos and Mann, communication is not directly related to patient-care.

Even if one is not concerned with improving patient-care, but only with better, more efficient functioning in the hospital, the kind of communication must be clearly specified before one can say that communication will improve functioning. Using three factors as criteria of nursing functioning – the performance of nursing personnel in different roles, nursing department co-ordination, and commitment to or identification with the work group – Georgopoulos and Mann found that it was (a) the extent of task-relevant information exchanged between non-supervisory registered nurses and their superiors, (b) the extent of communication up or down the hierarchy, and not horizontally, and (c) the extent of communication via formal channels (with the immediate supervisor) and not via others, that were important for nursing functioning. Not all communication is beneficial. To reiterate Georgopoulos and Mann, 'too little or, less frequently, too much communication, communication of the wrong kind or with the wrong people, may well be dysfunctional for the organization and the performance of its members'.

This is not to say that communication is of little use. There is considerable evidence that, in hospitals as well as in organizations more generally, communication in the broad sense is associated with staff satisfaction and with the results of satisfaction such as low absenteeism.[5]

But only particular kinds of communication are related to patient-care in hospitals, and then only by means of some intermediate factors, such as better co-ordination or shared expectations. If communication in this more limited sense is to be studied or utilized, then perhaps a better term might be 'influential communication' or even 'influence'. This is not to say, however, that communication (or information) is of little value in a change effort. It can be a starting-point or perhaps a tactical element in the strategy for change, and, in fact, we shall provide some reasons below for using communication in this way.

We have argued (see also Chapter 11) that the H.I.C. Project was an attempt to improve hospital functioning through hospital staff learning how to use surveys to obtain information. Available data-based models of organizational characteristics in relation to patient-care have not shown any direct relationship between communication and patient-care,[6] and thus, in this respect, the attempt by the H.I.C. Project to improve care by implanting survey techniques in hospitals was a venture into the unknown. We turn now to a consideration of how this kind of change might affect hospitals and their functioning.

## ASPECTS OF ORGANIZATIONS

To facilitate our examination of the H.I.C. Project, we shall utilize an analytical model by Leavitt (1965) of the basic characteristics of organizations. First of all, one may characterize organizations by their *task* or their goals. What is it that they are doing or attempting to do? We are assuming that patient-care is the task of hospitals. Then there is the *technology* of the system, the machinery and other physical elements utilized by individuals to perform the task: technology also includes procedures and routines (often written in manuals) to be followed in the organization.[7] Next, organizations are composed of *people*, human beings with their values, habits, needs, feelings. Finally, organizations are characterized by *structure*, the relationships between parts of the organization: there are a number of different kinds of structure – communication, authority or other kinds of role relationships, as well as work-flow structures.[8]

Now, one may look at the technology, the people, and the structure and see the relationships between these means and the end of goal attainment. There are some scientific studies of organizations, including hospitals, that are of help in this matter. The idea is to diagnose the organization and assess how it is doing in achieving its task or goals. Norms from other similar organizations (including perhaps some from industry) may facilitate this task (Holloway and Lonergan, 1968). Even better is information about the factors differentiating effective from ineffective organizations.

Depending on the diagnosis, one may come to some conclusion about the needs of hospitals for change. Is the technology adequate for goal attainment? Are, for example, the pathology laboratories properly equipped? Is there an adequate technology (set of techniques) for treating mental retardation, for treating heart disease, etc?

Are the kinds of people appropriate? For example, do they have the proper values to fit in with hospital goals? Do they have appropriate attitudes? One may ask what kind of human needs there are, and how these fit in with the organization and its needs.

Regarding structure, one may ask about the communication system, or the work-flow system, and whether they are sufficiently developed. Just as important is the question of how well different aspects of structure are articulated with one another.

It is the joint operation of technology, people, and structure that produces the outcomes, and so it is not a matter only of the adequacy in each of the three areas, but also of how the three areas are linked with and complement one another. If one focuses on a manager, for example, one may initially ask whether he has the proper skills to gather information. Furthermore, is the communication system adequate to provide him with the information for which he asks? Are there regular meetings of department heads, for example? Does the authority system give the manager sufficient power to act in areas where he has obtained information and made decisions for actions? What about the technology of the information system? Are patients' records computerized? Are there routine procedures and times for exchanging all relevant information?

Having diagnosed the areas in which problems seem to occur, the next task is to plan the change programme. First of all, this requires a change target, which need not be the same as the ultimate goal for the change programme. Ideally, one would attack a problem directly so that the full brunt of the change effort is brought to bear on the problem situation. That is to say, if there are problems in the technology, then one would try to build up a better technological system directly by bringing in new technology or by improving the existing system.

However, there may be a number of difficulties in attacking a problem directly. The client, or those being helped, may be reluctant to make changes in that particular problem area because of certain risks involved. In another case the client may not see the need for any help in that particular area. Alternatively, conditions may be so poor that an inordinate amount of effort is needed before even small-scale tangible results are possible. Similarly, there is the question of change-agent (i.e. helper) resources in the target area under review. Does he have sufficient time to create the required changes, or does he have sufficient staffing and financing? For these various reasons a change agent may begin work on certain aspects of an organization (a change target) and then work through one or more areas in order to reach the focal point of the problem, which in turn affects the task or goal of the system as a whole.[9]

Let us now turn to the H.I.C. Project to examine its strategy regarding the initial target and the ultimate ends of change. Basically, it would seem that the immediate target of the change activities was the *technology* of the organization's information system. That is to say, the H.I.C. Project provided a new technology for distributing information in the hospital. This new technology was the survey, or project. Details on the methods and procedures of survey research were given to certain selected members of the hospital organization. A subsidiary means of change, also aimed at the information system, was the provision of some temporary *structures* – a central team linked to the hospital members who were organized into a hospital team. In addition, some temporary *people* with distinctive values and skills, the members of the central team, were brought into the hospital system to help improve the functioning of the information system. In sum, hospitals were expected to obtain a better distribution of information by means of survey technology to be operated by a hospital team with the help of a temporary central team.

These temporary people helped to work the new technology, but they also seemed to have an important function in facilitating the change of attitudes and behaviour in the organization. That is to say, the central-team members spent time talking with, and working with, hospital-team members on other matters besides the survey methods themselves. The temporary structure, on the face of it, seemed to be intended to facilitate usage of the new technology, the survey, but it also may have affected the communication structure in the hospital. In other words, in the H.I.C. Project a great deal of effort was expended on the working of some new technology, namely, surveys or projects in the hospitals, which presumably had an effect on the behaviour of people in the hospital by providing them with greater amounts of information. In addition, this provision of survey information by means of a central team and a hospital team also had a potential for altering hospital structure and the characteristics of people in less obvious ways.

An improved information system, however, was not the ultimate aim of H.I.C. efforts, according to Revans. Improvements in information were expected to reduce the anxiety levels within people in the organization and this was expected to open up communication structures (reduce 'parataxis'), and ultimately improve functioning in the task of patient-care (Revans, 1964b).

Revans's approach to organizational change seems to be unique in starting basically with technology, and then moving towards changes in structure and people.[10] Generally, organizational change programmes that are focused on changing the organization as a whole, including technology, people, and structure, tend to start either with changes in people and move to structural changes (e.g. see Likert, 1961) or to start with structure and move on to people, such as changes currently flowing from the Salmon Report (see also Chapple and Sayles, 1961). Technology usually comes last, if at all, in these general programmes of planned organizational change (see Leavitt, 1965, for further details).

On the other hand, programmes emphasizing the modification of technology tend to omit active consideration of changes in either people or structure as concomitant or subsequent strategies. Most technological approaches seem to aim solely at the technological system; apparently it is felt that changes in this system are sufficient to change the task, or provide better goal achievement. Thus, work study or operational research may provide better ways of doing work by introducing new machinery, or providing new programmes for the use of existing machinery. Alternatively, new methods of doing the job may be provided for workers, in which case workers are treated as machines.

The consequences of planned technological change for people and structure have been studied by a number of investigators. Mann and Williams (1960), for example, observed the consequences of the introduction of a computer into an organization. Similarly, investigators have observed the consequences of shifting from single-place to long-wall coal-mining, and, on the basis of the observed adverse effects on people and structure, subsequent modifications in the technology were suggested (Trist and Bamforth, 1951). However, these studies did not include a programme of planned change of structure or people by means of technology. The closest comparison with the H.I.C. Project, in terms of Leavitt's typology, is the Ahmedabad experiment by Rice (1958), in which both technology and social structure were simultaneously modified to improve productivity.

A technological approach, such as that of Revans and the H.I.C. Project, typically emphasizes cognitive and objective orientations at the level of the individual and one-way influence in the relations between individuals. We shall examine each of these characteristics, and its alternative, in order to consider subsequently (Chapter 19) whether the rather unusual technological approach in this project enhanced or detracted from the results obtained, and whether further studies utilizing this approach or some modified version of it may be useful.

## COGNITIONS AND EMOTIONS

Probably the most basic dimension of the H.I.C. Project, or any similar project, is the extent to which cognitive or emotional aspects of people are emphasized. The ultimate aim of the H.I.C. Project was to affect people's behaviour, the usual aim of most change projects. However, the target of the change efforts is usually not behaviour directly but the cognitive or emotional aspects of people. By 'cognitive' aspects, we mean thinking as opposed to emotions or feelings. Cognitions or thoughts are influenced by providing information. Emotions may be influenced by emotional experiences (exposure to affective stimuli or to stimuli producing responses in the autonomic nervous system.[11]

Focusing on cognitions instead of emotions is likely to have advantages. Most people seem to want to learn, and if, in fact, they lack information, it is an easy matter to supply it and to gain acceptance of information in the place of ignorance. The provision of information is generally viewed as an efficient means of change. Even if there are conflicting beliefs present, it is easier to change or reorganize them than to change people's feelings, or even their behaviour. Feelings are irrational and illogical and are consequently unpredictable and hard to handle. On the other hand, information and 'communications' are popular and acceptable topics of discussion. Information is usually valued; it is 'a good thing'. It is commonly believed that people are eminently rational and that the more information they have, the better decisions they can make and the better their resulting behaviour.

Another reason for a cognitive emphasis is that if people do not understand or know why they behave differently, there is not likely to be as enduring a change as when they do understand. Even more important, understanding facilitates transference of learning and adaptive and flexible use of the learning obtained from any particular change programme.

In other change programmes emotional change or emotional learning is emphasized because it is 'deeper' or more basic. Emotional reactions are not readily amenable to change, but once changed they are more stable. Furthermore, it is believed that behaviour is often more closely linked to emotional stimuli than to cognitive stimuli. Thus, in psychoanalysis, the patient must re-experience the emotional situations and stimuli that are the source of his current maladaptive behaviour, and by working through them and emotionally relearning (which is more than merely acquiring cognitive insight), he is able to behave differently and more adaptively.

Having looked at the arguments for changing either cognitions or emotions, let us turn to the possible arguments against a focus of change efforts on one or the other. One danger in over-emphasizing cognitions is that it often entails under-estimating the importance of emotions. In addition, one may be lulled into a false feeling of success by the great ease with which large amounts of information may be transmitted, and by the facility with which clients may change cognitively without concomitant behavioural changes. We shall return to this notion of 'ease' (in Chapter 19).

The dangers in concentrating on emotions are, in part, the opposite of the foregoing. Firstly, cognition may be ignored, yet cognitive input should play some part in any change programme, if only because of the easiness with which such material may be provided. Furthermore, change programmes emphasizing emotions must face the problem of their relative intractability, and the greater resources needed to change them. To get at 'deep' emotions is not easy. In addition, it is a risky matter, requiring great skill as well as much time and effort. Things may go wrong because less is known about emotions and emotional change, than about cognitive change, and when something does go wrong it will have greater and more pervasive, as well as more enduring, effects on the client.

## OBJECTIVE AND SUBJECTIVE ORIENTATIONS

Another dimension, somewhat related to the cognitive-emotional dimension, is the degree of subjective-objective orientation of those participating in the change programme, including both change-agents and clients. This dimension refers to the locus of events or objects studied, examined, or considered. At the individual level, there are behaviour, cognitions, and emotions. Should one study the behaviour, cognitions, and emotions of *other* people, or of *oneself*? At the organizational level, an individual may study technology, structure, or people. Should he study other people, other structures, other technologies, or should he study people, structures, and technologies with which he is involved himself?

The subjective-objective dimension is subsumed by a more general dimension – the internal-external. Subjective is internal to the individual system, and objective is external to it. Thus, one may conceive of a group, rather than an individual, looking at matters 'subjectively' or as internal-to-the-group, instead of 'objectively' or as external-to-the-group.

It is probably easier to be 'objective' and study others, rather than oneself. One can of course readily introspect, but to look at oneself accurately is something more; it requires considerable skill and probably is most easily done with the help of others.[12]

It would appear that studying others or taking an objective approach is, at least initially, a 'safer' or a 'low-risk' approach to change in the eyes of the change-agent and of clients and sponsors. Study of oneself may be emotion-provoking. Including oneself in the purview of change efforts is likely to produce anxiety and to call into play some of the defence mechanisms available to the subject. The objective approach, furthermore, is based on the widely held assumption of our Western science-based culture that studying others facilitates an objective and scientific approach without distortions and error due to personal involvement and self-interest.

There are, however, some arguments in favour of a subjective approach. In this view science is not completely 'objective', and one should take advantage of the motivating and insight-producing qualities of subjective study. Theories often come from highly personal flashes of insight or even from the marshalling of facts by biased and prejudiced observers. Studying matters with personal relevance, and studying one's reactions to these matters, can certainly be interesting, and if there is a relatively low degree of anxiety, it can be, no doubt, quite productive.

If change of one's own behaviour is the criterion, then there is less of a transfer problem when one studies one's own behaviour rather than that of others. Alternatively, if the focus of the change programme is to 'set right' the problems of others, then the study of others does have some immediate value, assuming that one's own capabilities are sufficient to solve the problem and it is merely a matter of diagnosing the situation in order to solve it. But this would seem to be the exception rather than the rule. In addition, studying others probably facilitates cognitive learning, but studying oneself facilitates 'whole-person' learning, that is to say, changes in emotional as well as cognitive understanding, and changes in behavioural potentialities.

We have mentioned the difficulties in a subjective focus for change – the difficulties for those in a change programme (whether change-agent or client) if they include themselves as a focus of change. The difficulties arise because one cannot be as 'objective' about oneself, and because examining problems of one's own functioning and contemplating changes in it are anxiety-provoking activities. Nevertheless, there are strong reasons for persevering and dealing with these difficulties. In terms of scientific arguments, we are coming to realize that change outcomes are a function of change inputs and one must therefore study these change inputs – namely, the nature of the change-agent. Furthermore, the change-agent is often the recipient of change actions from the client, and how the former handles these actions, and whether in the process he changes in certain ways, are important to the change-agent, to the client, and to the outcomes of the change process as a whole. In terms of practice, or practical actions that are likely to be successful in producing change, one can argue similarly. Study by the change-agent of his own place in the change process gives him greater power to predict, and even control, the change process, than would a simple objective focus on the client. In short, a transactional view of change relationships suggests that both change-agent and client need to look at themselves as well as others in the situation.[13]

## INFLUENCE RELATIONSHIPS

So far, we have examined some possible psychological or individual-level emphases of an organizational change project such as the H.I.C. Project. We move now to a consideration of a social-psychological dimension – the influence relationships characterizing individuals, groups, or an organization. Change comes about by means of influence, and different kinds of influence relationships characterize organizations of varying degrees of effectiveness. By influence, we mean simply the extent one unit can affect another unit in some way.

A pair of units may be characterized by one-way, or by mutual, influence relationships. In the former case one unit influences the other to some significant degree, while the reverse is not true. In the mutual influence situation, both units influence each other to some significant degree; there is two-way influence.

The central team report that they had a strong and clear brief from the advisory committee, from Revans, and from the hospitals, to permit and encourage decisions by hospital-team members about the directions to be taken in Project work (see Chapter 5). Central-team members were not to influence these matters or to be 'directive'. There was to be 'self-direction' by hospital-team members. Only in one limited area were the central-team members to be 'experts' and to exercise influence – namely in deciding on the scientific methods used to collect and analyse data. In other words, the balance of influence of central-team and hospital-team members on each other was to be, by and large, in favour of the hospital team over the central team.

It can be argued that client self-direction is desirable because it facilitates the involvement of the client. If clients know they will have an important say in the direction of the programme, they are more likely to volunteer and join a project. In addition, self-direction is believed to encourage a continuing high level of motivation, and a commitment to carrying out actions initiated by people directing both themselves and the programme.[14] Furthermore, if instead of self-direction there is directiveness by the change-agents, there is the possibility of the directions being based on less than full knowledge of the local situation in the clients' organizations, and that clients would not be motivated to apply their full knowledge of the situation to the task in hand.

These are the arguments available to the H.I.C. Project to support the degree of influence accorded to clients and change-agents in the Project. This view of influence is based on a commonly held assumption – that influence is available in limited quantity, so that if one person in a relationship has more influence over a matter or over another person, then the other has less. This assumption may or may not be valid. But there is some research evidence that the total amount of influence in an organizational system is variable, and that some organizations may have high degrees of influence at a number of points in the organization, while other organizations may have very small amounts of influence at many of these points (Tannenbaum, 1962).

This research suggests an alternative approach to the question of the balance of influence between change-agent and client. Organizations with high degrees of mutual influence (i.e. with high influence at a number of points in the organizational system) tend to be organizations that are effective in reaching their goals. An H.I.C. Project with high influence for both change-agents and clients (i.e. more 'directiveness' from the central team) similarly may be quite effective in reaching its goals, i.e. the behavioural changes envisaged. (We shall examine this concept of influence further in Chapter 19.)

## CLARITY OF PROGRAMME

Somewhat related to the problem of influence relationships in the change programme is the extent to which programme ends and means are clearly stated and programmed. If there is ambiguity or an absence of information, then targets and programmes provide guides and thereby influence behaviour.

Clarity or structure may be assessed in a number of ways. First of all, one may assess the clarity at any one point in time. Is there something to focus on, or are there a number of different and perhaps even conflicting points, or is there nothing at all? Next, one may inquire into the relationship between events, or portions of the programme, at different times. Is there a relationship or a connection between events (e.g. between subgoals, goals) at different times, or is there no relationship, or are there conflicts between the implications of events at different times? Finally, what is the goal of the project; what is its end-point?

From the earlier chapters, the reader can see that the H.I.C. Project did not in fact specify the precise ways in which patient-care should be better at the end of the Project, although this lack of a clear end-point is not untypical of action projects. There seems to be, however, considerable variation within the Project in the extent to which the means or sub-goals were specified, and related to the ends of the Project. Certainly, the immediate steps in the Project were most clearly specified and programmed – the carrying-out of hospital projects on morale, using certain recommended survey procedures, down to even the use of certain kinds of survey instruments. But a model for the effects of this activity on aspects of the organization and its functioning or for the further ramification of these effects on patient-care was not formally specified. Neither was a model specified in terms of the previous informal experience of central-team members. The nature of 'communication' was not specified, for example, nor was it linked to other similarly specified organizational characteristics. There was no model for relations between technological, structural, and behavioural changes and task attainment. In other words, H.I.C. was to be a new change venture and there was, with the exception of the survey methodology, little definite preconceived notion of how changes would result in better patient-care.

What are the relative merits of diffuseness or lack of clarity instead of a relatively clearly specified model and programme for the change activity? The arguments for diffuseness or obscurity are, in part, similar to those for self-directiveness by hospital-team members. A diffuse project encourages willing participation by allowing people to project their own desires into the change programme. But if a specific, structured programme is proposed, there may be a conflict between the means or ends desired by hospital-team members and those specified by Project staff.

Perhaps as important as these positive reasons for devising a diffuse or unclear programme, are the situational constraints that may dictate such a programme. There may be, for example, insufficient time to work out a specific programme, even if one is desired. Similarly, the change-agents, the central-team members in this case, may not have sufficient previous experience to enable them to bring along a ready-made structure derived from earlier activities of a similar kind.

There are, of course, potential advantages for a clearer and less ambiguous (more structured) H.I.C. Project. A clear programme enables the client to examine his view of what the programme should be; it eliminates confusion, and facilitates the emergence of an integrative programme reflecting the aims and intentions of both sides. More clarity could also have been beneficial for the functioning of the central team. It would have given them guidance in a complex situation. That is to say, it would have simplified an extremely complex situation for the central team (and for the hospital teams, too), and by providing an 'external' structure, with clearly stated relationships between means and ends, would probably have given the central team more influence in running the change programme. Finally, greater structure would have provided more support in a highly emotion-provoking situation.

## ORGANIZATIONAL STRATEGY

We move now to the question of the client organization and the different focuses of change-agent attention within that organization.

If a change programme is to create change in an organization, it must somehow effect change in the various elements that make up the organization. We have mentioned before the rather unusual approach of the H.I.C. Project in starting with technology and then moving to (or trying to change) people and structure. We have also indicated above that the links between technology (use of surveys) and 'people' and structural change, and between them and the goal, were not clearly specified in the Project.

Other change projects are often equally unspecific, however. Particularly those change methodologies emphasizing 'people' change have a tendency to assume that such change, if achieved widely enough throughout the organization, is sufficient in some obscure way to produce organizational change. There is usually no explanation of how informal structure (e.g. organizational norms) or formal structure (roles and positions formally specified) would be changed by, for example, the attendance of members of an organization at T-groups (see Katz and Kahn, 1966).

One way of comparing the H.I.C. Project with other change projects is to examine how the change efforts aimed at different organizational components (such as technology, people, and structure) are specified, and in fact, carried out. Are different components systematically covered? Furthermore, what is the sequencing of these efforts? Efforts that are properly sequenced so as to support one another and to link together outcomes are probably more likely to result in enduring change for the organization as a whole.

Thus an integrated or a closely sequenced effort at changing the characteristics of technology, structure, and people in a particular segment of an organization, such as the H.I.C. efforts at changing these aspects of the hospital team in each hospital, is probably more likely to succeed in changing one or all three of these aspects than are efforts aimed at diverse segments of the organization. However, this raises the question of further strategy to bring in other segments, and eventually the organization as a whole. Since the 'top' people in an organization have a strong influence in determining organizational characteristics such as goals and various norms and rules, it is likely that change efforts at the top may be of strategic value. By starting at the top one has at least covered an important point of resistance to change, a source of 'veto-power'.

However, even if efforts at changing some aspects at the top are successful, there still remains the strategy for diffusing change throughout the organization as a whole.[15] This problem is particularly acute in an organization that is segmented or has barriers between different portions (Stanton and Schwartz, 1954). One way of dealing with it is provided by Floyd Mann

(1957), who, in the use of his survey feedback method, advocates taking change efforts sequentially down the hierarchy, level by level.

Blake and Mouton (1968) operate at various levels in the organization, including the top, but emphasize direct change of an organizational characteristic, namely the goals of the organization. The strategy is not to change first top people and subsequently people at other levels (Mann), or to change technology and then other aspects of the organization (Revans), but rather to work directly on organizational goals with an obvious bearing on organizational effectiveness.

## THE SEQUENCE OF CHANGE

One final set of concepts may serve to elucidate the H.I.C. Project and its results. We have for the most part conceptualized the Project in an essentially static way. Alternatively, one may view the change effort in a temporal or a dynamic, sequential fashion. While theoretical development in this area has not yet progressed far (Bennis *et. al.*, 1961; Bennis *et. al.*, 1969), such an approach to change is most useful, particularly for practitioners (as opposed to scientists) with certain definite goals in mind (Chin, 1961).

For the practitioner, and the scientist as he studies the process of change, Lewin's (1952) model of unfreezing the old structure, changing to a new one, and refreezing the new structure, is most useful. The structure of behaviour, as seen by Lewin, is maintained by a balance of forces, which must be modified (unfrozen) to a new equilibrium in favour of the desired change direction by either adding or (more usually) subtracting forces appropriately. After forces adequate to produce a sufficient amount of movement have been applied, then a new equilibrium must be established (refrozen) so as to maintain the newly changed position or status.

Lewin's model is also useful for understanding the diffusion of change efforts through an organization composed of various sub-systems. If one of these systems is unfrozen or efforts are made at changing it, this system will affect other systems which are linked to it or interdependent. These other systems may well show resistance (see Barnes, 1967). One way of dealing with the unsettling effects on adjacent systems is to take advantage of this unfreezing (or 'resistance', see Barnes, 1967) of adjacent systems and to pursue change efforts at the new points, thereby diffusing change further through the organization. To some extent these subsequent change efforts may also facilitate the earlier ones. That is to say, change in adjacent systems may also serve in part to unsettle and unfreeze further the first system, assuming that it is still relatively open and not refrozen. Alternatively, the subsequent efforts in adjacent systems may serve to create forces that will support the refrozen changes in the system initially changed.

In order to operate in this fashion, large resources are needed to provide adequate coverage across various sub-systems. To some extent, the programming or structuring of change activities may compensate for the absence of resources. Although there are disadvantages in the loss of flexibility, a programme frees change-agents from having constantly to improvise, invent, and decide. If the structure is appropriate, then change-agents are also given support against various pressures and strains.

Revans suggested that the hospital projects should be limited and have a definite end-point. One could interpret this in part as a programming and specification of the end of a change effort and the beginning of refreezing efforts. This is one way to make sure the limited resources of the H.I.C. central team are not overextended. However, a strategy must be specified for the focus of subsequent projects. If subsequent hospital projects were chosen as suggested above, it might be possible to integrate change activities in the subsequent sites with changes in the earlier sites, and enhance activities at both points. A thorough organizational diagnosis ideally provides some guidelines for selecting project focuses with appropriate levels of interdependence as well as guidelines for the pacing of efforts by the change-agent through adjacent sub-systems.

As we shall show below (Chapter 11), the design of the evaluation did not permit measurement of the sequential characteristics of the H.I.C. Project so as to provide a systematic, objective picture of this dynamic aspect of the change programme. However, Lewin's rather general model of change, which has been applied to 'brainwashing' (Schein, 1958) as well as to psychotherapy and community development (Lippitt *et al.*, 1958), seems useful for at least a subjective, judgemental analysis of Project events and their outcomes (see Chapter 19).

These, then, are some of the dimensions one might use to characterize the H.I.C. Project or for that matter, any similar change project. In examining the detailed descriptions of the H.I.C. Project given below, it will be useful to focus on the extent to which the means for, and targets of, change were cognitive or emotional, subjective or objective, and, turning to the change-agent and client system, the extent to which the influence relationships were one-sided or mutual. The degree of clarity in various aspects of the Project and the nature of the strategy for covering the whole organization to be changed, are also potentially useful in evaluating the Project and possible alternatives. Would some differences in emphasis within the Project provide greater success, and if so, at what cost? Or comparing the H.I.C. Project with other alternative possible change programmes, which kinds of emphases would seem to make desired changes easier? These are the questions examined in the evaluation report (Chapters 10 to 18 and especially Chapter 19).

NOTES

[1] Revans (1946b) most impressively demonstrated that variability in communications, morale, and patients' stay differed systematically by hospital. Analysis of variance showed that variability between hospitals was greater than the variability within hospitals – that these were organization-level phenomena.

[2] See Bennis *et al.* (1968, pp. 58-59) for a diagrammatic presentation of the evolution of planned change efforts.

[3] See Barnes (1967) and Greiner (1965).

[4] For further details on the aims of the H.I.C. Project, see Chapter 11. In addition, the following statement by an advisory committee member (Butterfield, 1968) provides a succinct statement of the Project courses and the overall aim of the Project:

> 'The intention was to encourage the members attending the course to pay special attention to communications between the three branches of hospital staffs which they represented and to try to improve communications by setting up research studies in their own hospitals, studies which would give good opportunities for two-way communications between various levels of staff, and thereby increase the insight into the hospital's workings and its problems. The overall objective was to improve the performance of the hospital not only in terms of staff relationships, but also in terms of medical care' (p. 186).

[5] For a survey of work done in hospitals see Wieland (1968b); also see Likert (1967) for information on organizations generally.

[6] Revans did show a correlation between some measures of communication attitudes and the length of stay of medical patients, but no other objective explanatory data were provided to amplify or interpret the relationships.

[7] Perrow (1965) defines technology as 'the techniques necessary for the execution of the task' (p. 914), or again as 'a technique or complex of techniques employed to alter "materials" (human or nonhuman, mental or physical) in an anticipated manner' (p. 915).

[8] To use the definition of organization given earlier, we might say that organizations have purposes for whose achievement they take *people* and organize them (*structure* them) so they can use *technology* to work on the *task* or goals.

[9] It should be noted that the efficacy of this roundabout way of creating change in the task of an organization need not depend solely on the change-agent ultimately reaching the problem area and directly operating on the problems. The parts of an organization are interdependent to a greater or lesser degree, so if one were to institute some major beneficial changes in, say, the nursing department, it would be bound to have (hopefully beneficial) effects on the pathology laboratory or the X-ray department. Changes in technology or structure or people may operate in an analogous fashion. Each is interdependent with the other, and with the task. Thus a change introduced in one will have effects on the other, and vice versa. In such a fashion a major change in one system may have ramifications throughout the organization, without the direct step-by-step intervention of the change agent. However, it is probably just as likely for the interdependent nature of relations within the organization to provoke the rejection and undoing of change. Changes in technology, for example, may create changes and subsequent problems in structure that are in turn solved by undoing the structural changes and reverting to the former state. For further discussion on the interdependence of organizational sub-

systems see, for example, Perrow (1965), Leavitt (1965), and Hage and Aiken (1970). Below in this chapter we shall begin the examination of the 'organizational strategy' in the H.I.C. Project, and further attention to this coverage of organizational sub-systems will be given in Chapter 19.

[10] In characterizing the H.I.C. Project as a technological project, it should be clear to the reader that we see the Project as focusing on technology and attempting to change that system in the organization. This should be differentiated from those projects which utilize technology as a means of changing people but do not change the technological system in the organization as a way of subsequently obtaining changes in people. Thus there are a number of highly 'instrumented' (Bennis, 1965) approaches to changing people, such as the questionnaires and programmed events utilized by Blake and Mouton (1968) and the survey questionnaires, data analysis manuals (including normative data from other hospitals and industries), and manuals and procedures for feedback utilized by Holloway and Lonergan (1968). The highly instrumented change programme relies on technology to produce changes in people, but once the project has been carried out, the technology is removed from the organizational system. Technology is a means to changes in people, but these changes are more or less immediately attempted, and subsequent change is a ramification of them, not a continual reiteration of the instruments or technology (although at some distant date the instruments may be applied once more as a 'booster').

[11] Of course, different kinds of information affect emotions differently, as well, and different emotional experiences (and the emotions elicited) may affect one's thinking, but the most economical efforts in either area would appear to be direct actions on cognitions or emotions, whichever kind of change is desired. In other words we assume that information facilitates cognitive change, and emotional experiences, emotional change.

[12] The principle of the T-group is based on this – the aim being to get one to use others, to use 'feedback'. Studying others is likely to be easier than studying oneself, when the focus of study is 'problems', difficulties, or other negative aspects of functioning, and when the aim of the study is to eliminate the factors causing problems.

[13] See, e.g., Schein (1969) and his emphasis on 'process consultation'.

[14] This, of course, is the basis for the emphasis on 'participation' in industry. In a sense, one might view the H.I.C. Project as an attempt to take these arguments derived from Lewin's studies of participation in discussion groups and apply them to organizations – organizational change as a result of organizational participation (self-study).

[15] See the 'Aims and Intentions of the Project', section 4d (reproduced in Chapter 1).

PART TWO

# *Central Team Report*

# 4 *Selection of hospitals and the initial training courses*

*HILARY LEIGH*

## INTRODUCTION

We open this chapter with a brief outline of the introductory meetings from which evolved a plan to carry out the Hospital Internal Communications Project, in which ten hospitals agreed to participate. This is followed by a description of the selection of members of the hospital teams, consisting of two senior representatives from each of three professional groups, and of the initial training provided. The supporting-team members (a matron, a group or hospital secretary, and a senior consultant from each hospital) attended a three-day appreciation course. Their deputies, the operational-team members, took part in a one-month training course.

In the remainder of the chapter the objectives of the Project and the purpose and content of the courses are described together with the methods used and some evaluation by the participants. Finally some recommendations are made which stress the importance of (a) identifying individual hospital needs before selecting the people to be involved and (b) building a relationship between the participants and the central team in the very earliest stages. A number of suggestions for additional training methods and for some modification of those used are also made.

## SELECTION OF PARTICIPANTS

The problem of finding a number of hospitals willing to take part in a Project based on the theme of communications was tackled in six stages over a period of twelve months. Firstly, through discussions involving representatives of The King's Fund Hospital Centre and Revans, it was decided to focus on London area hospitals, and to enlist the help of the regional hospital boards and the boards of governors of teaching hospitals. The Ministry of Health agreed to provide financial support provided that a number of hospitals could be found to take part.

At the second stage, the secretaries of the four metropolitan regions were invited by the Hospital Centre to discuss with Revans the Project proposals and to suggest hospitals likely to be interested in participating.

Approaches were also made to a few teaching hospitals. A list of hospitals was drawn up; some were suggested by the regional boards and others by the Hospital Centre.

At the third stage, over a period of five months, twenty-nine London area hospitals accepted invitations from the Hospital Centre to meet Revans to hear about and discuss his proposals. Eighteen hospitals were represented by the matron, a senior consultant, and (usually) the group secretary, as suggested in the invitation; the rest sent only one or two people. The actual length and intensity of the initial training was worked out chiefly during these meetings, and the result was a compromise in favour of what the hospitals felt would be practicable.[1]

Eventually, it was agreed there would be a two-tier team from each hospital: a supporting team consisting of the matron, the group or hospital secretary, and a senior consultant; and an operational team made up of their immediate deputies. The former would take part in a three-day appreciation course to discuss objectives, implications, and their own roles in the Project. The operational teams would undergo a one-month training in practical techniques to prepare them for undertaking projects in their own hospitals with the active co-operation of their senior colleagues, and would devote up to one-third of their time to the task. The selection of team members was to be the responsibility of individual hospitals. It was stressed that the hospital teams would themselves select the problems they wished to tackle and direct their own project activities.

During the clarification of these plans a number of major problems were discussed, although no wholly satisfactory solutions to any of them could be found. Involving doctors, particularly for the operational teams, was seen as one of the most serious difficulties. The non-clinical nature of the Project and lack of time were given as the main reasons. The feasibility of the operational teams devoting a third of their time to project work was seriously doubted. The delegation or reallocation of some of their normal work was said to be impracticable. Perhaps because of the emphasis on self-set objectives and on project activity as an essential part of the professional development of the operational teams, some hospital representatives agreed to discuss how the problem might be overcome. Revans promised to ask the regional boards to consider favourably any requests for temporary additional staff. The difficulties arising from team members leaving for higher positions elsewhere seemed soluble by the provision of training designed to meet the needs of replacement members.

At the fourth stage, the Hospital Centre followed up these meetings by writing to each group secretary inviting his comments, and asking if he wished to take any further part in the Project and what he saw as the major difficulties. Although many described problems such as the ones mentioned above, about two-thirds of the hospitals expressed continuing interest.

The fifth stage in the hospital selection process was a meeting between Revans and representatives of the hospital management committees of eighteen hospitals together with their group secretaries and regional board representatives. Revans described the progress of the attempts at collaborative planning with the potiential participant hospitals and invited support for the scheme from those present.

It was difficult at that stage to define exactly what 'support' might mean, other than goodwill and general encouragement. However, it was specifically requested that favourable consideration be given to hospitals requesting temporary staff to enable them to take part in the Project. The hospital management committee and regional hospital board representatives agreed to help, but pointed out that the extent to which the hospitals joined in the scheme rested with the hospital officers. A typical comment was: 'Those of us outside the hospitals can only provide support if they invite us to do so. Nevertheless we wish the venture every success.'

At the sixth stage the Hospital Centre followed up this meeting, writing to the group secretaries asking for reactions and inquiring whether they would be able to form teams in their own hospitals. Eventually ten hospitals agreed to join the Project, eight as a result of the meetings plus two who were approached subsequently.

In the preliminary stages the selection of hospitals was controlled by the organizers.[2] Subsequently, as intended, the process became one of self-selection by the hospitals themselves.

It seems important to ask why certain hospitals withdrew at this stage. We can glean some information from the letters written by the hospital representatives after the initial meetings. Whilst a few explicitly stated they did not think the Project would be of value to them, the majority indicated either that they could not raise enough interest among their colleagues (this certainly applied to most of the eleven hospitals who sent only one or two representatives to the introductory meetings), or that they would have liked to join if the timing of the courses could be changed. This would have enabled them to send an appropriate team.

Turning now to those who did volunteer, the following extract from the central-team director's[3] report after his initial visits to the ten hospitals gives some idea of their reasons: 'Their motives for doing so were very mixed. They included, in varying degrees, a willingness to experiment, a consciousness of some imperfections, a sense of obligation to the Hospital Centre, a wish to promote inter-disciplinary co-operation and a susceptibility to Professor Revans's eloquence and enthusiasm. Their (the group secretaries, matrons, and consultants) ideas about the possible outcomes of the experiment were, understandably, of the utmost vagueness.'

Revans designed the Project and played the leading role in meetings with hospital staff during the selection stage, working closely with Janet Craig[4] of the Hospital Centre who undertook the major part of the correspondence with the hospitals. Once it became evident that a number of hospitals were willing to take part, money was made available to recruit a small group of staff to constitute the central team, the purpose of which was to assist the hospitals throughout the Project. As Revans's main responsibilities lay in Brussels, he appointed a central-team director to organize the training courses and co-ordinate Project activities. Although remaining Project director, Revans subsequently acted chiefly as a consultant to the hospital teams and the central team.

## THE PARTICIPATING HOSPITALS

*Table 4-1* shows the ten hospitals which finally nominated teams to attend the initial training courses. Seven were general hospitals and, with two exceptions, were similar in size with between 561 and 934 beds.

TABLE 4-1 *The Ten Participating Hospitals*

| *Hospital* | *Type* | *Size (no. of beds)* |
|---|---|---|
| Edgware | general* | 673 |
| Hillingdon | general | 772 |
| Lewisham | general | 570 |
| The London | teaching | 717 |
| Mayday | general | 571 |
| North Middlesex | general | 702 |
| Queen Mary's Hospital for Children | paediatric | 720 |
| St Nicholas, Plumstead | general | 350 |
| Severalls | mental | 1620 |
| West Middlesex | general | 934 |

* Defined as 'general' or 'mostly general' by the Department of Health and Social Security.

One of the aims of encouraging a number of hospitals to become involved was to facilitate learning through the sharing of problems and progress amongst similar types of institutions. The organizers would therefore have preferred to see more than just a single teaching hospital, a single hospital for the mentally ill and a single paediatric hospital among the volunteers.

With one exception the hospitals were geographically scattered in a rough circle surrounding the Greater London area. The fact that the hospitals were located many miles apart, and that no two hospitals came from the same administrative group, probably also hindered the development of inter-hospital communication.

One of the first tasks of the central-team director was to visit each of the hospitals (once they had indicated they could form a team) to get to know something about them and discuss the selection of team members and preliminary arrangements for the training courses. Each hospital was also asked to provide certain statistical information which would be used on the courses. Usually the discussions took place with the group secretary. Sometimes the matron also took part. Only occasionally did a consultant appear at these meetings. This was in some ways a portent of subsequent team functioning.

The initial training for hospital-team members consisted of two kinds of courses repeated in two waves. Each wave comprised a three-day appreciation course for the supporting teams and a one-month course for their deputies in the operational teams. All courses were residential. The first appreciation course was held in London but the other three took place in a hotel on the seafront at Hastings.

## SUPPORTING TEAMS

*Table 4-2* shows that, with very few exceptions, the matrons, group secretaries, and senior consultants constituted the supporting teams as envisaged by Revans. About half the medical members had had some administrative experience, for example, as chairman of a medical staff committee or a medical advisory committee, although these are temporary appointments.[5] Apart from those from the London and West Middlesex Hospitals (who had been approached later) many members of the teams had represented their hospitals at the introductory meetings. A few doctors learned of the Project subsequently, for example, at a medical advisory committee meeting. One matron newly appointed was drawn into the team

TABLE 4-2 *Members of Supporting Teams*

| *Hospital* | *Medical* | *Nursing* | *Administrative* |
|---|---|---|---|
| 2 Edgware | consultant (pathology) | matron | group secretary |
| 2 Hillingdon | consultant (surgery) | matron | group secretary |
| 1 Lewisham | consultant (phys. med.) | matron | group secretary |
| 2 The London | consultant (psychiatry) | dep. matron | house governor |
| 1 Mayday | consultant (anaesthetics) | matron | dep. group secretary |
| 2 North Middlesex | consultant (anaesthetics) | matron | group secretary |
| 1 Queen Mary's Hospital for Children | consultant (paediatrics) | matron | group secretary |
| 2 St Nicholas, Plumstead | consultant (surgery) | matron | group secretary |
| 2 Severalls | consultant (psychiatry) | matron | group secretary |
| 1 West Middlesex | consultant (surgery) | matron | hospital secretary |

1 Hospital represented at the first appreciation course
2 Hospital represented at the second appreciation course

by the group secretary. Thus about half the supporting-team members had been involved in discussing the development of the Project since its inception and half knew comparatively little about the initial stages.

## OPERATIONAL-TEAM MEMBERS

The operational-team members were usually selected by the supporting teams after they had attended the appreciation courses. No hospital felt it had senior talent to spare, yet all the hospitals wanted to be involved. They experienced difficulty in finding staff to nominate and eventually sent the most senior individuals they could get.

During the introductory meetings Revans had stipulated that 'potential members should have gained from their superiors some understanding of the Project's aims, should appreciate the need to work as a team, and should want to participate'. He also suggested that 'should it not be possible for the deputies to join the operational team, then promotion potential, a reasonable level of education, and the capacity to work with colleagues selected for the team should be the criteria for selection'. Despite the difficulties arising from the non-clinical nature of the Project and the demands it would make on their time, Revans suggested that the most appropriate medical staff would be young consultants or senior registrars from the mainstream of hospital activity.

In all instances the matrons and group secretaries made their own nominations to the operational teams. Some of the administrators selected were deputy group secretaries (with responsibility for several hospitals), and others were hospital or deputy hospital secretaries (with duties in a single hospital). This was possibly in part because some of the hospitals housed the group headquarters and in part because the Project attracted interest from more than one hospital in a group. One administrative member had group and hospital responsibilities combined in his appointment.

The situation was rather different for the nurse members in that they all worked solely in their own hospitals. However, within the hospitals they functioned at widely differing levels, ranging from supervision of one department to deputizing for the matron. The nature of their work also varied considerably; for example one was in charge of the nurses' home, another was in charge of a ward, while another fulfilled a wide range of managerial functions affecting the entire nursing staff. Many matrons revealed that their nominees were selected by circumstances rather than choice.

In contrast to the nurses, the senior medical staff (see *Table 4-2*) frequently practised in more than one hospital, and sometimes in more than one group of hospitals, since they are appointed by regional hospital boards. When selecting their operational-team members, the doctors in the supporting teams usually sounded out a few people or put the problem to the medical staff committee. One doctor proceeded to choose the newest junior as 'the one who could most easily be spared – and my nominee was quite happy with that'. Where these methods were unsuccessful, the administrators felt it became their task to find medical team members. As one administrator put it, 'There was an additional difficulty in selling the Project to the doctors because we didn't understand ourselves quite what was going to be involved once the courses were completed.'

An examination of the operational medical members in *Table 4-3* shows that the largest number were psychiatrists, with anaesthetists a close second. This may be because the nature of the Project attracted individuals in these specialties. It may also be that the medical members selected were those who could most easily be released from their duties without disrupting the hospital routine; for example in at least two instances members had just taken up new appointments. A third reason may be that these members were from the more 'course-minded' groups of hospital staff. A fourth reason might lie in the fact that, in general, the medical profession does not seem to encourage aspiring doctors to involve themselves in social medicine projects.[6] This is sometimes viewed as a peripheral or deviant activity. In this Project one physician was given a 'friendly warning' by a senior colleague that he might damage his chances of a better job if he continued to devote time to H.I.C. activities.

The outcome of the selection process seems to indicate that the selectors had been influenced more by expediency in choosing their operational teams than by the need to build a balanced team fulfilling the stated requirements of the H.I.C. Project.[7] In failing to develop a sufficient understanding of what their operational teams were going to do, the appreciation courses compounded the difficulties for both teams. In many instances the courses and subsequent project activities were seen as an additional task for senior staff to undertake rather than as an integral part of hospital management.

The wide range of levels of responsibility and the different functional areas from which they were selected also made it difficult for some team members to work together and to implement their project findings. Thus the make-up of some teams created new relationships that did not match or fit with the individual members' actual work relationships. Consequently any development of effective group functioning could not be easily built upon during their normal daily work in the hospital. Despite this and many other problems, the hospital teams did solve some problems and did improve some of their communications practices (see, for example, Chapter 16).

## THE OBJECTIVES OF H.I.C.

The Project aimed to improve communication[8] among those most concerned with related hospital problems. Co-operative problem-solving by small multidisciplinary groups was a stated primary goal.

TABLE 4-3 *Operational-team Members*

| | Course members | | | |
|---|---|---|---|---|
| *Hospital* | *Medical* | *Nursing* | *Administrative* | *Notes* |
| 2 Edgware† | senior hospital medical officer (geriatrics) | deputy matron | deputy group secretary* | |
| 2 Hillingdon | consultant anaesthetist | deputy matron | deputy group secretary* | |
| 1 Lewisham | consultant surgeon | ward sister | hospital secretary* | |
| 2 The London | consultant psychiatrist plus a lecturer in social medicine | assistant matron | deputy house governor | additional medical member accepted at the request of the hospital |
| 1 Mayday | consultant anaesthetist | home sister | deputy hospital secretary | medical member also attended appreciation course |
| 2 North Middlesex | consultant psychiatrist | deputy matron | assistant group secretary* | |
| 1 Queen Mary's Hospital for Children | consultant psychiatrist | deputy matron | deputy group secretary* | medical member based at another hospital in the group |
| 2 St Nicholas, Plumstead | consultant anaesthetist | assistant matron | hospital secretary and group administrative officer | group administrative officer and medical member based at other hospitals in the group |
| 2 Severalls | assistant consultant psychiatrist | assistant matron | hospital secretary | |
| 2 West Middlesex† | senior registrar (gen. medicine) | assistant matron | deputy hospital secretary* | |

1 Hospital represented at the first training course
2 Hospital represented at the second training course
* Group administrative offices located at these hospitals.
† The supporting teams from these hospitals participated in the first appreciation course.

During the introductory meetings and again during the appreciation course Revans suggested that two of the most important contributions to improved communication were:

(a) more accurate information on how the hospitals functioned:
(b) the collection, analysis, and interpretation of this information by the people most concerned with its content, who would then act upon it and evaluate their actions.

In the process of carrying out (b) team members would have an opportunity to learn about the interlocking nature of their work and about their interactions in ways that would enable them to tackle subsequent problems better. The purpose of the courses was to equip the team members with a sufficient appreciation of certain tools of social science to enable them to start this process.

Therefore the kinds of change aimed at included not merely improvements in work methods or organization but changes in the process of problem-solving and changes in individuals, particularly team members, leading to better communication and improved hospital functioning (see Chapter 5, part one for a discussion of these goals).

## APPRECIATION COURSES

The object of the three-day appreciation course was not so much to exhibit the techniques of social inquiry as to discuss the problems of starting it, maintaining interest once it had started, and of adjusting to the stresses and strains that any ensuing action would inevitably create.

Thus, in planning the courses the central-team director defined two specific goals:

1. to explain the aims of the Project and to encourage discussion of the implications for each hospital,
2. to encourage the members to second appropriate deputies for the one-month course.

Attempts were made to reach these goals through reviews of relevant findings in current research on organizational change followed by group discussions concentrating on how the results might be applied in hospitals. A management consultant described his work in hospitals and other fields. Another session was devoted to examining recent developments in the hospital service. Small groups of team members talked about the kinds of problems they would like to tackle in their own hospitals. The feasibility of tackling these problems was then discussed with all course members and course staff.

It was stressed that an immediate aim was to create a team of six in each hospital. The function of the appreciation-course members (i.e. the supporting teams) would be to provide leadership and active assistance to their operational teams in whatever ways particular situations might demand. For example, it was the task of the supporting teams to ensure that their operational-team members would be freed sufficiently from their normal jobs to enable them to carry out Project work. It did not seem possible to define specifically the kinds of support that would be required except in these very general terms.[9]

Both supporting and operational teams jointly would select projects, which the operational teams could then plan and execute. The one-month training course aimed to help the operational teams gain a serviceable understanding of certain methods of social analysis. Using these methods to tackle specific problems would hopefully provide the participants with an opportunity for increased understanding of their own interactions and also help in developing a greater awareness of how their organizations functioned. It was hoped that the number of staff involved in the process would increase as confidence developed through successful attempts at co-operative problem-solving. The techniques of social analysis were seen merely as one approach towards the ultimate goal of improving hospital functioning.

In trying to foster the development of the process described above, the need to keep in close contact with participating hospitals nearby was stressed. In Revans's (1965c) view, 'Such contact will be essential for success since the problems of running an exercise of this kind will be novel and each hospital should be glad to learn from the experiences of others'.

At this point it seems appropriate to quote from the then Minister of Health's remarks to the appreciation course members. He described the Project as 'partly a research project, partly an experiment in education, partly a management adventure ... "enterprise" in both senses of the word seems most fitting. Professor Revans has said quite frankly that he can offer no guarantee of success or forecast precisely what he will discover. Like Christopher Columbus and his company you are quite likely to reach America when looking for India and to believe that it is India you have found, and some of you may quite easily feel inclined to mutiny on the way.'[10]

## ONE-MONTH COURSES FOR OPERATIONAL TEAMS

Three operational teams attended the first one-month course in the autumn of 1965, two months after the first appreciation course for the corresponding supporting teams. Seven operational teams attended the second course at the end of November 1965,[11] about a month after the appreciation course for their supporting teams (see *Table 4-3*).

The month's course aimed to provide an introduction to some methods of social analysis that might help the teams in their attempts to identify, analyse and ameliorate difficulties of communication within their hospitals. 'Their introduction to these methods should combine the maximum of practice with the minimum of theory and this theory should consist, as far as possible, in the records of successful research projects in parallel fields' (Revans, 1965c).

The central-team director designed the courses with the following goals:

1. to develop an increasing awareness of the nature, extent and implication of communication problems,
2. to provide experience in multidisciplinary team activities,
3. to introduce
   (a) group dynamics and group discussion methods,
   (b) survey procedures (interviews, questionnaire design, elementary statistics and their application in hospitals, report-writing),
4. to emphasize the relevance of communication to the organizational and economic problems of hospitals,
5. to encourage the development of inter-hospital contact during subsequent Project activities.

Two sets of papers compiled by the central team's information officer were circulated to each participant shortly before the course. The first set summarized some relevant research reports including the Hawthorne experiments (Roethlisberger and Dickson, 1947) and more recent work (Georgopoulos and Mann, 1962; Revans, 1964b; Bendall, 1965). The second set contained outlines of techniques which would be introduced on the course itself; these included statistical sampling techniques, questionnaire design, and critical notes on different types of interview.

The content of the first two weeks of the course can be classified into three broad areas.

1. Background topics: (a) problems of organization in the hospital service, (b) the role of operational research in hospital management, (c) a critical evaluation of the contributions of the social sciences to management with particular reference to different kinds of surveys, (d) the problems of communications generally, including perceptions, awareness, and the individual's reaction to change.

2. Research findings from studies concerned with (a) length of patient stay in hospitals, (b) staff stability and turnover, (c) the problems of professional and technical staff, (d) the measurement of ward sisters' attitudes, and (e) student nurse wastage.

3. Introduction to some analytical techniques with emphasis on (a) elementary methods and applications of statistics, (b) sources of statistical information, (c) interview and questionnaire design, (d) studying interactions in working groups and group discussion techniques, (e) work study, and (f) report-writing.

*Table 4-4* shows the number of hours given to each of these areas. About half of the time ($26\frac{1}{2}$ hours) was spent in learning about techniques through lectures and practical exercises. Background topics occupied just under a third of the time (16¼ hours), and hearing about research findings approximately one-fifth (11 hours).

TABLE 4-4 *Number of Hours given to Topics during First Two Weeks*

| | *Background topics* (hours)* | *Research findings (hours)* | *Introduction to analytical techniques (hours)* | *Totals (hours)* |
|---|---|---|---|---|
| First week | | | | |
| Monday | 4½ | | | 4½ |
| Tuesday | | | 5 | 5 |
| Wednesday | | 4½ | 1½ | 6 |
| Thursday | 1½ | 4½ | | 6 |
| Friday | 3 | | 3 | 6 |
| | 9 | 9 | 9½ | 27½ |
| Second week | | | | |
| Monday | 1* | | 3 | 4 |
| Tuesday | | | 6 | 6 |
| Wednesday | 1 | | 4½ | 5½ |
| Thursday | 2¼* | 2 | 1¾ | 6 |
| Friday | 3 | | 1¾ | 4¾ |
| | 7¼ | 2 | 17 | 26¼ |
| Total hours | 16¼ | 11 | 26½ | 53¾ |

* Including preparatory discussions on project exercises.

During the third week each team carried out a practice project in another Project hospital without direct supervision from the course staff. Whenever possible the hospital was the one nearest to that of the visiting team. With the help of a statistical profile and discussions with the home team, a particular group of staff was selected for investigation by the visiting team. A supporting-team member at the host hospital was asked to meet the visiting team on arrival. Subsequent arrangements for collecting data and interviewing staff were made directly between the visiting team and the home supporting team. Through analysing records, constructing a questionnaire, interviewing staff, and holding group discussions, each team set out to examine the turnover and recruitment problems of their chosen group. The results were then analysed and each team produced a written report.

During the final week of the course these reports were discussed and evaluated. Visiting and home teams exchanged views on each other's reports and reacted to the content. Subsequently members of the course staff commented on individual reports with each pair or trio of teams and discussed the problems encountered by the teams in carrying out their projects. Later three speakers who had lectured earlier in the course commented on project design, including methodology and the use of statistics.

Towards the end of the week, the supporting-team members arrived to learn how their operational-team colleagues had found the course and to read the project reports on their own hospitals. As this was the first time that all six members of each hospital's teams had met together since the courses began, they were given an opportunity to discuss the future of the project in more depth.[12] The final day of the course was devoted chiefly to a presentation of a management project in which hospital staff and a research team were co-operating. Some of the situations and problems relevant to the H.I.C. Project were emphasized.

One of the most unusual and exciting elements of the course was the mixture of participants. Senior doctors, nurses, and administrators are rarely found (in this country at any rate) attending the same course, although the situation is changing. The major challenge lay in providing appropriate course content at a level that would meet the different needs of members of such a heterogeneous group, particularly in terms of their ability to cope with the material and the recency of previous course experience. For some nurses it was many years since they had attended courses. A few administrators held university degrees, some held professional qualifications, others had learned on the job. The doctors were the most experienced attenders of courses. Another challenge lay in trying to help senior hospital staff, who are traditionally trained in professional isolation, to become integrated teams.

To help solve some of these problems the participants worked together as hospital teams in practical exercises, such as constructing interview schedules. Probably the most potent method of learning how they could work together was the practice project undertaken in another hospital. To foster the development of inter-hospital contact the teams from geographically close hospitals were placed in the same discussion groups whenever possible.

However, as *Table 4-5* shows, over half the course material in the first two weeks was presented in formal lectures. Over the whole course, lectures occupied about one-third of the total time. A smaller proportion would have been preferable,[13] but since the central-team director was obliged to recruit visiting speakers to staff the course, it was difficult to ensure the use of teaching methods that would involve maximum active participation by the course members.

With the ending of the courses, the initiative for starting specific hospital projects lay with the hospital teams. A date was agreed for the teams to meet the central team to discuss which projects, if any, they intended to

TABLE 4-5 *Teaching Methods used during First Two Weeks*

| | *Lectures** (*hours*) | *Syndicate discussions* (*hours*) | *Participative exercises* (*hours*) | *Totals* (*hours*) |
|---|---|---|---|---|
| First week | | | | |
| Monday | 3 | 1½ | | 4½ |
| Tuesday | | | 5 | 5 |
| Wednesday | 3 | 1½ | 1½ | 6 |
| Thursday | 4½ | 1½ | | 6 |
| Friday | 3 | 3 | | 6 |
| | 13½ | 7½ | 6½ | 27½ |
| Second week | | | | |
| Monday | 4 | | | 4 |
| Tuesday | 1½ | | 4½ | 6 |
| Wednesday | 5½ | | | 5½ |
| Thursday | 4¼ | 1¾ | | 6 |
| Friday | 1¾ | 3 | | 4¾ |
| | 17 | 4¾ | 4½ | 26¼ |
| Total hours | 30½ | 12¼ | 11 | 53¾ |

* Including questions and answers after lectures.

undertake and to define the nature and extent of assistance they would need.

## DISCUSSION OF THE COURSES

In his review of the courses, the central-team director commented as follows:

'Since the appreciation courses lasted only three days it was difficult to do more than paint a general picture of the very complex nature of the Project. Real feedback and considered criticisms of the month courses which had been planned was hardly possible. It might have been better to have held further short appreciation course after an interval of a month or so and before starting the training courses. Such an interval might have enabled the senior hospital managers to discuss aims and responsibilities with their colleagues and hence send appropriate representatives as operational team members to the training courses.

'In the event, the operational teams were diverse in character. In almost every instance, they arrived with the sketchiest of briefing, saying that they had not had time to read the background research papers. Many were surprised to hear they would be expected ultimately to undertake projects in their own hospitals. As the subject matter was entirely new to most of the course members, it would have been astonishing had they mastered the skills outlined after four weeks' training, including a week spent on a group project. In the event, the stimulus of three weeks' residence during which members of the medical, nursing, and administrative professions worked, ate, and drank together, proved to be of considerable value. In particular, the unique experience of working out a team project in another hospital inspired considerable confidence and enthusiasm.'

In order to obtain another view, we talked to a number of hospital-team members, approximately one third of the total course membership (20 out of 62). Six of these had attended the appreciation courses and fourteen had taken part in the one-month courses. As the purpose of the courses was to prepare the participants for undertaking projects in order to improve their work we chose some of those members who had been most active in initiating, planning, and working through problems. Usually their project work had involved contact with the central team. The interviews took place during July and August 1968. The sample of active team members is therefore selected so that it offers an opportunity to show how the courses were at their potentially most useful (participants' perceptions may become distorted over time but also, more importantly, are tempered by experience of the usefulness of the courses). Furthermore the sample does not attempt to say whether the consequences of the courses were good or bad (the sample is not representative), the purpose being to understand the process of the Project.

There was no single reaction to the appreciation courses. Some of the respondents had developed expectations from the introductory meetings and were irritated by the amount of repetition of earlier material. In any future Project it would be important to ensure all senior staff experience a common introduction even if it does take longer. The most well-received lectures were those concerned with reports of hospital research. However, in general, many of the respondents said that most of the lectures were too theoretical, and that they wanted more speakers with hospital experience.

Some found discussion groups helpful, while others described a lack of enthusiasm for discussing topics that had been talked about at the introductory meetings. This could have been due to insufficient material presented in the lectures or difficulty in relating the material to their own hospital situations. Different professional loyalties, different previous experience, and varied expectations also made it difficult for some members to adjust to discussion groups (Sofer and Hutton, 1959, p. 67). Some would have welcomed more information about the content of the month's course, whereas a few said that too much discussion was devoted to planning these courses.

At the end of the course the respondents said they were still unclear about what was expected of them. They were also concerned firstly about the problems of finding appropriate deputies, and secondly about the amount of time the Project would require. A few felt the course should have been longer; others said they learned enough to be able to work with those who attended the one-month course.

Joining up with their operational teams towards the end of the one-month course was described as valuable both in expanding appreciation-course members' knowledge of the process of the Project and in enabling both teams to get to know each other better before returning to the hospital environment.

Many of the above criticisms of the appreciation course were also made of the one-month course, and we shall attempt below to deal with them in more detail. Overall the chief benefits were intangible and related to incentives. Many said the course created an 'in-group feeling' among team members, 'provided impetus' and generally engendered enthusiasm to go ahead with the Project.[14]

Whereas many of the appreciation-course members had taken part in discussions from the very beginning, operational-team members were generally not well prepared for the one-month course. Most were told about the course by their immediate superiors and very few had taken part in the introductory meetings. Some did not realize that their project activities would continue after the courses. About half said they had not wanted any more information beforehand but, among those who did, there was a general feeling that their superiors were equally confused. Even central-team members were not able to give them satisfactory information. The background papers were generally felt to be difficult to understand: the statistical papers and the Georgopoulos and Mann study were particularly mentioned. Just under a third of the respondents said they had not had time to read them, partly because the papers were not received until a week before the course.

Lectures about actual research in hospitals relevant to the goals of the Project were better received than the theoretical lectures, such as those on statistics. In addition many respondents found it difficult to learn from lectures and felt little allowance had been made for this. More popular were the teaching methods that involved active participation by course members, for example interviewing, designing questionnaires, and studying the functioning of working groups.

The comments about syndicate discussions fell into two groups. Firstly they were recognized as potentially valuable learning situations, but inhibited either because participants did not feel sufficiently knowledgeable to discuss the topic constructively or, because of the multidisciplinary structure of the group. Secondly, many described the syndicate groups as valuable both in lowering barriers of status and profession and in improving behavioural skills, for example, by encouraging members to contribute more confidently to the discussion. Some tutorial guidance might have made the syndicates more beneficial but as the central team hardly existed at that time it was not possible to give it.[15]

The most successful part of the course, from the respondents' viewpoint, was the practice project undertaken in the third week. There was unanimous agreement that this was useful in promoting interdisciplinary co-operation, learning about other hospitals and the similarity of their problems and in discovering the kind of information the methods they had used could yield. A few mentioned that although the experience provided insight into problems, they collected too much information and found it difficult to define what was relevant. Many said they worked very late into the night most of the week yet they had little time to discuss the material properly. This might have been another opportunity for members of the central team (had it been formed) to learn about the kind of functions they would subsequently need to perform.

The respondents were most critical about the final week of the course. The evaluation and discussion with course staff of their reports fell far short of their expectations. They would have preferred a staff member to spend more time working closely with each team critically evaluating their individual reports. Guidance was also desired in interpreting the value of reports made by other teams on their own hospitals as well as in coping with the reactions of others to their own investigations. Thus the participants wanted not only skills that would help in appraising the content of the material, but also help in dealing with the process of giving and receiving feedback (Sofer and Hutton, 1959, pp. 55-58). These points were stressed again in the suggestions, made by some respondents, of ways in which the content of the course might be improved; for example, 'more about people's reactions to threatening situations' and 'more about the problems caused by delays in taking action on findings'. In other words, communication with hospital staff (outside the team) and the human problems associated with actually changing situations were felt to be areas in which the training provided did not meet the subsequent needs of team members.[16]

However, most respondents admitted that, in general, the course was helpful in teaching them how to work together as a team, and in developing a greater appreciation of the problems of other professional groups in the hospital. Informal contact between team colleagues and between teams from different hospitals was described as 'very helpful' by most respondents, although the latter type of contact was not made much use of afterwards.

In judging the course overall, the respondents were unanimous in saying they had gained a better understanding of 'what social science was about'. Most also said that while they had learned how certain techniques could help in tackling hospital problems, they were also aware of the superficial nature of their knowledge.

The administrators apparently learned something about social science methods that they could use to increase their efficiency, while most nurses felt that their perceptions of their own jobs and those of others had changed and said this had made them more tolerant. The doctors found the technical information useful and felt that the course had made them more critical. One or two doctors suggested that the course had helped in developing 'a greater potential for understanding my job in the hospital'.

On being asked about the extent to which the course had affected them in the execution of their normal daily tasks, nearly all respondents felt it had helped them become more 'analytical' in tackling problems and increased their willingness and ability to 'explain things more to other staff'. All respondents felt the course had demolished 'status and professional barriers' among team members. Some said they had learned something about different approaches and different techniques, which had influenced their attitudes and methods of dealing with people.

Finally, there was a general feeling among those interviewed that there was 'too much in the course'. Most of all the respondents would have liked a clearer definition of Project objectives.

## CONCLUSIONS AND RECOMMENDATIONS

As we have shown, there were many positive reactions to both types of course. The most useful lectures concerned hospital research and communication. Also popular were the participative exercises such as designing questionnaires, carrying out interviews, and studying working groups. The practice project seemed to be most successful in promoting team identification, providing new insights into problems, and developing a recognition of the similarity of hospital problems. But perhaps the most important achievement lay in the fact that the course generated considerable enthusiasm among team members for undertaking projects in their own hospitals.

However, the courses were also heavily criticized in many ways. As this training was a major influence on the nature and conduct of the thirty-eight projects carried out during the next three years it becomes extremely important to consider how it might have been improved. The following suggestions for changes are based partly on the sample evaluation of the H.I.C. courses and partly on the subsequent experiences of the central team and the hospital teams.

To facilitate the development of inter-hospital contact it might have been better to concentrate on recruiting hospitals from the same or adjacent administrative groups. Our experience suggests that problems are not easily shared among staff from different hospitals. Technical difficulties are willingly discussed, but specific problems of organization and management seem to be viewed as matters for internal discussion and resolution, and not for more public examination. An alternative approach might be to provide small groups of hospitals with a highly structured opportunity to work through a commonly felt problem in an atmosphere designed to create psychological security.

Now let us consider the selection of team members. The advantage of the H.I.C. team structure lay in emphasizing the participation of doctors, nurses, and administrators at a senior level in the hospital, thus directly tackling communication problems among representatives of these three groups. But with this emphasis, some of the disadvantages also became apparent. The focus was on the holders of particular offices, and perhaps insufficient consideration was given to the specific issues they would study and the process by which such activities would improve hospital functioning. As we have seen, some of the operational-team members selected did not meet the suggested criteria, and this was to have consequences for subsequent project activities (see Chapter 6). Nevertheless it was hoped the participants (in their roles as senior managers) would act as agents of change and improvement throughout their hospitals, both in solving problems and bettering communication.

An important conclusion, as Revans has pointed out (see Chapter 1), is that the supporting teams needed a more thorough preparation than was provided by the introductory meetings and the appreciation course. In any future Project, for example, a first step could consist of discussions between individual hospitals and the central team for the purpose of clarifying the nature of their interest, and the extent to which it was shared among top management. They would need to discuss specific issues that might be tackled in their own hospitals, the kind and number of people who might participate, and what criteria of success would be used. The implications of tackling different problems would then become clearer and attention would be focused on the type of problem that was of major common concern, systemic in nature and likely to benefit from a multidisciplinary approach. The relationship between the problem selected and the hospital activities the project was intended ultimately to affect would also need to be spelt out. These meetings should also raise questions about the implications of commitment, such as the resources and the time required, and the feasibility of participation at that particular period in the life of the hospital.[17]

During the appreciation course, it was difficult for the organizers to specify either a programme of activities to follow the initial courses or the amount of time that the operational-team members would need to devote to the Project, as particular problems in each hospital had not then been defined. The supporting-team members wanted greater clarification of their roles than could be given and most wanted more information about the content of the month's course.[18]

The suggested preparation described above would reverse the order of two of the early stages in the H.I.C. Project. The individual hospital needs would be ascertained first, and then the key staff to be involved would be identified.[19] Participation need not be restricted to the deputies of the top three although they might well be included. In this way, some of the uncertainties expressed by the appreciation-course members about the objectives of the Project should be overcome. Subsequent activities might then be accepted as an integral part of hospital management[20] and to a lesser extent of the professional development of managerial staff, rather than as an additional task for subordinates to undertake.[21]

As for the content and teaching methods used on the courses, there are a number of conclusions to be drawn. Participants in both courses valued the material concerned with organizational change, communications, and relevant research findings, but found more theoretical material, such as statistics, difficult. The practical exercises and the practice project, which emphasized 'learning through doing' were described as the most useful part of the one-month course.

In view of the difficulties experienced by course members with the lecturing methods, it seems desirable that any future course should employ a wider range of teaching methods and a smaller number of trainers or lecturers presenting better integrated material.[22] For example, with regard to training methods Bass and Vaughan (1968) in their evaluation of training techniques suggest (among other things) that case studies, simulation exercises, and programmed group exercises are all superior to the lecturing method in the extent to which they make use of certain basic principles of learning and give a better chance of the knowledge being applied in work situations.[23] Role-playing sessions might help in overcoming some of the problems mentioned earlier arising from the multidisciplinary structure of the group.[24]

From the evaluative discussions with course members it seems evident that information-gathering techniques were over-emphasized in the month's course compared with other stages and processes involved in carrying out surveys, solving problems, and implementing findings.[25] In addition, any future programme would need to include more emphasis on interpretation and critical appraisal of results. The actual content and training techniques used would be determined by the needs, experience, and educational background of participants in the light of the activities they would subsequently undertake.

A potentially important conclusion about future training may be inferred from the discussion of the course evaluation. Team members wanted more help in giving and receiving feedback and in learning how to develop constructive co-operative relationships with other hospital staff whose work was being investigated. Learning about some techniques for preparing staff and discussing findings, such as feeding back to groups systematically down the hierarchy, might have been helpful here (see Mann and Likert, 1952, p. 57). The problems of diffusion, of working with and through others, require skills of a different kind from information-gathering. To help others make adaptive changes in perceptions and behaviour in their work implies that those helping must be able to understand the processes involved. It is necessary to remember that although the teams were multidisciplinary, they came from highly compartmentalized institutions.

One possible approach might be to consider some kind of sensitivity training. Some important goals of sensitivity training are concerned with helping participants make adaptive changes in their perceptions and behaviour in the work situation through improved self-understanding and an increased capacity to develop meaningful, productive relationships.[26] While the evidence for this recommendation is somewhat tentative nevertheless it should be seriously considered by those who embark on a project with aims similar to that of the H.I.C. Project. However it is not suggested that such training should be used in isolation but that it should form part of an organizational change programme.

In conclusion, there are two major points to be made about the courses. Firstly, a primary concern during the early stages should be to build up a close working relationship between the hospital teams and the central team in which mutual confidence and shared influence can develop[27] (see Chapter 5 for more discussion on this point). Secondly, it seems desirable that the training sessions should be distributed throughout the whole Project period and not concentrated at the beginning as in the current Project. This suggestion is based on our experience that further doubts, problems, and training needs arise in the hospital as a result of project activity.[28] It might be better to provide initial training in relatively small amounts, increasing and varying the amounts to meet the needs of particular hospital situations within an overall framework mutually agreed at the outset.

Finally, it should be pointed out that the H.I.C. courses had many beneficial effects on the course members. The suggestions outlined above are based on the invaluable experience gained during the Project.

(For the evaluation viewpoint of the initial training courses, see Chapter 15.)

## NOTES

1 For a fuller account of the first introductory meetings see Human Relations in Hospitals (1964); Hospital Internal Communications (1964); Internal Communication in Hospital (1964); H.I.C., Conference at the Hospital Centre (1964); Further Communications (1964).

2 Revans, the chairman of the King's Fund Hospital Centre Committee, and the director and assistant director of the King's Fund Hospital Centre. Later they were joined by the central-team director.

3 When we use the term 'director' we shall mean Revans. This should be distinguished from the 'central-team director' who was appointed in 1965 to take charge of the Project on the spot in London.

4 Assistant Director, the King's Fund Hospital Centre.

5 Throughout the book we shall include doctors when referring to hospital-team members as managers; it has been urged that doctors should be considered as managers (Ministry of Health, 1966b) although they are not formally designated as such. For further evidence on this point see Ministry of Health (1967), and Scottish Home and Health Department (1967).

[6] At that time (1965), for example, there were, with one exception (St Thomas's), no departments of social medicine in the twelve medical schools of the University of London.

[7] For some views on the problems of training staff with heterogeneous backgrounds, see Adlington (1969).

[8] 'The term communication in this context is broadly defined. It suggests not only the physical means of communication, such as telephone and standard forms, since these are not unimportant; it connotes the interpretation no less than the transmission of data and emotions. Communication, in this sense, is a two-way process; it teaches both the sender and the receiver; and the hospital is seen as a self-adjusting organism rather than as a fixed mechanical structure. Hence, though it must have its formal network of organization and procedures, the sensory nervous system of the hospital is constantly obliging its staff to examine their own performances: feedback is its essential characteristic' (Revans, 1966a).

[9] For a view on some of the difficulties encountered by administrative trainees attempting to learn within the confines of a working hospital, see Adlington (1969).

[10] For a full account of the Minister's speech, see Hospital Internal Communications: A Three-day Course Provided by King Edward's Hospital Fund (1965).

[11] For a description of the month's course by one of the participants, see Watson (1966).

[12] The importance for training of the relationship between superior and subordinate is highlighted by Beahan (1966).

[13] For a concise account of the limitations of the lecturing method, see Bass and Vaughan (1968, pp. 94-95). See also Levine and Butler (1952).

[14] Similar feelings seemed to be much more apparent at the end of the one-month course although this was not reported in the interviews.

[15] For one brief view of two contrasting approaches to syndicate work, namely, groups with a formal structure of chairman, secretaries, and delegated work versus 'leaderless' groups, see Schurr (1969, pp. 120-121). A full discussion of aspects of group functioning is provided by Thelen (1954), Klein (1961), Cartwright and Zander (1962). See also Maier (1950).

[16] Translating learning into action cannot be left to chance. The Tavistock Institute of Human Relations organize 'application' group sessions after their T-groups (see Rice, 1965). See also Miles (1959).

[17] The importance of carrying out a thorough diagnosis of organizational needs before attempting to make changes is emphasized by Lorsch and Lawrence (1969, p. 468).

[18] For a detailed account of the preparation of senior managers in a training project to improve interpersonal and interdepartmental co-ordination and communication, see Hesseling (1966).

[19] For views on the need for a thorough assessment of training needs before proceeding with training, see Bass and Vaughan (1968, pp. 76-84).

[20] The need for planned integration of the involvement of top managers and team problem-solving is illustrated in the use of the managerial grid (see Blake *et al.*, 1964).

[21] See notes 9 and 12 above.

[22] For an example of a European School using non-lecture methods of teaching, including the project method, see Rees (1966).

[23] More specifically these methods provide in varying degrees opportunities for active participation of learner; feedback of knowledge of results; meaningful organization of materials; practice and repetition; and conditions most

favourable for transfer (see Bass and Vaughan, 1968, p. 131).

[24] One research programme is currently directed to 'verifying the specific relationships shown between various teaching methods and the acquisition of managerial skills'. One hypothesis being tested is that role playing can improve the ability of participants to 'understand better the view of others, and hence communicate more effectively (see Hawrylyshyn, 1969).

[25] A number of recently developed participatory exercises are described by Beckhard and Hesseling. For example Beckhard's (1969) goal-setting exercise creates an opportunity for all levels of management to take part in setting organizational goals by having members participate in a series of different groups (heterogeneous, functional, etc.), defining problems, categorizing problems, and eventually setting their own goals in what he calls an 'organization confrontation' meeting.

Hesseling (1966) describes a communication exercise originally developed by Leavitt and later Bavelas. The purpose is to develop insights into communication problems through personal experience of trying to solve a puzzle, and subsequently exploring interpersonal behaviour, opinions, and feelings. A puzzle consisting of eighteen pieces is distributed amongst five participants sitting round a table. Each individual has to form a square composed of more than two pieces and moreover, as a member of a team, to do so in such a way that every other member can form a square of the same area. Some individuals start with pieces that suggest an individual solution but, if retained, would prevent the achievement of a team solution. Participants can exchange only written communications to solve the puzzle, but they can talk about team organization, the communication structure, problem-solving strategy, and analyse their own shortcomings. At the end of the time limit of one hour, each participant completes a questionnaire, rating the importance of each participant, stating who had the most useful pieces at the outset, how much co-operation had been received, etc. The results are then discussed with the participants. This kind of game, in which individuals actually experience a problem situation, work through it, and obtain feedback on the principles, must be expected to be better than merely having either understanding or experience, but not both together.

[26] For a concise description of T-group training, see P. B. Smith (1968, pp. 286-287); Bass and Vaughan (1968, pp. 119-127). A more detailed account is given by Whitaker (1965).

[27] Some factors to be considered in developing this relationship are discussed by Lippitt *et al.* (1958, pp. 115-126).

[28] For a brief account of a further two-day course for some new hospital-team members, see Chapter 5, part two.

# 5 *The central team, its functions and relationships*

*HILARY LEIGH*

## INTRODUCTION

In the first part of this chapter we shall describe the staffing of the Project, the guidelines for collaborating with the hospital teams and the functions of central-team members. Some of the conflicts and problems associated with the modification of these guidelines are discussed. Some recommendations concerning the skills needed by central-team members are also made.

The rest of the chapter is devoted to outlining the relationship between the central team and the hospital teams with brief comments on how the regional hospital boards and hospital management committees became involved. The various methods of collaboration are described together with some of the difficulties experienced by hospital-team and central-team members. It is suggested that the central and hospital teams need to establish a closer, more open relationship in the very earliest stages, and that the central team requires a wider range of skills among its members if it is to fulfil its complex role. Finally, suggestions are made about some conditions desirable for effective collaboration in order to improve hospital functioning.

## PART ONE: THE CENTRAL TEAM AS A WORKING GROUP

It might help the reader if first we describe in outline the staffing of the Project as it evolved. Initially there were four central-team members recruited during 1965, although they did not meet together until January 1966. The first group of five students arrived in the middle of 1966 to spend approximately six months working in Project hospitals, because some teams could not undertake data collection. At the end of 1966, owing to various difficulties, the director of the central team and the information officer resigned. Two new members joined the central team in early 1967 and one of these left three months later to work on a study that developed out of the H.I.C. Project. A second group of five students were attached to the Project in mid-1967 for approximately six months. In early 1968, numbers were much reduced. Only two of the original members of the central team were left, together with one later arrival who resigned in November of that year. Of the other two, one was mainly concerned with organizing the writing up of the Project and the other was working half-time. There were also two students who joined the Project for six months, until September 1968.

The H.I.C. Project can be described as an action-research project in which the emphasis lay on 'learning through doing' by both hospital and central teams. 'Action research' is used here to mean research focused on problem-solving with the ultimate objective of effecting social change. The process consists of defining objectives, planning the first step, acting on the plan, obtaining feedback on action effects, evaluating, planning the next step and so on. Thus action research attempts to contribute to both action goals and research goals, to the production of change, and to the development of theories of change (see Schein and Bennis, 1965, p. 29).[1]

The Project had a number of goals: namely, improved communication, problem-solving, and helping hospital staff learn how better to solve problems (see Chapter 1, Introduction). In effect, no one of these goals took precedence over the others, although better communication (as the Project title implies) was the major theme. The ultimate general objective was to improve hospital functioning.

Partly because of the general nature of the objectives, both the kinds of action or change desired, and the control of their direction were matters of major concern among the Project advisory committee,[2] the central team, and the hospital teams.

At the beginning it was evident that the Project was aiming at a variety of changes. With hindsight it is possible to classify some of the different kinds of change, as follows:

(a) changes resulting from problem-solving (changes in methods or organization),
(b) changes in the process of problem-solving (increased ability to solve problems),
(c) changes in the general attitudes and relations among all staff members involved in, or affected by, problem-solving Project activities (better communication).

In other words the Project aimed at changes in individuals (in their attitudes and behaviour) and improvements in their environment (in their relations amongst themselves and with others, including the solution of problems). It was hoped that these developments would lead to internal improvements in the hospital system that would in turn help to improve the general level of functioning of each hospital. Emphasizing improved communication, or increased constructive interaction amongst staff most affected by related hospital problems, was one way of approaching the general goal.

During the introductory meetings the hospitals had been assured they would themselves set their own objectives and direct their own projects. Therefore in the early meetings with central-team members the director emphasized the following 'guidelines' for collaborating with the hospital teams:

(a) the hospital teams must decide for themselves the projects they wished to undertake;
(b) the hospital teams should be encouraged to collect their own data wherever possible;
(c) it was for the hospital teams to decide what action, if any, should be taken on the findings of a particular study;
(d) no pressure should be exerted on the hospitals to do anything they did not wish to do;
(e) the hospital teams should decide the extent to which the central team should be involved in, or even kept informed about, their activities.

Contrary to the more usual practice in planned change projects (in which shared goals, in this case between the hospital teams and the central team, and mutual influence form essential features of the process of change (Bennis 1961, Chapter 4)), the central team was advised that its functions should be defined by the hospital teams, and the hospitals were told that they alone should select projects and take action.

The financing of the Project was conditional upon the recruitment of the hospitals, so it was not until most of the hospitals had committed themselves to participating in the training courses that the central team could be recruited. Thus during most of the very crucial first year of the Project there was only one central-team member present besides the Project director. Furthermore the director's main responsibilities lay in Brussels, and his subsequent support was confined to acting as an occasional adviser and 'trouble-shooter' both for the hospital teams and for the central team he recruited. Some of the difficulties described below may have been influenced by both these factors.[3]

Diversity was the chief characteristic of the four members of the central team, who were assembled in the last months of 1965. Management training, in particular through formal courses, and considerable experience of administration were the primary skills of the central-team director, while the group discussion organizer brought many years experience of therapeutic communities to the Project. Training in sociological research and practical experience of hospital research were the most relevant attributes of the information officer and the research assistant respectively.[4]

Apart from organizing the training courses, the central-team director was responsible for keeping in touch with the hospital teams, developing relations with the regional hospital boards, and co-ordinating the activities of the central team. The roles of the other members were somewhat less clear. It had been intended that their function would be to provide methodological advice when requested to by the hospital teams. But, as we shall see, they needed to carry out a more complex range of functions than the guidelines suggested.

Late recruitment (the training courses were already completed before the last member, the group-discussion organizer, joined in January 1966) meant that there was little opportunity for them to consider how they might work together, or for the clarification of individual roles before the hospitals began to ask for assistance.[5]

Almost without exception they had no experience of action research or of being involved in a programme of organizational change. The area of common experience was small, the area of common knowledge unexplored (Caudill and Roberts, 1960, p. 14). Although they were undoubtedly inexperienced and ill-prepared as change-agents, they were enthusiastic and committed both to the hospital teams with whom they worked and to the many ideas the Project aimed to put into practice.

The research assistant and information officer developed similar functions centring around the provision of technical help in planning particular studies. As no hospital team at the beginning requested specific help in using group methods, the group-discussion organizer found considerable difficulty in defining a satisfactory role for herself. This is one example of the difficulties encountered when the central team refrained from giving any direction to the hospitals. Despite these uncertainties, which meant that the central team as much as the hospital teams had a great deal to learn about how to function effectively, the Project gathered momentum.

The impact of the projects was immediate and confusing and led to different reactions. Whereas the central-team director tried to ensure that each hospital embarked on a project and that rapid progress towards completion was maintained, others saw the primary tasks differently (Luszki, 1960, p. 25). The following were variously emphasized: the need to know more about each hospital, about team members, and about the goals they were trying to achieve before tackling specific projects; more active participation by hospital staff; rigorous research design. Some felt the central team should have more influence; others felt it was important that the hospital teams should do what they wished with minimal influence from the central team.

The extent to which the central team could understand, appreciate, and act on the needs of individual hospitals was limited by the different emphases given by its members to the different goals of the Project. This in turn influenced the way each interpreted his own role. Those who emphasized communication and learning goals tended to help hospitals only on request; but when help was requested, they tried to work with team members on training and human relations problems as well as providing technical advice. On the other hand those who emphasized the goal of problem-solving occasionally bypassed the hospital team—they might, for example, help with collection of data on a problem defined by a senior manager. The former focused on the people making a request, and help was geared to the needs of the hospital teams. The latter were not so much concerned with fostering the development of the hospital teams as with solving the actual problems that existed and helping whoever in the hospital was worried about them.

The extent to which each member of the central team was able to pursue his aims was determined by the extent of his influence in particular project situations. This, in turn, was determined by the extent to which the official 'guidelines' were accepted by each hospital team, by the professional skills of the individual central-team member, his ability to communicate effectively, and whether he was working alone or with others of the central team.

The conflicts that developed over the degree of influence or direction exercised by individual members were not entirely due to the central team's inability to tolerate an ambiguous role. The small size of the central team in relation to the number of hospitals wanting assistance was a contributory factor. The conflicts also reflected problems of communication between team members themselves, due in part to the inter-disciplinary nature of the team but also to factors of personality.

All the team members had strong personalities, which made it difficult to unite them into an effective working group. In team meetings there was little difficulty in developing frank discussion, but understanding, mutual confidence, and trust were harder to achieve.

There were differences of opinion about the importance, and the method, of recording what was happening.[6] Few records were kept of the central team's meetings. However there was constant concern that all meetings with hospital teams should be written up. The accounts of these meetings were, of necessity, subjective descriptions. To aid understanding of each other's views and to counteract individual biases it was agreed that a report should be written by every central-team member who took part in a meeting with hospital-team members. In this and many other ways individual members learned from each other and developed their understanding.

The subsequent recruitment of social science students (for temporary attachments of approximately six months) eased the work pressure on the central team. The first group of these students joined the Project in mid-1966. However this did little towards resolving the basic conflicts concerning the development of acceptable and effective methods of collaborating with the hospital teams. With hindsight, it is easier to understand some of the influences that made these conflicts become acute, but at that time they were sensed rather than clearly expressed or resolved.

Perhaps one of the strongest influences was the desire not to lose any hospital from the Project because this would be seen as a failure on the part of the central team. The director had explicitly instructed that 'the hospitals must be allowed to make mistakes, it is from these that they will learn'. The strain of allowing this to occur and the consequences both for the hospital teams and the central team were such that the latter at least was not able to face the situation without serious misgivings and internal recriminations. In any future Project of this nature it would be important to define very clearly the areas in which 'mistakes' should be permitted in the cause of educational progress (for example, should senior hospital staff be encouraged to carry out surveys without adequate time or a clear idea of the goals they are trying to achieve, or to bypass middle management staff to interview their subordinates, a practice that rarely led to greater consultation between hospital-team members and middle managers).

Important exacerbating influences, such as the lack of sufficient knowledge about each hospital, the lack of defined areas of responsibility, the barriers of physical distance,[7] and the inevitable psychological stresses, only served to sharpen the recriminations among the central team. The conflicts about directiveness can be interpreted as characteristic of the defensiveness of the original members when faced with problems to which they could not easily see solutions. In addition, the difficulty of integrating their skills within a common policy, the application of which might differ in different projects at different stages, seemed too great to overcome.

The problems and difficulties described above, led finally, at the end of 1966, to the resignation of the central-team director and the information officer. These resignations, which meant the loss of its two most experienced members, led to changes in the structure of the central team. Subsequent members were more alike in their backgrounds, fairly recent graduates with little research experience (this was almost inevitable as the appointments could be for a short period only). The areas of responsibility and the relationships within the central team were more clearly defined (no member worked closely on more than two projects at any one time; each student was responsible to one particular member; regular fortnightly meetings were held to which all student members were invited). It seems probable that in the early conflicts, bitter and poorly handled though they were, some of the distorted perceptions and ill-defined role concepts were worked through. Thus new members came into a less conflict-ridden situation and could begin work with the hospitals more easily.

The new, slightly larger but much less experienced central team had a more uniform background that made communication between its members a little easier. The allocation of responsibilities lessened the difficulties of keeping in touch with the hospitals, but did not solve some of the problems associated with achieving effective collaboration with the hospital teams.

The logic of the situation forced the central-team members to become more involved whether invited or not, and its members learned to recognize the importance of being explicit about values, stating the kinds of changes they wished to see. However, learning how to diagnose problem situations and when to confront staff with the need to learn was a much slower process. Somewhat related was the problem of articulating and striking a balance between the technical demands of particular hospital projects and the general learning goals of the H.I.C. Project. To solve these problems and operate effectively required that hospital-team members be willing to accept greater influence from the central team, but often they were unwilling to do so. However, there were also opportunities to influence the development of particular projects, that the central team did not make use of because they lacked the necessary experience.

To begin with the central team attempted to abide by the guidelines suggested for helping the hospital teams. However, they found that providing methodological advice on carrying out surveys was only a fraction of the complex range of functions they needed to perform. The process of accepting that the central team needed to be involved throughout all stages of a project, that methods of collaboration could vary considerably, and that projects needed to include a greater emphasis on feedback and action, contributed to the difficulties of attempting to integrate the often different needs of individual operational teams and the demands of particular hospital problems.

Many of the difficulties experienced by central-team members may have derived from the ambiguous structure of the Project. The objectives of the Project had been decided before the team members joined, thus accepting a position on the team implied acceptance and understanding of both goals and methods of work. These, however, were quite unspecific.

Partly because the initiator and director of the Project was largely absent, partly because the central team was not intended to control the Project, and partly because it was assumed that all members would participate on an equal footing, it was important that the team members shared in defining objectives. In this way some of the ambiguities in the structure and direction of the Project might have been clarified.

In any future Project it would be vital, before work in the hospitals begins, to hold preparatory discussions so that the central team can explore and learn to appreciate its members' several skills. They need to discover those areas in which they need to integrate their skills and to find out how they can work together. There probably needs to be a substantial amount of theoretical knowledge in common if the frustrations of interdisciplinary team activity are to be minimized and effective work produced.[8]

Team members need to be able to tolerate a high degree of ambiguity, to be flexible in adjusting to unanticipated circumstances and to be able to learn from each other, particularly in developing new or unfamiliar methods. Also, members need to be aware of their own motivations and interests in joining such a Project. Personal characteristics are important in interdisciplinary teams but their importance seems to assume exaggerated proportions when the considerations just mentioned are not taken into account.

It is essential for individual central-team members to get to know particular hospitals as early as possible. It is important to build a continuing relationship between senior staff at each hospital and one or two members of the central team who can get to know their hospital well. However, without some mutually agreed, appropriate action goals, including some specification of stages, of staff to be involved, of methods to be used, and some plan for evaluative feedback sessions, it seems unlikely that much would be achieved despite a good relationship.

In developing effective collaboration it is extremely important to explore the goals the hospital staff want to achieve, not just the specific problem and how it arose but the overall goals and how they relate to particular hospital objectives. Is the object to be information gathering or change and improvement? Are the key people most affected drawn into the discussion? What are the alternative ways of achieving particular goals and how can these intentions be translated into action? The central-team member must be able to help the hospital managers answer these kinds of questions and show that he can identify himself with their needs sufficiently to be accepted as a member of the working group.

The central-team member must also know his own limitations and be explicit about the resources he has to offer. He needs to know when and where to obtain help in areas outside his competence. His ability to observe, analyse, and assess situations is as important as his awareness of his own behaviour and the forces operating in any given situation. Only then can he contribute and share influence, yet leave all decisions of substance to the hospitals.

Given the general functions of the central team as described in this chapter, the education and experience of members of any future central team probably needs to include:

1. a basic training in one of the behavioural sciences such as psychology, sociology, or anthropology;
2. a period of training and research in the field of organizational behaviour and the management of change in organizations. This would need to include education in concepts of change and in understanding the processes of change (Lippitt *et al.*, 1958; Leavitt, 1965; Beckhard, 1969) in addition to learning about quantitative methods of systems analysis.
3. sensitivity training, which has as part of its aims the development of self-awareness, tolerance of ambiguity, and improvements in communication skills. In addition, experience of the emotional mechanisms that operate in the development of a close working relationship;
4. knowledge of, and a substantial amount of supervised practice in, the techniques and procedures of providing help (gained, for example, through assisting with action research projects, management consultancy projects, working as a staff member of training programmes);
5. a thorough understanding of professional ethics and standards, and the evaluative functions of a change-agent's role (Lippitt *et al.*, 1958; Sofer, 1961).

It may not be possible to get such individuals. Nevertheless we have described how a central team might be internally organized and how it might relate to the hospital team in ways that would probably make the best use of the skills that are available.

(For further details about the central team, see Chapter 17, in the evaluation report.)

## PART TWO: EXTERNAL RELATIONSHIPS

### INTRODUCTION

The central team's chief obligation was to the ten hospitals and the major purpose of this section is to describe the relationship between the central team and the hospitals and the kind of activities the central team undertook. However, first we shall discuss briefly how the Project organizers took account of the network of authority relationships within which hospitals operate, with specific reference to the regional hospital boards and the hospital management committees.[9]

### REGIONAL HOSPITAL BOARDS AND HOSPITAL MANAGEMENT COMMITTEES

From the very earliest days, both the director and the Hospital Centre representatives emphasized the principle of starting at the top of the power structure and working with those in authority. Every effort was made to involve the regional boards and obtain their agreement and co-operation during the early stages (for details on the introductory stage of the Project, see Chapter 4). The initial approach to the hospitals was through the four metropolitan regional hospital boards, who were invited to select potential participants. At subsequent meetings, the organizers discussed the implications for the boards with their senior officers. The organizers wished to ascertain, for example, how the boards would view requests from hospitals for temporary replacement staff, such as doctors, to allow hospital-team members to devote sufficient time to their chosen projects. In the event, at least two hospital teams were successful in their applications for temporary medical staff.

The regional boards also helped in other ways. A regional board statistician lectured to the training courses and later analysed staff turnover data from the ten hospitals. He presented the results at one of the early Project meetings (described below). A senior administrative medical officer also took part in the training courses, outlining his view of the future pattern of medical care in hospitals.

Once the hospital teams had embarked upon specific projects, the director of the central team visited the secretaries and regional training officers of each board both to obtain some feedback and to keep them informed about what was happening. Copies of all newsletters (described below) were circulated to the boards and comments were invited. One board secretary attended one of the early inter-team meetings at the invitation of the host hospital. The boards' officers[10] were invited to attend the fourth series of Project meetings and a few took an active part in the discussion. Some comments on these meetings from a senior administrative medical officer are included in Chapter 7. Finally, each board received a copy of the final Project report in draft.

Although fairly close contact characterized the initial stages of the relationship between the central team and the regional hospital boards, later it became more tenuous. The central-team director had hoped that half-yearly meetings would take place between the central team and the boards' officers but for various reasons they did not occur.

Perhaps some of the regional hospital boards' reluctance to play any major role in the H.I.C. Project was because the boards' officers were anxious not to be seen as 'interfering' in the affairs of individual hospitals. The hospitals, on the other hand, seemed pleased to see tangible evidence of the boards' support for the Project, although they may not have desired the display of too close an interest.[11]

Direct contact between the Project organizers and the hospital management committees was initiated through one of the introductory meetings at which the Project's aims and intentions were discussed (see also Chapter 4). Representatives from each management committee and usually their group secretaries took part. Each member had to decide whether he would recommend that his committee pay for senior hospital officers to participate in the training courses. As intended by the Project organizers, much of the contact between the central team and the hospital management committees was through hospital-team members, most of whom reported regularly to their management committees on their activities.

In two instances at least, management committee members became actively concerned in particular projects. In one case the committee nominated members to participate in a study of the relations between the committee and its hospital executive officers (see Chapter 8). In the other, the chairman of a hospital subcommittee took part in project discussions concerned with improving the functioning of the hospital's accident and emergency department. Thus there were a number of contacts between the central team and the hospital management committees.

As in the case of the regional hospital boards, hospital management committees were consulted and actively involved by the Project organizers at the outset. Subsequent participation by the hospital management committees and regional hospital boards depended upon their interest and the extent to which the hospital teams drew them into particular activities (see also the data for item R218 of the evaluation survey, reported in Chapter 15).

THE TEN HOSPITAL TEAMS

Uncertainty was common to both the central team and the hospital teams in most first projects. The hospital teams were uncertain what specific skills the central-team members had to offer, how they should be treated when they visited each hospital, and how far they should be involved in its affairs. The central-team members were uncertain about the future. Were all the hospitals going to ask for help simultaneously? What would the hospital teams want of them? How was the work to be divided up? How far were the hospital teams really highly motivated, well-integrated groups, enthusiastic to disturb the equilibrium of their institutions in the cause of improved communication, however that was understood? Even at that time, it was evident to the central team that its resources might not be adequate for the demands likely to be placed upon it. It was necessary to resolve problems such as these if adequate working relationships were to develop.

There were two main ways in which the central team and the hospital teams collaborated with each other: (a) through activities organized by the central team for members of all hospital teams (e.g. training courses and Project meetings) and (b) through meetings with hospital-team members at their own hospitals to discuss individual projects. Both categories of activity took place concurrently throughout the Project period from late 1965 until the latter part of 1968.

The following account of the Project will include only those aspects necessary for the reader's understanding of the development of the relationship between the central team and the hospital teams. In the next chapter we shall discuss the hospital projects in more detail. The centrally organized Project meetings are described in Chapter 7, but the first of these meetings, which took place six weeks after the completion of the second training course in which seven hospital teams took part, is mentioned here because of the light it sheds on the early relationship between the hospital teams and the central team. The main purpose of the meeting was to give those hospitals who wished to do so an opportunity to define both the projects they intended to undertake and the kind of help they would like the central team to provide.

Although all three hospital teams who had attended the first one-month training course had embarked on projects, and one had received considerable help from the central team, there was some uncertainty as to whether the remaining seven hospital teams would undertake any further activity. The second training course had ended on an almost euphoric note, but the central-team director felt that, with a period of hectic Christmas activity and the inevitable accumulation of work to be cleared after a month's absence, the teams might well have decided that they had no time for project work. However, at that first Project meeting the hospital teams announced the problems they intended to tackle, and a lively, if wide-ranging, discussion ensued. Most teams said they would like to discuss their projects with central-team members although they were uncertain about the kind of help that would be required.

In order to draw attention to the most expensive item in every hospital's budget, each team had been asked to collect figures of staff turnover for all groups of staff. At the meeting a regional board statistician who lectured during the training courses presented his analysis of this information. To avoid any possible embarrassment hospital names had been replaced by code letters, but these were soon discarded by the teams themselves as each identified its own figures.

Almost inevitably, as comparisons were made, some teams were anxious to defend their own figures. It was suggested that a team from a hospital with a high turnover rate for a specific group of staff might learn how their own situation could be improved by working with a team from a comparable hospital, but with a low turnover rate for the same staff group. However, this often seemed to reinforce the need to explain why particular figures were peculiar to particular circumstances. A more positive reaction might have occurred had it been possible to circulate the information and the suggestion for collaborative study before the meeting, thus giving time for the teams to consider the implications before selecting their individual projects.

To emphasize the importance of evaluation the central-team director suggested that, if the teams continued to collect these data, another meeting six months later might be useful. The effects on the relevant groups of staff of the projects each team had chosen could then be considered.[12] However, the work involved in collecting this information drew complaints from the hospitals, since this additional task often fell on their already hard-pressed clerical staff. Because the central team did not wish to appear to be pressing the hospitals, the subject was eventually allowed to lapse until the evaluation team took it up again a few months later (see Chapter 13 in the evaluation report).

In retrospect, this early meeting attempted to achieve too many diffuse goals too quickly, but it did achieve its main purpose of creating an effective deadline by which the hospital teams had to define specific projects and it gave the central team an indication of which teams wished to collaborate with them and which wished to work alone (see also Chapter 7, first series of inter-team meetings).

Three hospital teams, The London, Mayday, and North Middlesex, worked on their first projects alone. Central-team members visited those of the remaining seven hospitals that had given any indication of wanting assistance. Usually the central-team director, sometimes accompanied by the group-discussion organizer, visited the hospitals first, and in five instances then called in the research assistant and information officer to help with planning and methodology.

Typically, the initial meetings took place in the office of the supporting administrative member, usually the group or hospital secretary. He would describe the project the operational team wanted to tackle and what kind of help they would like from the central team. Sometimes more specific project details would be contributed by the members of the operational team. Second meetings tended to be between them and the other two members of the central team.

The director was known to all the hospital-team members, both through visiting the hospitals and through organizing the training courses. For other members of the central team, most of these meetings were the first occasions on which they had visited the hospitals or met the team members. The atmosphere tended to be formal but friendly as each group explored the other's commitment, skills, and ability to contribute towards constructive progress.[13]

Collaboration between the hospital teams and the central team took several forms. The roles of individual team members varied according to the nature and stage of particular projects and the hospital-team members with whom collaboration took place. For example, in the first of all the hospital projects, an attitude survey of a cross-section of Lewisham Hospital staff, the information officer and three temporary recruits functioned chiefly as interviewers, after the initial planning discussions.[14]

A common function of central-team members in other first projects undertaken by each hospital was advising on carrying out surveys within a framework formulater chiefly by the operational teams. A rather unusual example was where the information officer and a nurse from the operational team met weekly over many months to construct and validate a questionnaire to be administered to the entire nursing staff of the hospital. In West Middlesex and Queen Mary's the research assistant collaborated with the operational teams in attempting to work through issues such as how to involve other appropriate staff, what kinds of publicity and preparation were necessary, reappraisal of goals, how to collect data, and who would be able to undertake data collection.

In St Nicholas Hospital the operational team, the nurse member of the supporting team and the departmental sister met frequently with both the research assistant and the information officer over a period of four months to attempt to clarify specific sub-goals (the general aim was to evaluate the functioning of the accident and emergency department and to discuss alternative practicable methods of achieving them, which included executing a pilot survey. Between the meetings, the central-team members surveyed the literature and other sources of information to produce an acceptable project design, while the hospital team staff collected preliminary statistical data about work loads and staffing. In Hillingdon Hospital, the group-discussion organizer and the central-team director worked closely with hospital-team members in organizing discussion groups with representatives from associated departments in order to identify issues of concern relating to the transfer of a large part of the hospital into a new building.

These issues were used subsequently as the basis for a series of internal management conferences devoted to the implications of the move.

Enthusiasm and anxiety characterized the efforts of the hospital teams, particularly the operational teams, in their first projects. There was enthusiasm to use their newly acquired skills to achieve success, not only to their own satisfaction but also in the eyes of their superiors, usually the supporting team. There was a desire to understand others better, and to improve the functioning of their hospitals. 'Communication' became an 'in' word. However, the translation of theory into practice was difficult.

Some meetings were ill-defined, frustrating occasions; often key hospital staff, such as departmental managers, had not been invited to participate in planning and some members' interest rapidly declined. Progress was slow and sometimes there did not seem to be any at all, particularly when meetings were spread out over a long period. Nevertheless, issues such as those mentioned above were worked through to some extent.

The operational teams were anxious about their ability to carry out their selected projects. Some members were apprehensive about involving other staff who had not been on the training courses (because 'they won't understand what we are trying to do'). Other members felt it was inappropriate for them to be involved in carrying out the projects they had helped to select, because, for example, it would involve crossing traditional professional boundaries to examine the work of others or, occasionally, because it would be difficult for a team member to take part as he was based at another hospital in the group.

Occasional attempts by central-team members to encourage consideration of other projects more closely associated with the normal work of the hospital-team members were not successful. However, sometimes it *was* hard to define projects that would be the appropriate concern of all three operational-team members.

The members of the operational teams often found it difficult to maintain their identity as working groups in the face of day-to-day pressures. Few members were given sufficient time to work on their projects, although it had been suggested that the operational teams should devote up to one-third of their time to this activity. Where supporting-team members were uncertain of their roles or sceptical about the value of the Project, the hospital projects were given low priority. Thus some operational-team members found themselves in a very frustrating position, unable to find sufficient time to work on their projects and unable to discuss how the problem might be overcome. Providing psychological support to individual members, chiefly through listening to their difficulties and exploring ways in which more effective co-operation with colleagues might be achieved, emerged as a major function of members of the central team. The fact that they proved unable to solve these problems sometimes caused resentment. It was often difficult to recognize how the hospital teams related their specific projects to H.I.C. learning goals. The educational strategy of the

Project emphasized that, in order to *learn* how to improve hospital functioning, the teams must both diagnose their own problems and implement remedial action. To help in diagnosing their problems the teams were encouraged to experience the functioning of their hospitals in a very personal way, through carrying out surveys. It was hoped this would increase the motivation to change both personally in terms of perceptions and behaviour and in terms of solving problems. In a sense the design of the Project, by stressing the involvement of the hospital teams in the information gathering aspects of project activity, gave less weight to clarifying objectives and to implementing changes.

Finding time to collect survey data became a major obstacle to progress for most teams. In fact, just over half the teams did collect their own data in their first projects. Although the experience was described as valuable, they felt they could not devote further time to it. This was not solely because they felt they could use their time better carrying out their normal managerial tasks. There were problems associated with a growing awareness of how their hospitals functioned and the limitations of the existing authority structure. Many team members said they gained greater understanding of the attitudes and problems of respondents. However, at the same time they described feelings of guilt about the content of interview material, because they did not possess authority to act on matters that arose, and also because they experienced difficulty in coping with their growing appreciation of the complex and sometimes threatening issues they had begun to raise. The central team attempted, unsuccessfully, to arrange a weekend seminar at which some of these issues could be discussed.

In certain cases the central team was not asked to help, and it was then faced with the problem of discovering what was happening where it had not been invited to participate. A major frustration of the central team, who sometimes knew too little about a given project, lay in trying to find the kinds of support needed to create and maintain constructive interaction and to increase its share of influence in the process.

It was not uncommon for central-team members to note down two general objectives from the initial meetings to plan a project, thus:

'(1) The specific objective for the hospital is to obtain information on X and to improve the working of the system. (2) Our overall objective is to involve the key hospital staff in defining the problem and solving it, thus helping them (and us) to learn something about the mechanisms at work in the organization.' The former objective was almost invariably voiced by the hospital team, the latter by the central team. While these two objectives could be complementary, and occasionally were, the fact remains that they were rarely worked through openly together with members of the hospital teams.

To resolve the problem of collecting data the central-team director recruited social science students, chiefly from Brunel University, in the summer of 1966.[15] These students were placed in various hospitals under the supervision of the hospital teams. In the following extract Ken Eason, a psychology student, describes his role in the hospital and his relationship with the hospital team.

'It became apparent quite quickly that my work was not to be controlled by a unified hospital team as I had expected, but that I would work from the hospital secretary's department. The lay administration is involved in all aspects of hospital life and this makes it the best location for a student involved in projects which cross professional boundaries. The hospital did not, at this time, have a full team but even with one it is difficult to see how I could have been controlled by a team when its members had offices widely separated throughout the hospital. The existing team met infrequently but again even the most hardworking team would not meet often enough to give detailed supervision to a student working full-time on a project.

'Within the administrative department the hospital secretary devised tactics that cleared the way for my work with other senior executives while I planned the project methodology. The deputy hospital secretary advised me on the practicability of my plans and introduced me to the relevant hospital staff. Relations with the rest of the team were distant. The hospital secretary convened meetings to consult matron and the senior consultants on matters which concerned them or their staff. The concept of an integrated team equally concerned with all hospital problems is false in my experience. Each person was intimately concerned only with those projects relevant to his normal work. Matron showed little interest in matters not immediately relevant to the nursing hierarchy; the surgical consultant was apathetic to the medical ward study and the medical doctors were uninterested in the theatre study.

'My relations with team members were friendly, the only real difference being created by our divergent approaches to the way changes should be introduced. While I emphasized the need to motivate lower level workers and to employ full consultation before making changes, the team emphasized the diplomatic and political discussions necessary to gain support from senior staff.

'I found in my work that I had the freedom to do more than act as a data collector. I was able to interpret the data I collected and present it so as to facilitate executive action. Despite this, to the team I remained a student and a data collector. They displayed little interest in my methods of collecting and analysing data and, although I am confident that some of the findings surprised them, in talking to me they were not able to admit this. It is interesting that they turned to the permanent central-team members when they wanted advice on the interpretation of data and its translation into action.'

The students had a very beneficial effect on the progress of individual projects in at least three ways. Firstly, they collected and analysed data for the hospital teams, thus accelerating the pace of the information-gathering stage towards problem-solving goals; secondly, they acted as 'publicity agents', explaining to respondents, peripheral participants, and other staff what the hospital teams were trying to do in particular projects; thirdly, they provided information valuable to other central-team members in their efforts to support the hospital teams.

The placing of students in the hospitals did not necessarily increase the amount of interaction amongst team members. Nor did it encourage the hospital teams to work more closely with key hospital staff closely affected by individual projects. The use of students and other central-team members to collect survey information was an acceptance of the fact that it was not feasible for most hospital teams to do this. Further groups of students undertook similar tasks during the remainder of the Project.

A few hospitals replaced team members as the original members left to take up more senior posts. Chiefly in response to suggestions by the central-team members, some new members were added to existing hospital teams, usually for specific projects, [16, 17] and the hospitals requested some training for them. The central team suggested a one-week training session followed by brief visits to other hospitals to work with the team members most concerned with a current project. However, the hospitals felt that this would be too time-consuming, and eventually it was agreed to hold a two-day appreciation course for fourteen participants from seven hospitals and the new members of the central team, including students.[18]

One of the main reasons for encouraging a number of hospitals to take part in the H.I.C. Project was to promote inter-hospital discussion of problem-solving activities. Inter-team meetings at Project hospitals were suggested by the central team to create opportunities through which this might develop. Occasionally hospital teams did consult each other outside these and other Project meetings, but there seemed to be a strong feeling that problems of stress and strain were matters for internal resolution, and not issues that might benefit from discussion with other hospitals. In addition, to Project meetings a newsletter, consisting of progress reports contributed by each hospital team, was circulated to all members at six-monthly intervals.

It had been one of the aims of the Project to establish links between each hospital and academic departments of management or social science in a local institution of advanced education. It was hoped that such relationships might provide a permanent source of mutual stimulus and help (see evaluation item, F102, Chapter 5).[19] Part-time management students assisted with one hospital project, and college staff collaborated with hospital- and central-team members in carrying out another project. In most cases joint discussions led to mutual agreement that 'it would be good to keep in touch'. Subsequently at least one hospital sought and received help on a work-study problem.

The collaborative projects seemed to work out reasonably well and no insurmountable difficulties arose. However, it is not always easy to match the needs of the hospitals with those of particular colleges. For example colleges are often anxious to find work placements for students but feel apprehensive about the time and resources they may need to invest in research or consultation on hospital problems. On the other hand hospitals often expect colleges to provide definite and rapid solutions to problems, without the management being much involved.

Despite these different expectations we believe these contacts were useful in some cases and should be encouraged among other hospitals and colleges. Often it will mean a few false starts until either the college or hospital finds an institution that can meet its needs. Like most other relationships the college-hospital link requires that both parties are willing to work through the implications (see Sofer and Hutton, 1959, Chapter 6).

The action stage of hospital projects was frequently marked by different characteristics from the earlier stages. Many hospital teams no longer felt dependent on central-team members. Earlier dependence lay in the need for advice (whether taken or not) and help in carrying out surveys. At the report stage hospital-team members often saw themselves as possessing sole responsibility for the direction, nature, and amount of action to be taken or changes to be introduced. In the early stages of the Project, central-team members accepted this view. In some later projects both hospital- and central-team members modified these views and in a very few instances central-team members were able to help hospital-team members in taking action on project findings.

Certain improvements in methods or organization did result from most projects. The few improvements that were of any size or structural significance had already been given some thought beforehand; the H.I.C. Project thus functioned as facilitator or enabler.

However for both hospital and central teams some meetings to discuss project reports left much to be desired. Where general conclusions had been drawn and the issues were fairly clear it seemed as though authoritarian attitudes and centralized decision-making came to the fore. One influential team member would make decisions and the others agree. In other instances, where changes required sanction and action by a number of individuals, delegated and divided responsibility seemed to be adhered to rigidly. There was understanding of the interdependent nature of the situation but uneven recognition of the need for shared responsibility. In other joint meetings where the problems were more complex and the issues less well understood, lengthy discussions seemed to result in the hospital teams selecting minor points on which to take administrative action. The more fundamental issues thus remained only partially clarified, if at all. Thus, despite the increase in the amount of information available, it was evident that central-team members were not notably effective in helping the hospital teams to work through difficulties in solving problems and implementing changes.

After seemingly interminable discussions within the central team about how these difficulties might be overcome, the central-team administrator recommended to the Project advisory committee that the central team needed to be strengthened by additional specialist staff. However, at that time (June 1967), the committee felt that the experiment was too near its planned conclusion (December 1967) to justify employing anyone to help, even if it were possible to find someone with suitable qualifications and experience.

In July of that same year, the King's Fund Hospital Centre's representatives on the advisory committee offered the hospital teams facilities to meet and discuss the future of the Project among themselves, with no representatives of the committee or the central team present.[20] After the meeting, the teams wrote to the advisory committee saying that they wished the Project to continue and that other regions should develop similar activities with the help of university management departments and other management training centres.

To clarify the reasons for this suggestion and, in particular, the way the hospital teams saw their own activities developing, the advisory committee invited representatives to meet them at Guy's Medical School in the autumn. The central team was not permitted to attend this meeting as the advisory committee felt that their presence might inhibit the hospital teams. As a result of the second meeting, the advisory committee decided to extend the life of the central team for a further year although the reasons for doing so were not very clear. However, it seemed reasonable to assume that several hospital teams had indicated that they benefited from the activities of central-team members.

On the other hand, central-team members were concerned about their lack of constructive influence in project situations and particularly about the gap that sometimes existed between their aims and those of the hospital teams. Whereas the central team tried to emphasize participatory data-collection methods, the consultation and involvement of appropriate staff at early stages, and the goals of individual and team learning in the process of solving specific problems, the hospital teams tended to lay emphasis on involving as few people as possible in getting more information about particular problems in order to take administrative action.

In the early stages the hospital teams and the members of the central team had held strongly to their respective objectives and methods of approach, however hazy these were. As experience was gained, some of them began to compromise, modify their views, and scale down their expectations to a more realistic level.

The following description, by a central-team member, Sheila Hillier, of one of the later projects in which the central team did increase its share of influence, illustrates some of the points discussed above. Although the project could not be considered an example of ideal collaboration, many managerial and supervisory staff below the top level in the organization collaborated in an exercise that affected their own work.

'The group secretary had noticed what he felt was an excessive number of staff walking the corridors. The aim was to find out where all these people were going and why.

'In response to a request for "observers" who would stop people in the corridors and ask where they were going, the central team suggested that departmental managers and ward sisters might be invited to discuss the purpose and problems of carrying out such a study. Eventually a working group, consisting of clinical service department managers, ward sisters plus hospital- and central-team members, discussed and agreed upon objectives and methods, namely to find ways of meeting the service needs of wards and departments and reducing congestion in the corridors. Each ward and department would record all "callers" and also all journeys made by their own staff. Forms were designed by the central team for distribution to all wards and clinical service departments for completion by staff members.

'Publicity plans were made and executed by members of the working group. Student central-team members helped to publicize the study by discussing the data sheets with key staff members in each ward and department. Central-team members also collaborated in discussing the project with portering staff and studied existing messenger services. Apart from a member of the senior medical staff who was convinced the scheme would not work, the response was enthusiastic.

'After a pilot run, the data collection sheets were amended and the main data were collected over a period of two weeks. Perhaps this was too long for collecting such detailed information as the data sheets for the second week were incomplete. There was almost immediate feedback by both central- and hospital-team members through normal meetings of heads of departments and of sisters to discuss the implications of this for the communication system in the hospital. These were lively meetings and after the meeting of the heads of departments the administrative member of the supporting team commented that it had been the most active meeting of its kind in his experience.

'When the data were analysed and presented in the form of large scale charts and diagrams, the hospital team, which had expected the central team to provide them with a set of conclusions on which to act, was disappointed. This refusal of the central team to co-operate and fulfil a prescribed role annoyed the hospital team and the atmosphere was very strained. The onus was thus placed on the hospital team to discuss the data with the staff who had provided it, with no clear idea of what decisions would be reached.

'When members of the original working group met two weeks later, it was evident that the data had acted as a catalyst in some of the preliminary meetings for the discussion of problems other than those strictly concerned with staff journeys. The first half of the meeting became a problem-solving session on a number of points that affected relationships between different departments and wards. There was a readiness to co-operate and take responsibility for introducing improvements. After several meetings and further analyses of the data by both hospital staff and central-team members, it was decided to experiment with a hospital-wide messenger service. A brief trial involving members of both teams showed that this seemed a practicable proposition.

'The management had promised the porters that there would be no redundancy as a result of the project, and, by gradual redeployment of staff because of normal wastage, they were able to keep this promise.'

The roles and functions of central-team members in this project were varied. In the initial planning meetings two members took part. The outline of each stage was developed by the hospital-team and central-team members, including students. The details were worked out amongst the central-team members and students. Two students and a junior central-team member worked on the publicity and supervised data collection. At critical stages and report-back sessions a senior central-team member took part as well.

In this project key hospital staff were involved in examining a common problem. Both the central team and the hospital staff took part in all stages of the project including experimenting with a possible solution. The project appeared to result in better understanding by nursing staff and departmental managers of each other's problems. Some team members also learnt that it was possible to involve a large number of staff and yet reach a satisfactory solution. In order to achieve these results a much greater investment of central-team time and skills was required than had been suggested by the original guidelines (for further details of the extent of participation by the central team, hospital teams, and other hospital staff in projects, see Chapters 17 and 18).

## CONCLUSIONS AND RECOMMENDATIONS

In the latter part of this chapter we have given some indication of the ways in which the central team collaborated with the hospitals during project activity, during further training, and in developing joint college-hospital relationships. Among the points we have tried to make is the need for a much closer and more open relationship with senior hospital staff in the very early stages. As Ken Eason's description shows, the concept of an integrated top-management team equally concerned with all hospital problems is unrealistic, particularly where a number of isolated projects are started in different parts of the hospital. Integrated teams are not feasible without some attempt to relate projects to the achievement of specific hospital goals in ways that highlight the inter-relatedness of different parts of the hospital system.

In effect, the hospital teams came to view the central team as an occasionally useful third party that enabled different professional groups to come together and tackle certain problems (see Chapter 9, Conclusions). Most often, central-team members were considered as an extra source of help in gathering information.

The lack of clarity concerning Project goals, the inhibiting nature of the guidelines for the central team, and the problems inherent in collaborative relationships in 'action research' all threw into sharp relief the inadequacies of the central team both in numbers and skills. The lessons learned suggest that the following conditions are desirable if a collaborative effort to improve organizational effectiveness is to have a reasonable chance of success.

(i) Motivation to change with as much intellectual understanding and emotional commitment as possible needs to be present among senior hospital managers.
(ii) The people and resources in both hospital and central teams must be appropriate for the task and they should have the sanction of other key hospital staff, both superior and subordinate, as well as active support from top management.
(iii) There needs to be some cohesion or potential cohesion among both the senior managers and among the central team to sustain both groups in the difficulties that will inevitably arise.
(iv) There must be as much agreement on, and explicit understanding of, specific goals and likely consequences as possible.
(v) A clear and acceptable programme specifying stages and timing (including evaluation) must be worked out between the hospital and the central teams in collaboration.
(vi) The programme needs a better balance of emphasis between emotional, and value-laden factors and informational factors. This implies consideration of different kinds of training integrated with other hospital-based activities.
(vii) Both parties must accept the need for mutual influence in the collaborative process; this implies the existence of mutual trust and appropriate skills in the central team.
(viii) Either party, or individual members of either party, must have the opportunity to withdraw from the relationship at any stage.

## NOTES

[1] In the view of the Project advisory committee, action and research were separate issues. The hospital and central teams were to emphasize the action side of the Project, while the research aspect was seen as the province of the

evaluator, who was appointed in mid-1966. Essentially his task was to work independently of the central team in assessing the effects of the Project without giving them any information (or feedback) or helping them. More usually action and research are seen as sequential but articulated and integrated activities carried out by the same staff. See Foundation for Research on Human Behaviour (1960, pp. 32-33).

[2] The members of the advisory committee are listed among the participants at the beginning of the book. Although their principal function was to advise the central team they often undertook executive functions in the absence of the director.

[3] An illustrative listing of the different roles consultants can play when they are only temporarily available is suggested by Beckhard (1969, pp. 106-110).

[4] For a discussion of some of the problems in interdisciplinary collaboration, see Caudill and Roberts (1960, pp. 11-18).

[5] The need for trainers to study one another before studying others is described by Harrison and Hopkins (1967).

[6] For example, how much attention should be devoted to recording project details and how much to the underlying dynamics? Different levels of understanding in both these areas constituted an additional problem.

[7] The difficulties of getting to know more about each hospital and of communicating with each other were made worse because it took, on average, one and a half hours to travel from the Hospital Centre (where the central team was based) to each hospital.

[8] For a detailed discussion of the training required by change-agents, see Lippitt *et al.*, (1958); Sofer (1961).

[9] For more information about the structure and functioning of the National Health Service see Lindsay (1962); Stevens (1966); Health Services in Britain (1968).

[10] The secretaries, nursing officers, senior administrative medical officers, and training officers of each of the four metropolitan regional hospital boards.

[11] It is often thought that the higher echelons in the NHS exert great influence on hospital management committees. That this is not always the case is indicated by a study of the lack of effect of a Ministry Circular on HMC behaviour (Stewart and Sleeman, 1967).

[12] For an example of this kind of use of turnover records to improve hospital functioning, see United Hospital Fund (1968).

[13] Organizations often regard with ambivalence the outsiders who have been asked to help. Both enthusiasm to learn and fear of having to face problems they prefer to avoid are characteristic elements of this type of relationship (Sofer and Hutton, 1959, pp. 60-62).

[14] The implications of providing this help were reviewed at a weekend meeting organized by the director at the request of the central team. It was decided that the amount of help given could not be repeated for other hospitals because it was not feasible to lend the whole of the central team to a single hospital for an extended period, and because it was too costly to recruit outsiders. It also appeared to contradict a basic tenet of the Project, that the hospital teams should execute their own projects. For the following few months, the central team encouraged the hospitals to collect their own data.

[15] For a description of some of the educational techniques, including student work placement, used at Brunel University, see Jahoda (1963).

[16] For a list of possible roles 'inside' change-agents may play, see Beckhard (1969, pp. 111-115).

[17] These individuals represented only a few of a much larger number, including departmental managers and ward sisters, who became involved in

projects. In specific projects often their major interaction was with central-team data collectors. They were usually consulted collectively by the hospital teams, but sometimes not drawn into planning studies, although this had been strongly urged by the central team.

[18] The course contained a description by the director of the aims and intentions of the Project; an example of another collaborative project discussed by the research workers and senior hospital staff involved; two sessions devoted to examining the goals and characteristics of hospital systems and sub-systems, illustrating the conflicts and compromises necessary for the achievement of effective hospital functioning; and a critical appraisal of situations in which survey methods might be useful. Finally, a panel of hospital-team members answered questions from participants and discussed their own project experiences.

Although the length of the course had been fixed by the hospital teams, most participants felt it had been too short. It had been assumed that participants were familiar with the activities of their own hospital teams, but in a few cases this was evidently not so.

In retrospect, the course could have been improved in a number of ways, even allowing that only a limited amount can be achieved in two days. For example, one or two hospital teams could have worked through specific projects they had undertaken, describing what had been learnt and whether problems had been solved. Finally the teams might have been encouraged to evaluate their efforts against other methods of tackling problems. Each participant on the course could have been helped to define the current project in which he was involved, describing how it affected his work and how, and to what end, he was working with others.

In any future Project, we believe training should take place over a much longer period with a greater emphasis on experience-based sessions including diagnosing problems, sensitivity training, and action projects involving participants' own work (for further details on the two-day course see also note 2, Chapter 15).

[19] By late 1967 the medical member of the Mayday hospital team had approached Croydon Technical College and four part-time senior management students were assisting in the 'ease of contact' survey. With the help of the central team, North Middlesex Hospital and Enfield College of Technology (Management Department) set up a working group which spent several months designing, executing, and analysing a staff opinion survey that formed part of a plan for introducing changes in catering facilities in the hospital. Partly as a consequence of Brunel University students working at West Middlesex and Hillingdon, both hospitals developed links with the school of social sciences at Brunel University. Through the central team, Queen Mary's hospital was put in touch with the management department of Kingston College of Technology, and St Nicholas and The London contacted Woolwich Polytechnic and the City University, respectively.

[20] On some of the problems of terminating a helping relationship, see Lippitt *et al.* (1958, Chapter 9) and Schein (1969, p. 129).

# 6 *The hospital projects*

*HILARY LEIGH*

This chapter concentrates on the different stages of the hospital projects in an attempt to understand the process of the Project and to draw some conclusions about the use of survey procedures by senior hospital staff in solving problems and improving communication.[1] These projects were not intended to be research projects; they were efforts by busy senior staff to improve the functioning of their hospitals. The picture presented is intended to reflect the 'average' project.

To facilitate analysis, the projects are arbitrarily divided into six stages: project selection; planning; publicity and preparation; data collection; analysis and interpretation; and feedback to respondents and other hospital staff.[2] For each stage we shall describe who took part, the methods used, some of the problems encountered, and the role played by the central team. Finally, we shall look at what the projects achieved in terms both of action taken to solve problems and of improvements in communication, describing what appear to be the determinants of success.

Between December 1965 and December 1968, thirty-eight projects were undertaken by the hospital teams. Every team carried out at least two projects, some carried out three, and one undertook nine. A list of each team's projects in the order in which they were undertaken is given below in *Table 6-1*.

TABLE 6-1 *Projects undertaken by the Ten Hospitals*

| *Project number* | *Hospital* | *Title* | *Number of staff involved as respondents* |
|---|---|---|---|
| 1. | Edgware | Survey of nurses' attitudes | 22 |
| 2. | | Study of the accident and emergency dept. | 43 |
| 3. | | Evaluation of internal management courses | 53 |
| 4. | | Study of causes of congestion in hospital corridors – 'traffic survey' | 500 |
| 5. | Hillingdon | Management conferences in preparation for moving into a new building | |
| 6 | | Decentralization of nursing administration | |
| 7. | | *Study of co-ordination between supplies and engineering departments | 18 |

| *Project number* | *Hospital* | *Title* | *Number of staff involved as respondents* |
|---|---|---|---|
| 8. | | Study of nurses' preferences for different duty rotas | 432 |
| 9. | | Study of staffing in relation to workloads and routine of wards | 60 |
| 10. | Lewisham | Attitude survey of hospital staff | 141 |
| 11. | | Study of medical records | |
| 12. | | Study of journeys, admissions, and discharges | |
| 13. | The London | *Emergency admissions project | 139 |
| 14. | | *Visiting hours project | 141 |
| 15. | Mayday | *Survey of ward sisters' attitudes | 17 |
| 16. | | *Survey of junior doctors' attitudes | 26 |
| 17. | | Survey of consultants' attitudes | 27 |
| 18. | | Ease of contact survey | 400 |
| 19. | North Middlesex | *Study of staff wastage in medical records department | 43 |
| 20. | | Survey of staff opinions on hospital amenities and welfare | 14 |
| 21. | | Study of staff attitudes towards catering facilities | 680 |
| 22. | Queen Mary's | Study of contact between a paediatric ward and departments | 50 |
| 23. | Hospital for | Study of contact between a 'subnormal' ward and departments | |
| 24. | Children | Study of contact between two wards and departments (in St Ebba's Hospital) | 39 |
| 25. | St Nicholas Plumstead | Evaluation of the accident and emergency department | 33 |
| 26. | | Follow-on inquiry in the X-ray, medical records, and out-patients departments | |
| 27. | Severalls | Survey of nurses' attitudes | 354 |
| 28. | | Survey of patients' attitudes | 96 |
| 29. | | Hospital management committee and senior officers survey | 11 |
| 30. | West Middlesex | Pilot survey of a paediatric and a medical ward | 64 |
| 31. | | Study of medical social work | 11 |
| 32. | | Project 'paper chase' | 114 |
| 33. | | Inquiry into the use of operating theatres | 60 |
| 34. | | Student nurse counselling | 50 |
| 35. | | Student nurse wastage survey | 39 |
| 36. | | Medical unit observation study | |
| 37. | | Study of patients' anxieties | 20 |
| 38. | | Opinion survey of domestic services | 135 |

* Central-team members not directly involved in these projects.

## SOURCES OF DATA

Most of the data are derived from descriptive records made by the central team while working on particular projects. In projects where central-team members were not involved some data have been taken from hospital reports written for newsletters or presented at meetings organized by the central team. Where the data are not concerned with facts, the information represents judgements made by the central-team members most concerned with the particular project. The results are presented in the form of figures and tables, which form the basis of the discussion.

## PROJECTS AND PARTICIPANTS

First let us look at the projects in terms of the extent to which the supporting and operational teams participated at different stages. *Figure 6-1* shows the pattern in the first projects undertaken in each of the ten hospitals. In general, some members of supporting teams and most members of operational teams took part in the preliminary stage of selecting projects and later spent some time discussing the results. As envisaged, the operational teams undertook the bulk of the active work throughout most projects. The central team played some part in seven of the ten projects, chiefly at the planning and analysis stages and to a much lesser extent in the collection of data.

*Figure 6-2* showing the participation of hospital-team members in second projects, is of the same general shape as *Figure 6-1*. However there are noticeable differences in second projects compared with first projects. There is a decrease in the numbers of operational-team members who collected data; for reasons discussed elsewhere (see below and Chapter 5) the central team eventually undertook much of the data collection because the operational team did not have sufficient time.

In first projects, the difference between the numbers of participants from supporting and operational teams was very marked at nearly every stage. In second projects, however, the difference is much smaller, which tends to suggest a greater similarity of roles between the two teams. There is also a decrease, in second projects, in the overall number of team members participating; this is not entirely due to a decrease in the participation of members of a particular professional group but reflects difficulties experienced across all three professional groups. Nevertheless (although this is not shown in *Figure 6-2*) other hospital staff became more involved in second projects than in first projects, a development in accord with H.I.C. aims.

*Figure 6-3* presents data for all the projects undertaken. The pattern suggests that the differences found in second projects hold good for subse-

FIGURE 6-1 *Participation in first projects*

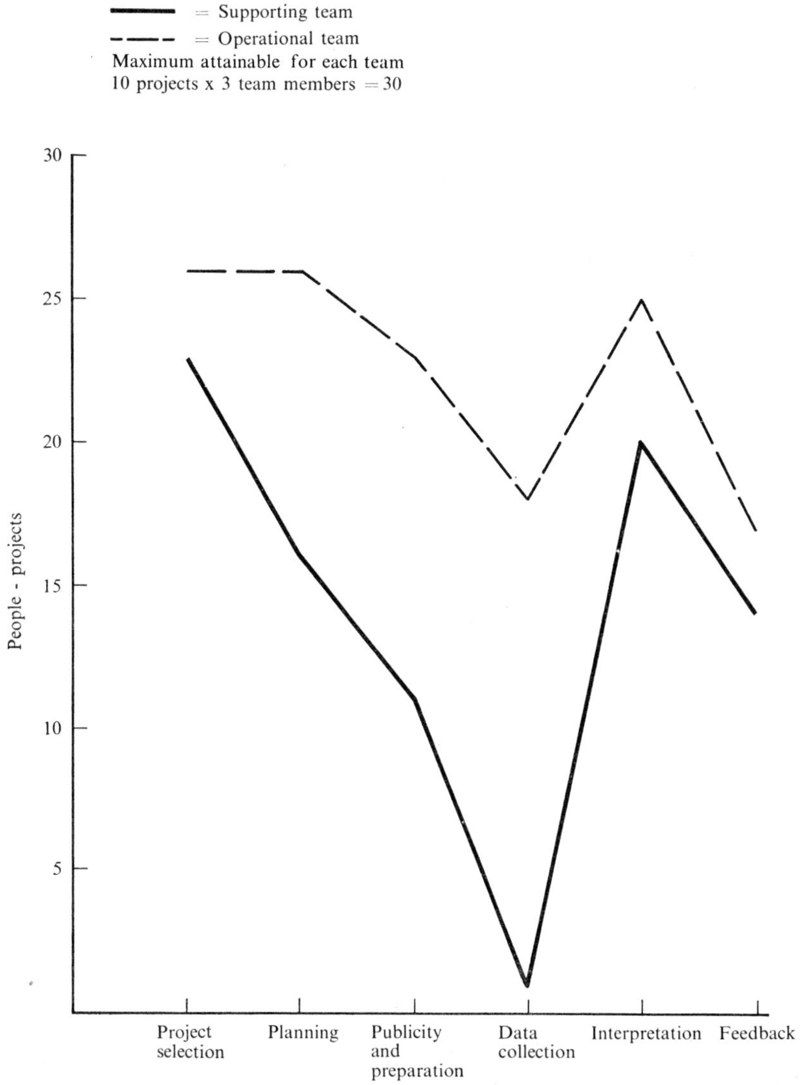


quent projects, but this conclusion should be treated with caution because nine of the thirty-eight projects were undertaken in one hospital while some of the other hospitals carried out no more than two.

The data allow a more detailed analysis of the amount of participation by the different kinds of team member. In terms of the most active and least active groups, the results are consistent throughout. Taking first projects and second projects separately, and then looking at all the projects together, the hospital administrators in the operational teams appear as

FIGURE 6-2 *Participation in second projects*

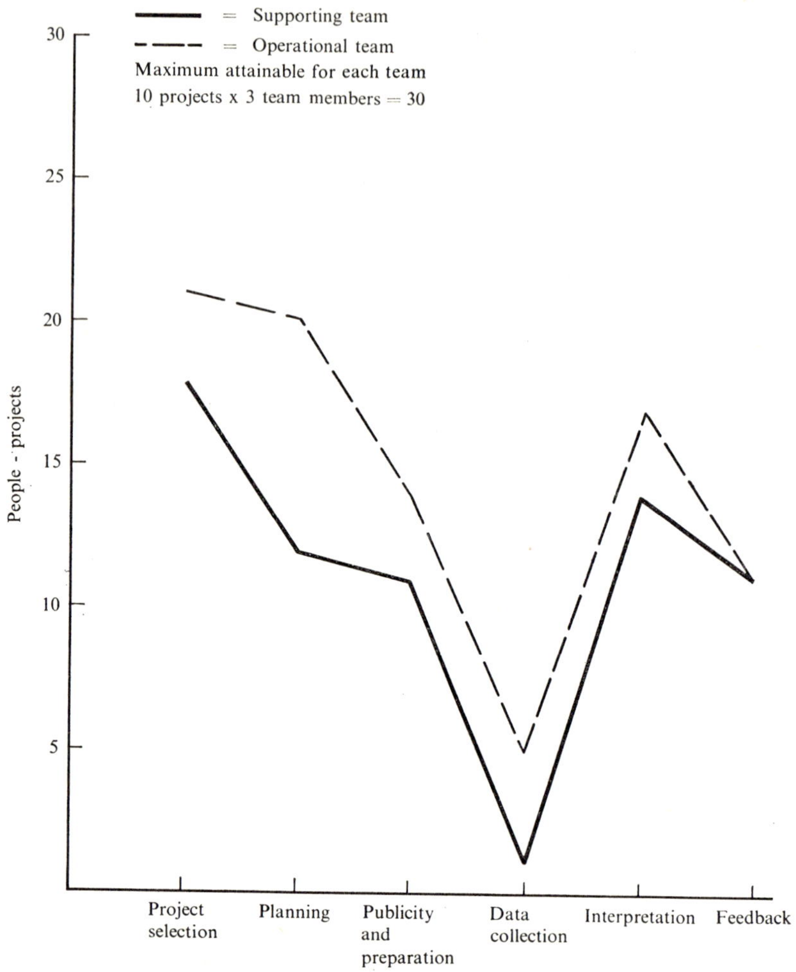


the most active group and the medical members of the supporting teams participated least often. The very nature of the administrator's role in the hospital meant that he, more than other team members, could be interested in almost any project the team decided to undertake, whether it was a first or subsequent project.

The medical members of the operational teams took part on fewer occasions than their colleagues; this may be explained partly by the fact that many of them became increasingly aware of the difficulties of contributing to studies in areas where they did not practise or possess formal authority. However nurses in the supporting teams became involved on an increasing number of occasions, perhaps because a large number of studies

FIGURE 6-3 *Participation in all projects*

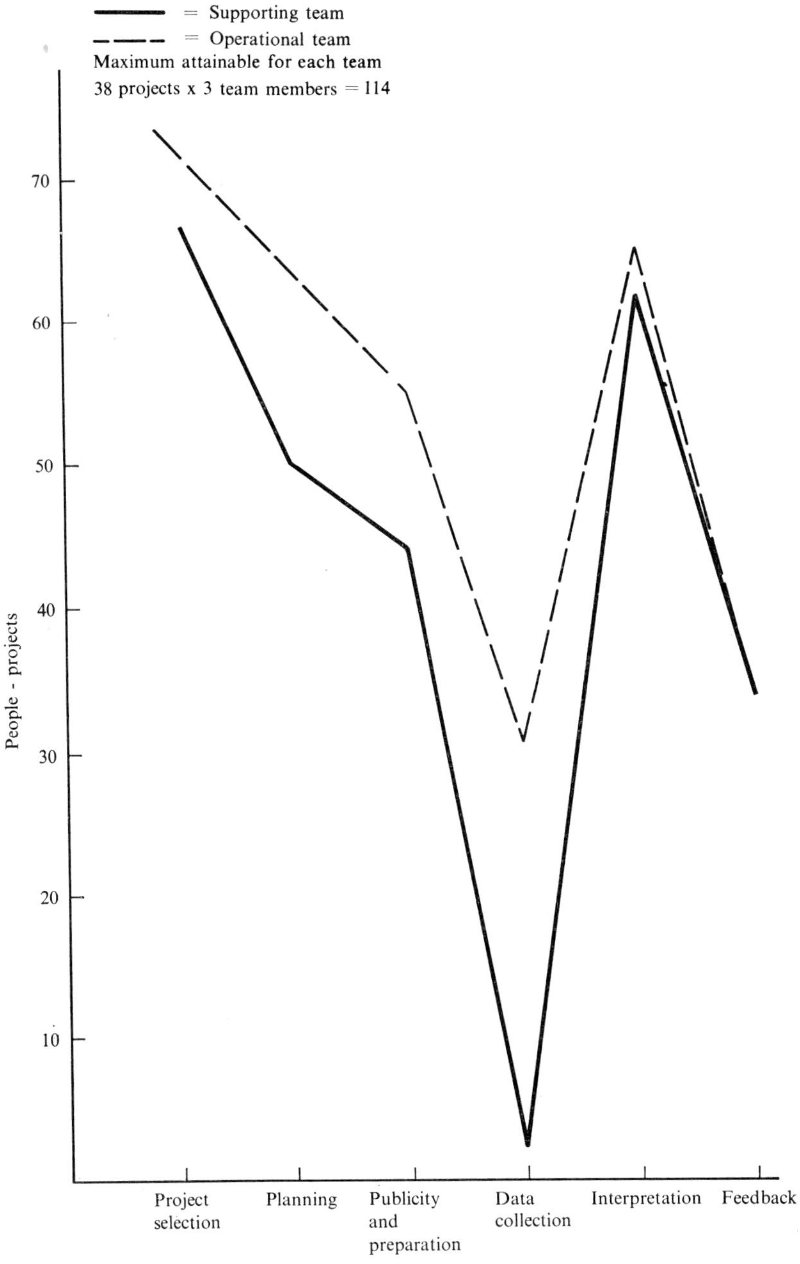

involved nursing staff for whom they were directly responsible. There was a wide variation in the pattern of participation in different hospitals, which changed over time. However, in the 'average' project, the group most concerned consisted of one member of the supporting team, one or two members of the operational team, and one other staff member, often a departmental manager. Although the administrators in operational teams took part on more occasions than any other group, our impression is that often they possessed little authority to act on survey findings.

A somewhat different question is the effect, as distinct from amount, of activity of different team members. In other words who were the 'leaders' or most influential members, either at all times or at crucial points, in initiating, organizing, and taking action on findings, and sometimes acting as spokesman for the team? Leadership functions were often carried out by different people at various stages. In projects where it was difficult to define a single overall leader, we have defined the leader as the person who intervened when progress was slow and tried to ensure that some action resulted from the project.

Despite the fact that the administrators in the supporting teams participated on many fewer occasions than their operational-team colleagues, they often seemed more influential in determining the progress of particular projects. In twenty-three out of the thirty-eight projects the administrators appeared to be the 'leaders'. Doctors seemed to be the leaders in nine projects, but this is tentative as one consultant (not a member of the original team) was chiefly responsible for five projects, and another consultant for three projects. The nurses led five projects. The single remaining project seemed to be led by a central-team member.

To summarize, initially the hospital teams functioned in their suggested roles, but subsequently as the central team took over data collection, the supporting and operational teams developed similar roles. It is evident that not all professional groups contributed equally to team functioning, and that the administrators emerged as the most active group overall. The administrative members of supporting teams often appeared as the leaders in particular projects (for the evaluation of team members' participation in projects see Chapters 15 and 18).

## PROJECT SELECTION

Most commonly the operational teams selected projects and then discussed their choice with members of the supporting team, usually in a meeting convened for the purpose. Sometimes members of the operational team consulted only the one or two supporting-team members whose approval was required for a specific project. Occasionally the procedure was reversed and a supporting-team member (usually the administrator or the nurse) decided that a particular problem could be tackled as an H.I.C. project.

In the operational teams, although doctors often took part, administrators were those most often involved in selecting first projects, a position they shared with their nursing colleagues in second projects.[3]

Turning now to the process of selection, it is possible to classify the projects in terms of what appeared to be the predominating influence leading to their adoption. As *Table 6-2* shows, previously recognized hospital problems were the chief single influence.

TABLE 6-2 *Main Source of Influence on Selection of Projects*

| *Main source of influence* | *First projects* | *Second projects* | *All projects* |
|---|---|---|---|
| (a) Known hospital problem | 4 | 4 | 15 |
| (b) Problems uncovered by previous H.I.C. projects | 0 | 2 | 5 |
| (c) Training courses | 6 | 0 | 7 |
| (d) Both (a) and (b) or not separable | 0 | 2 | 7 |
| (e) Other sources | 0 | 2 | 4 |
| Total number of projects | 10 | 10 | 38 |

Most operational teams found it difficult to choose a project of common concern involving their own work, partly because of the disparate nature of the functional areas from which they were drawn. Eventually, in choosing their first projects, many teams drew on their common H.I.C. training experience. During the one-month course it had been suggested that a central area of concern should be what happened at ward level. Thus, four hospitals focused on identifying ward staff problems. Another team chose to repeat their practice project (this time in their own hospital) and identify problems of staff of the medical records department. The teaching hospital team chose to carry out an attitude survey to supplement a current operational research project aimed at improving methods for coping with emergency admissions to the hospital (Webster, 1967). Two others tackled issues first raised at the introductory meetings before the courses began, thus building on earlier stages. For the majority of teams, however, it was not until after the courses were over that they considered which projects they would tackle. With one exception all the teams used survey methods that had been introduced on the courses.

The second projects tended to be more concerned with specific hospital problems, some of which were revealed or confirmed by first projects. The goals of the projects (see *Table 6.3*), reflect this change in influence. Whereas many of the first projects set out to identify problems, in nearly half of all the projects taken together the intention was to gather more information about problems that had been recognized for some time. There was some progression towards tackling problems that were of primary concern to at least one member of the supporting team.[4]

TABLE 6-3 *Major Emphasis in Project Goals*

| *Major goal emphasis* | *First projects* | *All projects* |
|---|---|---|
| (a) Identify problems | 6 | 12 |
| (b) Gather information about known problems | 2 | 17 |
| (c) Test a proposed solution | 0 | 3 |
| (d) Facilitate changes already envisaged | 1 | 5 |
| (e) Both (b) and (c) | 1 | 1 |
| Total number of projects | 10 | 38 |

On the whole, the projects selected did not set out to examine the roles and relationships among team members. Although the issues chosen were seen as important, they did not often directly affect the work of team members. When such an examination did occur as a consequence of a particular project it was often the nurse members who were affected. Sometimes this was because they had initiated projects involving nursing staff and because (unlike most other team members) in terms of formal authority the nurse team members were directly responsible for taking action.

## PLANNING STAGE

Planning consists of clarifying objectives, and deciding on methods and the content and sequence of steps to be followed in achieving project objectives. This includes deciding the staff to be involved, the amount of preparation required, as well as linking information with action. At the planning stage, we find that the pattern of participation of hospital-team members is in general similar to that of their participation in projects as a whole.

The time allocated by hospital teams for planning a study ranged from a single meeting to a period of seven months. The amount of joint planning in a project in which the central team was involved seemed to be determined more by the quality of the relationship between the hospital team and the central team than by the nature of the study. Where there was mutual trust and confidence, then meetings tended to be frequent and many of the aspects mentioned above were worked through jointly. Usually brief consideration was given to the possible implications for action to be taken (or changes to be introduced), and the methods that might be used to disseminate survey findings. Where the central team's function was seen as more mechanical, such as, for example, simply collecting data, there were generally few meetings. In other words, the collection of data rather than the purpose for which they were going to be used seemed to be of major importance.

It was usually at the planning stage that central-team members were first invited to assist: at this stage they were involved in varying degrees with eight of the ten hospital teams. *Table 6-4* indicates, within very broad categories, the extent of the role of the central team.

TABLE 6-4 *Central-team Role in Planning*

| *Central-team role* | *All projects* |
|---|---|
| None – central team did not take part | 7 |
| Offered suggestions only | 4 |
| Planned jointly with hospital-team members | 22 |
| Planned project chiefly alone | 5 |
| Total number of projects | 38 |

As intended, the hospital teams generally selected their projects alone and the central team was subsequently instructed to help, if at all, on request. No hospital team asked for help in clarifying objectives although they often received it as plans were discussed. In early projects, particularly, there was often some reluctance to examine this issue, which meant that it was difficult to know what hospital-team members wanted. Yet a clear understanding of the reasons for choosing particular goals, and of what the hospital-team members wanted to do with project findings, saved a great deal of frustration and effort in some later projects.

The central team saw its initial tasks as trying to ensure that the appropriate staff took part in planning and that some preparation of respondents took place, and sharing in discussions about data collection methods. In other words, to ensure that the opportunity to improve communication amongst those most affected was part of the process of any project as well as a goal.

In first projects, a major activity of central-team members was to give advice on matters such as the use of existing records, interview methods, the importance of accurate recording, and the pitfalls in analysis. In later projects these functions were rarely feasible because either the hospital team worked alone or central-team members collected the data.

In first projects particularly, some hospital teams were dismayed by the amount of time and effort required to prepare respondents and project activity generally. They were also reluctant to involve other staff, at least until survey data had been collected. The teams felt uncertain about their skills and apprehensive about crossing traditional boundaries to examine the work of others. At that time, however, it seemed foolish for the central team to press criticisms of methods and goals when relations among hospital-team members themselves were often uncertain and the relations between that team and the central team not yet established. For example, in one survey that was due to start early in 1966, the central team suggested that a more comprehensive plan was needed and that many other staff would need to be consulted before starting. In addition the central team felt that the questionnaire was a somewhat blunt instrument and would not give information proportionate to the vast input of effort and preparation. This resulted in the hospital team refusing to consider any further advice about that project.[5]

In the process of carrying out their projects, the operational teams were being encouraged to consult and involve subordinate staff in ways contrary to normal practice. In some cases, this was hampered by the fact that there had been no similar change in the nature of the relationship between the supporting and operational teams. Attempts were sometimes made to make the central team act on behalf of the operational teams and present their problems to the supporting teams. The central team offered to be present at joint discussion of problems (between the two teams) and where this was accepted, the meetings occasionally proved useful in developing temporary improvements in relationships. In later projects, as the roles of operational and supporting teams merged (and fewer members took part), this problem of relations between the two teams became less noticeable.

Now let us examine the projects in terms of the extent to which the hospital staff involved in their planning were appropriate to the specific objectives.[6] 'Appropriateness' is defined as the degree to which the people involved in making decisions about the depth, scope, and methods of the project

(i) possessed some effective authority in the area studied,
(ii) were staff whose work would be directly affected by the study and any action arising from it, or
(iii) were staff who could discuss the study and results from intimate knowledge of the area being studied.

In half the total number of projects, most of the appropriate people seemed to be involved. But in rather more than a quarter few or very few of the appropriate people seemed to have been included. This was due to a variety of reasons, such as staff shortages and team members' uncertainty about their ability to use newly-acquired skills. In addition, the difficulties felt in crossing traditional professional and departmental boundaries to examine the work of other staff were sometimes exacerbated by the lack of supportive relationships between the operational and supporting teams.[7]

An example of a project in which the planners seemed appropriate was one in which a group of medical social workers co-operated in analysing their own work-loads and their relations with other staff who used their services. The aim was to maintain the same service with a limited number of professional staff and to educate other staff about the ways in which the department's services could best be used. The project was initiated jointly by the medical social workers and a consultant physician. Almost from the beginning, they invited the hospital administrator, the matron, and a consultant surgeon (the supporting team) to discuss their plans. Subsequently, regular meetings to discuss progress were held with the supporting team, who later assisted in implementing jointly agreed recommendations (for further details of this project see Chapter 9).

Nearly all teams found it difficult to involve appropriate doctors in relevant projects, although it was comparatively easy to obtain their permission to study a particular ward or department. Beyond that point, most medical staff did not see the necessity for their own involvement.[8]

Some hospital teams became aware of the problems which arose about the involvement of appropriate people, in their first projects, and they were able to resolve them in planning their second. For example, one hospital team concluded that

(a) although the operational-team members had gained from the exercise, they could not be spared for interviewing;
(b) investigations should be carried out only where they had personal responsibility for taking action;
(c) methodological advice concerning design and analysis was necessary.

In their second project, concerning the accident and emergency department, this hospital team worked closely with the nurse in charge and the central team. To implement (a) and (c) above the central team collected and analysed the data, which were discussed together with the hospital team, and the nurses were the first to carry out some changes, thus partially implementing (b) above. However the agreed action by administrative staff took somewhat longer, in part because the changes required were relatively low on their list of priorities. The problems affecting medical staff led to some frustration, because the doctor in charge saw the problems differently and felt the proper place for resolving them was in a medical committee. Although previously consulted and invited to take part in the project, he had done so only to a very small extent. Thus, although some of the information-gathering problems had been rectified in executing this project, the results illustrated very clearly the difficulties of integrating the activities of the three professional groups in ways that would result in effective co-ordinated action for the department concerned.

As change and improvement were overall goals in the H.I.C. Project, it seems important to ask whether the intention to act on survey findings was evident at the planning stage.[9] In other words, what kind of connecting links between gathering information and acting on the findings were built into projects at the planning stage? Perhaps the closest link was evident in the five projects where the staff most affected were helped to collect their own information and to implement solutions. For example, the discussion by medical social workers of methods for rationalizing their work-loads (see above) eased the way for changes in work patterns.

Another project, which was considered to be action-oriented to a large extent, aimed to achieve optimum staff organization in the operating theatres. It was the urgency of the problem in the eyes of those whom it affected, combined with the setting up of multidisciplinary staff groups to deal with the problem at top and middle management levels, that determined the extent to which action was likely to be taken (see Chapter 9 for project details).

Thus motivation to act, plus evidence of involvement or intended involvement of affected staff, were the prime indicators of action-orientation. By these criteria, about a quarter of all the projects were highly action-oriented. At the other end of the range, a quarter of the studies evidenced little intention of acting on survey findings. Most often these projects lacked both the characteristics mentioned above. However, comparing earlier projects with later projects, there was some movement towards greater action-orientation. In very few first projects did other hospital staff share in planning and most usually there was little planning for report-back discussions with respondents. In later projects, usually those where central-team members took part, there was greater emphasis on including other staff in planning, preparing respondents, and scheduling of some feedback activities against a time schedule. But, in general, the improvement could hardly be described as very great.

In a few projects, the hospital team wanted to discover the possible reactions to a particular course of action that had already been decided. For example, the nurse members of one hospital team were concerned about the effects of removing split shifts from the duty rotas of nursing staff. They hoped to discover whether the relations between ward staff and senior nursing staff would be adversely affected.

In another project, when survey findings were discussed, it became evident that setting out to identify problems, using a small sample of staff, was one way a hospital team could set a limit to the amount of change it wished to provoke. In one hospital this occurred in two consecutive projects. The operational team decided to carry out a free-interview programme with the staff concerned. The findings raised a number of issues, some minor ones being dealt with by immediate administrative action. Investigation of deeper issues, however, was seen as involving 'possible major upheavals' which the hospital team did not wish to consider. Nevertheless, this could be one way in which a hospital might embark on a programme learning about itself.

In five projects the central team did the bulk of the work at the planning stage. Most of these projects arose from requests from administrative members of supporting teams. The central team acceded to such requests for various reasons. For example, they wished to avoid conflict in a delicate situation at an early stage when there still seemed an opportunity to promote subsequent constructive interaction among team members and other hospital staff. Where hospital-team members rarely met to discuss projects, planning a survey would provide (it was hoped) an opportunity to promote discussions both among team members and other hospital staff.

Our experience brings us to the conclusion that a policy of confrontation about issues such as the involvement of other staff, action goals, and commitment may be highly desirable but it needs to be arranged with great care.[10] Avoiding conflict at the planning stage did not promote constructive discussion later, neither did it necessarily lead to greater involvement of staff most affected by particular surveys. Even when the surveys did not create threatening situations, they raised hopes that 'something would be done' about problems raised; when 'something' was not seen to be done, cynicism sometimes resulted.

In conclusion, at the planning stage, when goals and implications are under discussion, the central-team members are in a position to influence the shape of particular projects. Clarification of methods and expectations by both hospital teams and central teams is essential. Equally important is the need to define each step in the process of achieving objectives, with emphasis on consulting those most concerned at the earliest possible stage. In this way, a more appropriate beginning may be made towards solving specific problems and improving communiciation. As envisaged, central-team members were rarely involved in selecting projects. The outcomes of problems experienced at the planning stage may be regarded in part as a reflection of the inadequacy of central-team skills. Yet, at the same time, it must be remembered that the relationships of the members of the central team with one another and with the hospital teams were tenuous and yet crucial. It was also the policy of the Project to 'follow' what the hospitals wanted; having started in this way it proved difficult to change that policy.

## PUBLICITY AND PREPARATION

As might be expected, the hospital teams and other hospital staff were more active than the central team at the publicity and preparation stage. The administrative members of the operational teams took part in nearly twice as many projects (sixteen) as any other team members.[11] This activity by the administrators is hardly surprising in view of their normal work in the hospitals.

The central team's principal contribution at this stage was to suggest methods and media that might be used, and to encourage discussion among team members of matters such as the content, extent, and timing of the publicity and preparation. Where the central-team members also collected data, they were introduced to staff by hospital-team members. Additional publicity was gained when central-team members, especially students, lived in the hospital for a time. Both formally and informally such student residents were able to explain to the staff what the hospital team was hoping to achieve.

More than one method of publicizing a study was used in most projects but the most common was normal staff meetings. This presented an opportunity for discussion and for clarification of any doubts among those present. That this opportunity was not always used may explain why members of staff below the level of ward sister or departmental manager sometimes did not know about particular projects until just before being interviewed or observed at work. However, the subsequent response rate was often reasonable, suggesting that the operational-team members, other hospital staff and, occasionally, central-team members found adequate informal methods of encouraging respondents.

Circular letters plus discussion at normal staff meetings could be effective in preparing departmental managers. Where managers were responsible for discussing projects with their own staff, then effectiveness was often determined by the existing communication patterns within the particular departments. It also reflected the clarity of the managers' own preparation for the project. Nevertheless, in our experience, special meetings are more useful, because the study becomes the main focus of attention and there is likely to be more discussion. In addition, it is helpful to circulate printed information.

The amount of effort involved in publicizing the studies depended on the number of media used, the amount of time expended on the task, the number of people involved, and the size of the respondent group. In ten projects a considerable amount of work was involved. For Lewisham's first project, an attitude survey covering twelve per cent of the hospital staff, the medical member of the operational team wrote an attractive one-page description of communication in the hospital newsletter. He explained that management was anxious to discover how good communication was in the hospital and how it could be improved; that some staff would be interviewed and that everybody would hear the results and would be encouraged to suggest and implement improvements. The administrative member arranged for notices to be inserted into staff pay packets. The administrative and nurse members of the supporting team publicized the study through normal meetings and also held special meetings of departmental managers (nursing, administrative, and medical) to discuss the purpose and methods of the survey and to introduce the central-team interviewers. Subsequently all the 141 people interviewed received individual letters.

In half of all the projects, non-team hospital staff were involved in preparing respondents or participants, sometimes jointly with a team member. They were usually heads of the affected departments, and were drawn into the projects at a fairly early stage. For example, in a study of an accident and emergency department, the sister-in-charge took part in planning the project with team members, and then held a series of discussions with her staff, inviting suggestions and co-operation.

## DATA COLLECTION

Data collection took from three days to as long as three to four months, the average period being about six weeks. In twenty projects, most of the data collection was carried out by the central team or by central-team students. The hospital-team members collected data in twelve projects. In three projects, other hospital staff collected the data. All these projects involved some kind of survey.

The most frequently used method was interviewing of one kind or another (seventeen projects), with questionnaires a close second and discussion third. Records and observations were used at times too, but generally as subsidiary methods. This probably reflected the relative emphasis placed on these methods during the initial training courses. *Table 6.5* shows the frequency with which various methods of data collection were used.

TABLE 6-5 *Data Collection Methods*

| *Method* | *Frequency** |
|---|---|
| Discussion groups | 7 |
| Free interviews | 10 |
| Interviews (open and/or closed questions) | 7 |
| Questionnaires | 13 |
| Records and/or observations | 11 |

* Since a number of projects used more than one method the total is greater than thirty-eight.

It was at the data collection stage in first projects that some hospital teams ran into major difficulties: that most frequently cited was lack of time. Some team members had officially been given one half-day per week or one day per fortnight to work on their projects, but their ordinary work-loads were not cut correspondingly. In some cases this resulted in a considerable amount of overtime, and working in the evenings and at weekends. A few doctors managed with a little less difficulty, by obtaining locums to cover their absence.

There was a strong feeling among some operational teams that their senior colleagues did not recognize their difficulties or take much interest in the projects once they had been selected and the outline plans drawn up. This tended to occur rather more in surveys that aimed at identifying problems than in those tackling known problems. However the whole situation confirmed to the supporting-team members the doubts expressed at the early conferences about the operational teams being able to devote sufficient time to H.I.C. activities.

As 'learning by doing' was a central tenet of the H.I.C. Project, the initial reaction of some central-team members was to question whether 'lack of time' and 'lack of adequate support from seniors' in fact reflected a lack of commitment. However, it seemed more realistic to accept that carrying out surveys was not a task that senior staff could undertake.

In later surveys, the central team collected some or all of the data in most of the projects (in eight of the hospitals), but it would be unfair to minimize the hospitals' contribution. In one-third of the projects hospital staff did collect, analyse, and interpret their own data, occasionally with assitance from the central team in the later stages. Almost without exception hospital-team members who had been involved in interviewing described the experience as valuable. They learnt about other staff groups, the nature of their work problems, and how they related to other staff groups.[12]

In withdrawing from the data collection stage, operational-team members lost an opportunity both to learn more about their hospitals and to improve communication. To the central team, the task provided a chance to move the emphasis away from doing surveys to acting on the findings. But as we have described in Chapter 5, central-team members rarely participated in helping the hospital team to take action on survey findings.

Survey methods had taken root in the hospitals and the initially prescribed role of the central team as giver of advice on how to carry out studies had been taken one stage further. However, changing the method of carrying out a project was sometimes as difficult as changing the role of central-team members. The following example illustrates this point.

An administrative member of a supporting team asked for interviewing help in an acute problem of relationships between domestic and nursing staff. The central team suggested that the domestic service as a whole might be discussed by the team and those responsible. Staffing, work standards, training, and supervision should be considered. However the hospital team said these issues were being dealt with and they did not wish to discuss them further. It was then suggested that a group of sisters and domestic supervisory staff might be helped to tackle the relationship problem among themselves. One such group was already holding discussions on procedures and work standards. The hospital team saw this as impracticable and likely to heighten the tension between sisters and domestic staff, without any certainty of constructive results. Eventually the central team agreed to interview the sisters on the understanding that the domestic staff would be included in the survey. The hospital team was not easily convinced that it would be of benefit to involve domestic supervisory staff in carrying out this exercise.[13]

The data collection stage highlights two main points. Firstly, the difficulties of the operational teams trying to carry out surveys without appropriate time, skills, and, in some instances, encouragement from senior colleagues. Secondly, in taking over the collection of data, the central team failed to persuade the hospital team that other methods might be more productive. This failure was due both to lack of skills and to the nature of the relationship with the hospitals teams.

## ANALYSIS AND INTERPRETATION OF DATA

The analysis of data and the writing of reports were usually executed by those who undertook the data collection. In thirty-six of the thirty-eight projects, a report or some data were available for consideration. On five occasions in different hospitals central-team members and hospital-team members worked together in analysing the data and writing the report. Twenty reports were written either wholly or in part by the central team. Fourteen were written by hospital-team members alone.

Most reports were issued within one month after the completion of data collection, but a few came out several months later.[14] The delays were due either to the sheer bulk of free interview material or to computer problems. When the central team alone was responsible for the analysis and reports, initially it deliberately refrained from spelling out conclusions or making recommendations because this was seen as essentially the province of the hospital team. It was believed that the hospital teams were more likely to feel bound by conclusions and changes decided by themselves than by those of outsiders, even it it had been possible for the central team alone to make recommendations. However, it became evident that most hospital-team members preferred a set of conclusions and recommendations (see Chapter 5, part two).

It was mainly in later projects that central- and hospital-team members began to work together more effectively in analysing and interpreting data. For example, in one survey among nursing staff the hospital team collected the questionnaires, and the central team coded them, prepared the data for a computer, and worked through the results with the nurses in the hospital team. A central-team member then wrote a report based on the results of the joint discussions.

Occasionally a report written by the central team was posted to the hospital after inquiring whether a joint meeting could be arranged to discuss it. Mostly, the hospital teams preferred to consider the report among themselves before any such meeting was arranged.

Sometimes a long gap ensued before the hospital team could find a suitable date for a joint meeting.[15] At the meetings, it became evident that few people had had time to read the reports thoroughly but that many had picked points, often different, on which they thought action should be taken. On some occasions hospital staff felt that the interviewers did not know enough about particular problems and that the material was not helpful.

It is necessary for central-team members to visit the hospital first and work through the report with hospital staff. Not only does this method ensure that the report is read, but it lessens the possibility of the material being misunderstood. It also offers an opportunity for immediate clarification of any points hospital staff wish to raise. Central-team members learn about the extent to which the data (and the way in which it is presented) meet the needs of team members. Finally, it offers an opportunity for both teams to work through possible courses of action that might be pursued.

The supporting and operational teams shared the consideration of reports on data fairly equally. Taking all projects together, the administrators often took the most active part in discussions and seemed to have most influence on decisions concerning what action should be taken (see also Chapter 5, part two). Slightly less often, the nurses from supporting teams took a similarly active role, particularly in the projects they had initiated. The nurses and doctors from operational teams, although they often attended meetings, took a less active part in the discussion.

In over half the projects, hospital staff other than team members were involved in interpreting the project data. They played a major part in the discussion in twelve projects, usually in conjunction with one or two hospital-team members.[16] This kind of development tended to occur where central-team members also played an active role and reflects the central team's policy of attempting to include all those whose participation was implied by the project's terms of reference.

In sixteen projects, as shown in *Table 6-6*, the hospital-team members and other hospital staff discussed and interpreted the data with little or no intervention from the central team. In twenty projects, the hospital staff discussed the data or reports with the central team at the hospital concerned. In six of these there was only a single meeting. Where more than

TABLE 6-6 *Central-team Role in interpreting Project Data*

| *Central-team role* | *Number of projects* |
|---|---|
| Played no part | 9 |
| Suggested some interpretations | 7 |
| Joint discussion with hospital-team members | 20 |
| Not applicable | 2 |
| Total number of projects | 38 |

one meeting was held, reports or sets of data were discussed but rarely were two meetings devoted to the same data. In fourteen projects, members of the hospital teams and central team worked fairly closely together in interpreting project data.

For example, in one survey of staff problems, the operational team completed the interview programme and asked the central team to help in analysing the data. Two central-team members worked on the data at the hospital, but the operational-team members found they could co-operate only spasmodically because of the urgent demands of their work. Whereas both the operational and the supporting hospital teams and the central team all agreed on the list of problem areas that emerged, most hospital-team members disagreed with the principal conclusion that many of the specific problems were symptomatic of the fact that, although the unit concerned had changed its function, the organization was still geared to its former role. No one disagreed that the role had changed, but not everyone recognized the relationship between this and the problems raised in interviews. Some hospital-team members blamed the difficulties directly on the head of the unit. Such communication difficulties, where one group interprets problems in situational terms and another in terms of personalities, were a not infrequent occurrence in the hospital projects.

In some instances, managers of departments were seen by their superiors as incapable rather than as victims of the circumstances of their work. The managers themselves, on the other hand, were more likely to talk about lack of staff or facilities, the difficulty of persuading the departments they served to conform to certain routines, and the lack of understanding among their superiors of the problems they had to cope with. At the same time, they expressed fears for their jobs; in other words they felt threatened, sometimes with justification. When they were not invited to participate fully at the planning stage, this feeling was reinforced.

Discussions of departmental difficulties between central-team members and hospital-team members frequently had the unintended effect of confirming the hospital-team members' tendency to interpret problems in terms of personalities. However, nobody was in fact dismissed in circumstances such as these, and often some of the problems were resolved through joint discussion and action. The solutions to conflicts of this kind are not clear, but at least it is more difficult to consider superficial solutions, such as the dismissal of individuals, when all the parties involved are members of the same working group. However this restraint tends to be short-lived because the attitudes may persist after the task is completed and the group disbands. For more lasting effects, it might be better in some cases to identify more carefully the training needs of departmental managers and provide training designed to meet them. Concurrently the hospital might provide opportunities for them, and for their peers and superiors, to participate in temporary working groups set up to tackle specific interdepartmental problems. In other instances a more systematic approach might pay better returns. The most maligned groups seem to be those concerned primarily with circulating clinical information and those concerned with some 'hotel' aspects of hospital functioning.

These examples illustrate some of the communication problems between the hospital teams and the central team in their joint efforts to interpret survey findings. However, most commonly, the team members and other staff involved themselves decided what action should be considered and in some instances outlined plans for discussing the report with the staff concerned.

## FEEDBACK

Feedback is considered here to be the discussion of results with respondents and others not directly involved in the planning and execution of the study (Mann and Likert, 1952; Chestler and Flanders, 1967). It should not be taken to imply a one-way traffic of information at a particular stage, but one step in a two-way process of potentially mutual benefit, which should take place throughout a project. Where a considerable amount of preparation and publicity had been carried out, more effort was invested in feedback and more than one method tended to be used.

At this feedback stage, most of the work was undertaken by hospital-team members. Taking all the projects together, the number of times the supporting teams and the operational teams were involved is equal, but there were fewer projects in which this activity occurred. Again the administrators, particularly those in operational teams, took part most often. Nurses participated on fewer occasions, but those from supporting teams participated equally as often as those from operational teams.

In seven projects it is inappropriate to describe feedback within the hospital in the context discussed in this section. In five other projects, no feedback activities were planned.

*Table 6-7*, based on thirty-one projects, shows the staff groups who received information from one or more members of the hospital team or other hospital staff, sometimes in conjunction with those central-team

TABLE 6-7 *Recipients of Feedback*

| *Recipients* | *Frequency (based on thirty-one projects)* |
|---|---|
| Respondents or respondent groups | 25 |
| Respondents' superiors | 17 |
| Some other hospital staff | 13 |
| All hospital staff | 2 |
| Hospital management committee | 16 |

members who collected the data. Often several groups received the information simultaneously in normal staff meetings. In sixteen projects, hospital management committees are known to have received a report, sometimes in summary form.

Where the anonymity of respondents had been guaranteed it was difficult to ensure that each received a report or heard about the findings, but attempts were made to reach them either through meetings with their superiors, or with representatives of particular staff groups or, in a few cases, through information circulated in hospital newsletters. *Table 6-8* indicates the media through which feedback was carried out in the thirty-one projects.

TABLE 6-8 *Media used in Feedback*

| *Media* | *Frequency (based on thirty-one projects)** |
|---|---|
| Special meetings | 16 |
| Normal staff meetings | 16 |
| Normal day-to-day activities | 17 |
| Publication of report or results | 27 |

* Since some projects used more than one medium the total is greater than thirty-one.

Of the special meetings, twelve concerned small groups of staff, usually within a particular department or professional group. The example quoted below (written jointly by hospital- and central-team members) describes an elaborate procedure set up by very enthusiastic team members to discuss the results of a questionnaire on nurses' attitudes towards their work (see also Chapter 8).

'Because of computer delays, the team postponed writing a full report, and published results in the weekly newsletter as they came to hand. The nature of the material suggested to the team a feedback strategy that would involve weekly meetings.

'At first this was done through the regular formal meetings of senior nursing staff but the team saw that in some areas no discussion took place. They developed a new series of meetings with senior nursing officers. These went well, but there was still reluctance to discuss the issues at ward level. Thus four months later the team set up eight small groups of ward sisters and charge nurses, and these met each week with a team member as convener. Statements containing highly controversial attitudes towards other groups of staff were held back until the meetings had begun to function effectively. During this period other hospital staff, mainly nurses, had become involved, and the hospital team was enlarged to nine, only four of whom were original team members.

'Eventually controversial issues affecting other professional groups were raised. The publication of results concerning critical nursing attitudes towards social workers resulted in the latter discussing and implementing changes to remove misunderstandings.

'Subsequently, criticism concerning doctors published in the newsletter drew a defensive reaction from the medical staff. A paragraph explaining medical staff problems was published in the newsletter. Attempts by the team to involve medical staff in discussing the relevant issues were unsuccessful.

'After functioning for approximately six months, the feedback meetings were terminated upon a vote by some of the participants.'

While the feedback in this project seemed successful, there were three areas in which more could have been done. Firstly, it might have been more appropriate to provide summaries of data on particular topics combined with encouragement to establish objectives and evaluate progress towards them. Secondly, the medical staff probably would have felt less threatened if the results had been discussed with them before more general release. Thirdly, and perhaps most importantly, members of top management were anxious that existing communications should not be upset. They did not try to prevent the project developing but neither did they actively encourage it.

In seven projects, special meetings with larger groups of staff were convened. This was sometimes in addition to the use of other methods, as in two studies concerned with accident and emergency departments. In both projects, respondents received copies of the report before meeting team members. In one case, two feedback meetings were held within a month of the data collection, and most of the hospital team and the departmental staff concerned took an active part in the discussion. In the other case, chiefly as a result of pressure from the central team, a meeting chaired by the departmental sister was held after a gap of several months. A very formal atmosphere prevailed, and discussion was inhibited. After the meeting, it was learned that several earlier informal discussions between the sister and her staff had led to procedural changes, and suggestions for improvements in facilities had been made by the staff. Thus the formal meeting was quite unnecessary. There were other occasions when long gaps occurred between data collection and the reporting of results to respondents, sometimes because of delays in analysis. However, in other instances the delay was the result of other factors.

Some hospital-team members regarded H.I.C. activities as part of their normal function and discussed the results informally and routinely. This occurred in nearly half the projects. Differentiating between the discussion of the content of studies and the discussion of possible ways of making changes in 'normal' functioning is often difficult, and it is not particularly beneficial to try to do so.

On some occasions, senior staff discussed problems arising out of surveys with individual departmental managers. Although this may enable a team to take action on specific problems, it does not appear particularly useful for generating better communication at lower levels in the organization. That the teams nevertheless acted in this way could be because they saw themselves as facilitating communication through direct action.

*Table 6-9* indicates the general character of the central team's relationship with hospital teams in feedback meetings with respondents and other staff. In twenty-one projects, feedback meetings were organized. In six of the seventeen projects where no formal feedback meetings were held, the central team attempted to intervene and suggest how they might be carried out. In some instances suggestions were turned down because the hospital teams wished to use such meetings to announce changes or solutions already agreed among themselves. Where these changes or solutions required ratification by the hospital management committee, which often took some time, the hospital team were in no hurry to arrange meetings of any kind. Conversely, some hospital teams could see no evident solutions to the problems that had been raised and were not convinced of the benefit of holding discussions with staff. At least one team decided the most appropriate method of improving communication in their hospital was to circulate survey results among the respondents.

TABLE 6-9 *Central-team Role in Feedback Meetings*

| *Central-team role* | *Number of projects* |
|---|---|
| None – no known feedback meetings | 17 |
| None – the hospital team worked alone | 5 |
| Observed hospital team carry it out | 4 |
| Shared equally with hospital team | 4 |
| Presented most of the data with hospital team observing | 8 |
| Total number of projects | 38 |

Where the central team was involved, members usually made suggestions about the procedures for the meetings. Sometimes the meetings took the form of explanation by a central-team member of the details of the analysis, with the main findings being discussed by a hospital-team member. Where the hospital team felt apprehensive about presenting technical details they asked the central team to do it. Where the hospital-team members were more confident in their understanding of the data and its implications, they played the major part, and the central team's function was chiefly to observe what happened and answer any questions about the way in which they had collected and analysed the data. This situation, with minimum intervention in the meeting from the central team, was seen at one time as being in keeping with the policy of the Project. Nevertheless the central team wanted to be involved; they had collected the data and knew most about it. It was often difficult to generate discussion and not infrequently hospital-team members or departmental managers were anxious for the central team to report on the findings. The latter, although willing to help, were apprehensive lest a dialogue should develop between the respondents and the central team rather than between the respondents and their superiors (usually members of the hospital team).

In a few later projects less effort was given to deciding who should present the data and attention was focused on how they should be discussed. For example, it was suggested that some positive findings should be presented first, and the material arranged in small logical steps, each one shaped into a question about implications for action. More time was spent in working through the data with hospital-team members beforehand, exploring the extent to which they wanted the staff concerned to work out solutions to various problems. Sometimes this resulted in central-team members presenting the data. On a few occasions the task was shared equally. In other words, despite this change in emphasis, greater central-team participation at the feedback stage seemed a better policy to pursue.

If the purpose of a feedback meeting is to encourage the respondents to work through some of the problems they have raised during the survey, then more than one meeting needs to be arranged, small enough in size to permit some participation by all present. Probably the respondents' immediate superiors need to be the ones with whom the respondents discuss the findings. It may be desirable (but not necessarily so) for those who collected the data to present the findings.

While it is easy enough to describe some useful hints for organizing such meetings, putting them into practice in the hospital situation is far from easy. However much senior staff may want to generate discussion, the structure of hospital meetings seems to be designed to preclude it. Firstly, the seating is often arranged in serried rows with some barrier (either a table or raised dais) between the audience and the speaker. Secondly, meetings are primarily used as opportunities for senior staff to give information or instructions to subordinate staff. To develop collaborative, open discussion as a permanent feature just cannot be done in a short time. It needs constant fostering, and several different methods may have to be tried over a long period of time.[17]

## PROJECT ACHIEVEMENTS – DISCUSSION AND CONCLUSIONS

Taking decisions on specific actions and implementing them was effectively the province of the hospital teams, and sometimes the central team found it difficult to discover what actions or changes, if any, had taken place. The fact that actions 'fan out' in the hospital and become part of normal adjustments in functioning also made it difficult to discover the extent to which actions or changes derived from particular surveys. Finally, while some projects resulted in fairly immediate action, in others action was not taken until considerably later, if at all.

However, we shall now look at the known achievements of the projects with two criteria in mind, firstly, solving problems and, secondly, improving communication, in each case describing what appear to be the determinants of success. We can then compare these determinants with the characteristics suggested as desirable in an H.I.C. project (see Introduction).

In terms of solving problems, some action was known to result from well over half the total number of projects. Very few projects led to the solution of major problems and much of the action taken consisted of minor administrative adjustments. Nevertheless, some projects were more successful than others in terms of the amount of action taken.

The following are examples of action taken in two of the more successful projects (see Appendix 6B for further examples):

1. The setting-up of meetings for departmental managers where none existed previously; the arrangement of an extended network of meetings between senior and junior nursing staff; improvements in the system of requisitioning maintenance work.
2. Improvements in physical conditions and facilities in the accident and emergency department together with clearer definitions of areas of nursing responsibility and changes in staffing patterns.

At the other end of the range there were a number of projects that apparently resulted in very little action, or none at all.

Let us first examine projects in terms of their success in solving problems. The following factors seem to discriminate between the most successful and the least successful projects in the extent to which they were found together in any project. Most often the project was concerned with a problem (not necessarily clearly specified) recognized by at least one member of top management (often the group or hospital secretary or the matron) who had some effective authority in the problem area and wanted to take some action to improve the situation. In other words there was some pressure to change, either on those whose work was affected, on top management, or on members of both these groups.

Although not necessarily the initiator, or the most active in executing a project, the same top manager devoted some time and effort to supporting it. i.e. to a varying degree, shared in planning, ensured progress, obtained necessary co-operation from other senior managers, discussed the findings with those who collected the data, and assisted in taking action on the results.[18] Sometimes the initiators, or top management, had some administrative action already in mind and saw the project as providing an opportunity to facilitate changes.

A further discriminating factor seemed to be the extent to which the central team was involved in project activities. In a majority of the relatively successful projects, central-team members took some part in planning with the hospital team, collected most of the data, analysed it, wrote a report, and spent time discussing the findings with hospital-team members.

Other hospital staff also took part in these relatively successful projects, but not necessarily at the planning stage. Often the staff affected by the project were drawn in to discuss the findings and try out solutions. In the relatively successful projects, closer attention was given to preparing staff and carrying out feedback activities. All of these factors together seem to be necessary to facilitate more successful problem-solving results in the H.I.C. Project. In the less successful projects some, but not all, of these factors were missing.

Other factors that we thought might discriminate did not seem to do so. Clarity of specific objectives seemed to be of less importance than studying a problem that was communicated and understood by those involved in carrying out the project.

Neither did the existence of reliable and comprehensive data discriminate clearly between the more successful and the less successful projects. There were instances when the data were not comprehensive or reliable yet some administrative action resulted when the other conditions mentioned above were present. While better data did characterize some of the most successful projects, they did not do so to the extent of discriminating clearly between them and less successful projects. Finally, the size of projects did not seem to be a determinant of success, although bigger projects offered more opportunities for taking action.

Perhaps one of the important findings, in view of its emphasis in the design of the Project, is that it does not seem important to use the H.I.C. team structure to get problems solved: all members of the supporting and operational teams did not have to be actively engaged on the projects they chose to tackle. Usually only two, or perhaps three, team members would play a very active part in the early stages, and some part in later stages.

It seems doubtful whether even the relatively successful projects gave rise to the development of more refined self-correcting mechanisms for organizational functioning. In a very few instances, mechanisms for dealing with specific problems of a recurrent nature were set up (for example, one project led to the introduction of a seven-day prediction system to regulate admissions (Fairey *et al.*, 1970)) and the activities of the teams were occasionally progressive, leading from one project to another (see Chapter 14 for the evaluation of problem-solving outcomes).

Now let us look at the projects in terms of the second criterion, improved communication. Katz and Kahn (1966) have defined communication as 'the exchange of information and transmission of meaning'. Did those most involved in particular projects become more aware of the effects of their own behaviour, more open to influence by others? What were the effects on respondents? Did the projects lead to more open constructive interaction among those concerned with specific or related hospital problems?

Central-team members made no attempt to measure changes in team members in any scientific way but relied on their observations during different stages of projects. The stage at which changes might have been most noticeable was during feedback meetings and follow-up discussions with hospital staff, but since central-team members were not present at all of them it is difficult to know.

Primarily, the Project was intended to change the hospital-team members, and it was hoped they would be able to improve communication in their hospitals through carrying out projects, involving other staff in the process. Thus solving problems and improving communication were seen as being inextricably interwoven, part of the process of carrying out any project as well as a goal. However, as we have shown, with few exceptions, the projects selected did not directly set out to involve the work of team members. Most teams found it impracticable to collect survey data and in many projects few other hospital staff became closely involved. Thus the desirable qualities of an H.I.C. Project suggested by Revans were rarely evident.

Nevertheless some team members did change more than others. The evidence consists in most cases of changes reported by team members themselves. Our belief is, although we cannot prove it, that the number of people who changed and the extent to which they changed is not very great. Most often it was the nurses, particularly those of the operational team, who said they had changed, usually in the sense that they had learnt it was important 'to explain things more' to their subordinate staff. A few said it was important to 'listen more' and find out what other staff were thinking. These were the people whose work had been most affected by projects and, since a preponderance of studies involved nursing staff, it is perhaps not surprising that nurses, more than any other group of staff, reported changes.

Sometimes active involvement in projects developed relationships created during the training courses and led to improved communication among team members. Perhaps the most commonly reported behavioural change among operational-team members was that of consulting each other directly in matters affecting their own work. For example, one administrator said, 'Dr X (operational-team member) will now call in and discuss problems rather than send a memo. This saves a lot of time and makes for a better relationship.' Yet in one hospital there was reported improvement in communication among team members whose work rarely, if ever, brought them into contact. This meant that the improvement was irrelevant in any direct way to bettering the functioning of the hospital.

There is some evidence that changes arising directly from particular projects occurred where the participants involved their own work in a project that also had the characteristics found in the more successful problem-solving projects. The first example above of a more successful project in solving problems can also be cited as improving communication. For example, the matron had felt for some time that there needed to be some direct contact between junior nurses and herself. When she discovered from the survey that the nurses also felt a similar need she organized an informal meeting to discuss this and other problems with them. Subsequently, similar meetings were arranged on an experimental basis. The fact that the junior nurses began to raise and discuss problems that could be solved suggests that meaningful new communication links were in the process of being established.

In another project, the managerial, clerical, and technical staff in three departments worked with a central-team member to improve the co-ordination of services they provided to a fourth department. As a result, those involved understood each other's problems better and worked out and implemented changes in procedure that met the needs of the consumer department. Some months later the hospital administrator who had initiated and supported the project reported, 'It now takes a much shorter time for problems from the departments concerned to come up the line to me. I get to hear about them before they become too serious.' Other examples of individual learning are given in the evaluative discussion of the training courses in Chapter 4 based on interviews conducted after two years of project activity (for another view of communication outcomes see Chapter 14).

However, most hospital-team members saw communication as a nebulous concept of little utility compared with the practical problems with which they had to deal. While the central team tended to look for changes in attitudes and behaviour, they had very little success in bringing this expectation into open discussion with the hospital teams. While this can be said in part to be a consequence of the policy governing the relationship between the hospital teams and the central team, failure to examine communication issues is perhaps also a reflection of the central team's lack of skills and experience in organizational change activities. It also reflects the different understanding and, consequently, emphasis given to the various Project goals by hospital-team and central-team members.

At the end of 1968 there was a little evidence to suggest that certain aspects of the H.I.C. approach might become more permanent. For example, one hospital was experimenting with thrice-yearly interviews of a small random sample of staff carried out by team members; so-called H.I.C. committees had been tentatively set up in two hospitals to follow up project activities. Towards the end of 1969 only one hospital was continuing to use survey methods (Revans, in press, Chapter 5).

Taking the more successful projects as a guide, it would appear that, to improve on the problem-solving and communication results, the following are desirable:

(a) At least one member of top management must want to change or improve a situation and be willing to be involved in the process to some extent.
(b) Key staff affected need to be consulted and involved at an early stage.
(c) More is needed in the way of preparation of respondents.
(d) A greater emphasis needs to be placed on feedback activities.
(e) A much greater input of outside assistance would seem to be required not only for data collection but for all stages of project activity.

However, it should be remembered that these specific changes would seem to be especially desirable in the context of a project that had the specific features of the H.I.C. Project – namely, hospital teams carrying out project work with a relatively small central team with little influence. If any of these features were changed, then the suggested modifications described above might well be rather different.

At this point it is perhaps appropriate to review points made in the two previous chapters and see how these modifications relate to those suggested here. In Chapter 4, it was suggested that more emphasis was needed on diagnosing individual hospital needs with senior hospital managers, exploring the extent to which they wanted to change their hospitals, and identifying the key staff who would need to be involved. It was also suggested that the initial appreciation courses would need to devote more attention to helping managers examine their roles and relationships. All of these points would seem to be helpful preliminaries for achieving modifications (a) and (b) mentioned above. Where the aim is to help hospital staff carry out action programmes involving participative problem-solving, then some of the suggestions for other changes in the training courses would seem to be congruent with modifications (c) and (d) above. For example, the wider use of participative learning methods with more emphasis on feedback activities and problems of implementation, integrated with hospital based activities. As the reader will see in the next chapter, the recommendations concerning inter-team meetings would also seem to provide a contribution towards improving intra-group and inter-group relations.

Increasing the size and range of skills of the central team and employing central-team members before work in the hospitals begins, as suggested in Chapter 5, would also seem to be in line with the recommendations made here. Not only does such an increase in the size of the central team meet with the apparent needs of central-team members themselves, but it also facilitates the collaborative efforts required in the early stages, and meets training requirements and particular project needs as well. In sum, then, we see that the recommendations made in these last chapters more or less complement one another.

## NOTES

[1] The reader interested in exploring further the problems involved in doing survey projects expected to produce action may consult Festinger and Katz (1953), Selltiz *et al.* (1962), and Katz and Kahn (1966, pp. 416-425).

[2] See Appendix 6A, the Hospital Projects Chart, which indicates the different stages of projects over time.

[3] The central team had some influence on the selection of four projects out of the total thirty-eight. The projects suggested either arose out of current projects or from hospital problems mentioned by the administrative members of supporting teams in discussions with the central-team director. On other occasions, central-team members tried unsuccessfully to influence the choice of projects, because, for example, the hospital team seemed to have chosen too broad a goal for the resources they were able and willing to invest.

[4] Over twenty of the thirty-eight projects involved less than a hundred people, usually as respondents. Larger projects involving more people seemed to have a greater chance of success both in terms of some objectives being achieved and attracting commitment from team members.

[5] See Festinger and Katz (1953, p. 609) on the problem of getting acceptance of the problem statement and objectives of the research.

[6] Mann and Likert (1952, p. 58) recommend that all those possibly involved in actions following from the research should be involved from the beginning (see also Festinger and Katz, 1953, pp. 608 and 612-613; Selltiz *et al.*, 1962).

[7] For example, a project in which few of the appropriate people were involved and for which, through force of circumstances, a poor design was adopted, concerned a pilot survey amongst ward staff. Owing to a shortage of nursing administrators, the nurse member was withdrawn from the operational team. Advice was sought from the central team on designing an interview programme that could be undertaken over two months, working one day per fortnight (this being the time allocated for H.I.C. activities). The team members were very enthusiastic but did not feel they could alter their plans or discuss them further with their supporting team.

> 'It's impossible to get a nurse member, include more wards, or obtain appropriate time. We have to prove we can get useful results within these limitations before our seniors will consider extending anything.'

They felt that discussion groups were impracticable as they could not possibly take staff off the wards, and that they could learn more from individual interviews. This project also illustrates the difficulties in developing 'open' supportive relations between the supporting and operational teams in situations where the latter see the relationship as being paternally authoritarian and where the supporting-team members do not see the particular project as a real problem.

[8] The position of medical operational-team members in the hospital projects was a curious one. In part, their degree of interest seems to be a function of their specialities. Generally, the projects did not affect the medical members directly (fields such as anaesthetics and psychiatry were over-represented), and they had little authority in the areas studied. Usually it was not the medical member of the operational team who contacted the other doctor or doctors concerned in particular projects. Either the nurse or administrative member asked the medical member of the supporting team to do it, or, if this was unsuccessful, the nurse or administrative member would make a direct approach

to the doctor concerned. The influence of doctors over other staff is probably a function of their position in the hospital and their method of working. They often have little influence over medical colleagues from other firms and little inclination to exert any (Goss, 1961).

The more senior medical members of supporting teams might be expected to possess greater influence over their colleagues, but with few exceptions they showed less interest in the H.I.C. Project, if participation in meetings is taken as the yardstick. However a few consultants were extremely active. They tended to be those who worked almost entirely at one hospital and had done so for some years. Usually, they had also held some administrative position, such as chairman of the medical advisory committee or medical staff committee.

[9] Some of the problems encountered in setting survey objectives so as to provide useful data are described by Festinger and Katz (1953, pp. 608-611).

[10] There is considerable recent research activity on arranging confrontation situations that result in subsequently improved interpersonal functioning (Walton, 1969).

[11] In second projects, nurses in the supporting teams were as active as the administrators in the operational teams, probably because of the large proportion of projects involving the nursing staff.

[12] A more positive example of a potentially useful role for a data collector from outside the hospital is a project in which the central team was asked to help in an attempt to interest hospital management committee members in other projects in the hospital. The initiator was the operational team, which supported the project and eased its passage. Semi-structured interviews with executive officers (some of whom were operational-team members) and five committee members were designed, carried out, and written up by a central-team member, who also chaired the report-back meeting. Understandably the report was restricted to those interviewed, and the rest of the hospital was not informed of the project's existence. Planning and preparation took six months, and there was an interval of a month before the report-back meeting to discuss the results, which had previously been circulated.

[13] The activities of two other hospital teams illustrate possible outcomes where survey methods are used by operational teams. In one case, the team carried out two projects already defined by their superiors, and the team had access within the hospital to methodological advice. From these projects, sufficient information was obtained to improve both situations. In the other case, the operational team chose to carry out opinion surveys among different professional groups. Both these teams invested a great deal of time and effort in their projects and hoped the results they circulated would be used. Neither team saw acting in the findings as their primary concern. Both teams viewed themselves as hospital survey teams.

[14] See Selltiz *et al.* (1962) on the need to avoid delays after data collection.

[15] Also see Selltiz *et al.* (1962) and Mann and Likert (1952) who stress the need to structure presentations according to the audience – 'positive' finding first, pacing of results with change implications, etc.

[16] For details on the advantages of using groups for data analysis, see Mann and Likert (1952).

[17] For a detailed comparison of successful and unsuccessful feedback situations, see Chestler and Flanders (1967).

[18] These points are similar to some of the conditions described (Barnes, 1967) as generally present in successful organizational change projects: (1) The organization is under great pressures for improvement both from inside and outside the organizational unit. These pressures precede change attempts. (2) The head of the organization assumes a direct role in implementing changes.

Some of the other conditions specified include external assistance, initially to top management, from individuals with experience and reputation in the field who introduce new methods and recommendations for problem solving. Many parts of the organization are involved in collaborative fact-finding and diagnosis and later in implementing changes after they have first been tried out on a small scale.

# 7 *Project meetings*

## *ELIZABETH BARNES*

### INTER-TEAM MEETINGS

Between January 1966 and December 1967, there were four main series of meetings. The first three are best described as inter-team meetings; the fourth were formal presentations by the hospital teams before an invited audience. The common, and explicit, purpose of all of them was to provide an opportunity for hospital teams to learn from and support each other by sharing information about their projects (for the evaluation of the various meetings see chapters 15 and 16).

With hindsight, it can be seen that the form each series took depended, apart from practical considerations, on how far the central team could understand and act on the needs, spoken or not, of the hospital teams. The information offered for discussion depended on the stage individual hospital teams had reached in their understanding of the aims and intentions[1] of the Project as a whole, and also on the progress they had been able to make in their own projects. The content and nature of discussion illustrated the quality of communication between hospital teams and the central team. The development of this communication, then, closely follows the central team's groping towards a definition of its own role, both in the inter-team meetings and in work with individual teams. This, in turn, gave a specific, though not always universally known or stated, purpose to each series of meetings.

The specific purpose of the first series seems to have been to keep up the spirit generated at the training courses.

#### FIRST SERIES: JANUARY–JUNE 1966

The first meeting after the training courses was a semi-formal occasion one evening in mid-January at the Hospital Centre attended by members of the seven teams[2] who went on the second training course, some members of the advisory committee, the central team, one or two people who had given lectures on the courses, and the Parliamentary Secretary[3] to the Minister of Labour, who gave a short address of encouragement. The Centre's chairman took the chair and the audience sat in rows facing him.

Spokesmen for the seven teams, usually the administrative members of the supporting teams, briefly outlined plans for their first projects. Discussion was generalized and short. The meeting was too big, the time too short, some members too new to each other, and the teams' tasks too unformulated at this stage for any discussion in depth. Two problems still being felt, however, were the need for more instruction on interview techniques and statistics, and the limits of the doctors' involvement. The central-team director's suggestion for a combined project that could involve all the doctors, which was being designed by a doctor member of one of the three teams that attended the first training course, was rejected, possibly because the teams were too preoccupied with their individual projects to consider a combined one. Also, since the courses had finished, the seven teams had not met the three who attended the first course.[4]

A few days later, these three teams met the central team and some advisory committee members at Lewisham Hospital. The administrative member of the host hospital's supporting team ran the meeting, and everyone sat around in arm-chairs.

This group felt themselves to be the real pioneers, the first people to try the H.I.C. approach. They had been back in their own hospitals for nearly four months and were in the throes of their first projects and beginning to come up against feedback problems, some trying to explain to colleagues what they were doing, others already worrying about how their reports should be circulated and how they would be received.

They wanted to preserve the in-group developed at their course and to continue meeting in each other's hospitals. Though curious about the other seven teams, they were not yet ready to meet them.

Revans reminded the group of the four points he felt a well-designed project should have: team work and the participation of staff involved in the area or problems to be studied, an attainable goal that could lead elsewhere, action rather than mere recommendations, and, finally, a need for outside help. He also mentioned his idea that all ten teams should present their projects at a series of formal meetings with outsiders during the next year (this fourth series of Project meetings is discussed below in this chapter). The prospect provided the teams with a common and comfortably distant goal. But at the time, they, like the other seven teams were preoccupied with the immediate problems of their individual projects.

The cosiness of the meeting contrasted with the more competitive and intellectual tone of the seven-team meeting and led the central team to believe that the smaller group, with fewer outsiders and with one team as host in its own hospital, provided a better opportunity for discussion in which not only problems in designing projects, informing staff, and collecting data could be dealt with, but also some self-learning about communication could occur. But an evening was not long enough, perhaps even a day would be too short.

The operational-team members, the central team believed, were the ones having the most difficult time. Some of their difficulties, however, came from the nature of their communication with supporting-team members who, for reasons varying from under-developed personal insight to organizational and practical difficulties, could not define or play the roles required by H.I.C. All the members of both supporting and operational teams from all the hospitals would need to meet long enough in the kind of setting conducive to sorting things out.

A circular letter proposing a weekend conference sent to the administrative members of the supporting teams as a feeler, met with an unenthusiastic response, backed by practical impossibilities. There was no weekend during the next six months when enough team members would be free. The idea was dropped and the central team decided to continue the evening meetings of three or four teams in the same geographical area, about once a month in one of the hospitals. Four more meetings were held on this pattern, with the administrative member of the hospital's supporting team or the central-team director as chairman, each team giving a progress report followed by a short discussion.

The type of discussion that many members of the central and hospital teams felt was needed never seemed to get far, partly because of the formal limitations of the meeting itself – for example, shortage of time, the increasing amount of material to be discussed and the presence of outsiders invited by the central team – but also because some of the data being collected in individual hospitals and the implications of the H.I.C. Project as a whole were beginning to be felt by team members as a personal threat that could not be dealt with, or even verbalized, either in the meeting itself or, at that time, within individual teams.

The operational stage of the project had been running for six months. Communication problems, between the central team and hospital teams, within individual hospital teams, and within the central team, were becoming more sharply prominent. All were involved in the beginnings of a change process that no one knew how to guide (for a discussion of the central team's problems and some of the conflicts mentioned below, see Chapter 5).

There were unresolved conflicts in the central team over who should be involved at what stages in the hospital projects, and how far should that involvement go. In one incident, for example, two central-team members taking discussion groups in different departments of a hospital, in preparation for one of the first projects, had differing ideas on how to run the groups. One perceived his role as that of a trouble-shooter who collected complaints from the group and conveyed them to the hospital secretary, urging him to take action. The other took a less active role in the group, listening and trying to draw out issues for clarification mainly by asking questions; she did not report back to the hospital secretary, believing this to be incompatible with the confidentiality of the discussion and to cut across and perhaps damage the normal communication line between the department and the hospital secretary. The central team's own meetings at the time did not allow examination of these differing viewpoints either before or after the two members began their work in the hospital, and the disagreement exploded into a row in the hospital itself – luckily out of earshot of the discussion groups and the hospital team – which was never resolved.

Such incidents accumulated, as did the residual feelings, and were not seen as ordinary and inevitable parts of a change process but as personality clashes to be avoided or played down.

The central team's reluctance to examine its own problems of role definition gave it little chance to help the hospital teams with their similar problems. Thus, the central-team members tended to perform their jobs as if only the hospital teams had problems – a false approach which the hospital teams could see through and which, though never verbalized and perhaps not clearly understood but merely vaguely felt, must have contributed towards their reluctance to share their own problems with the central team and with each other. The only examination of this situation took place secretly, outside meetings, in one-to-one discussion which in itself added to the general distortion of perception, though it might offer temporary relief to the two people involved at the time.

In a period of uncertainty, confusion, and change, when distortions and misbeliefs flourish, the arrival of an important newcomer is often anticipated with unrealistically high expectations. He is seen as the 'saviour', the one who will point out the right way and miraculously solve all the problems. The evaluator, who was due to join the Project at this time, was seen in this light. He was also seen as the inquisitor who would show up the perceived inadequacies. This additional threat to personal stability distorted communication even more.

There remained the one certain fact that the central team's job was to help the hospitals. In its most useful form during this period, the job consisted of technical advice and practical help on research design and methods of collecting data. The problem of learning how to help the teams to develop a feedback system in the hospitals was not touched on, chiefly because the central team was bypassing its own feedback problems. Shared examination of personal and group functioning as a method of correcting distortions of perception and maintaining a feedback system in the organization is entirely foreign to most hospital people. Only a few Project members, mainly in the Severalls Hospital team, and the writer had any experience of it. The introductory glimpse given during the month's training courses could not be followed up and developed in syndicate and other discussions because of lack of resources in the course staff. Yet something of the same nature, modified to suit hospital attitudes generally and the current stage of understanding within the H.I.C. Project specifically, was needed if those involved in the Project centrally and in individual hospitals were going to attempt to touch the group of guidelines on self-learning laid down by Revans (see Aims and Intentions, Chapter 1).

So far the teams had not requested help in this area – had, indeed, probably neither felt the need for such help nor believed that it could be available. There was strong ambivalence about 'psyche-probing', as it was called, among the hospital and central teams. Furthermore, even if individual teams had asked for help of this kind, it could not have been adequately supplied by the sparse resources of the central team and would probably have been regarded as too expensive to be supplied by specialists from elsewhere.

Help in learning about self-awareness, then, was neither requested by, nor offered to, individual teams. Instead, a research colleague in the central team and the writer devised a new form of inter-team meeting.

### SECOND SERIES: JULY–AUGUST 1966

We believed that a small group, composed of hospital-team members, might provide an opportunity to explore through undirected discussion the problems of feedback in the individual hospitals. The idea was explained by the writer to the administrative members of the hospital supporting teams in a letter:[5]

'The plan is to run a series of discussions at the Hospital Centre, during the summer months, a one and a half hour's session on one afternoon per week for six weeks. Each team could select one of its members to join this group – one of the six members, that is, because everyone will be involved with feedback and implementation, certainly in the planning of it. I visualize a self-help, self-teaching group for team members to present feedback problems to each other and generally to exchange and sort out ideas. If the team in your hospital is interested in the idea, I would be glad if they would select one member, two if they like, to join the group. . . .'

Response was good; most teams thought the opportunity would be useful. One doctor complained angrily of the 'non-English sociologese' in the letter and felt such a group would be a waste of time. His spontaneous honesty, though uncomfortable, was a welcome change from the usually guarded exchanges that seemed to be the only possible form of communication at that time between hospital and central teams.

Members from eight operational teams attended the first meeting, one each from four teams (Edgware, Hillingdon, The London, and the West Middlesex) and two each from the other four (Mayday, the North Middlesex, Severalls, and Queen Mary's) with the research colleague as participant observer and the writer as convener, making fourteen in all. No supporting-team members attended. The operational-team members were four nurses, five administrators, and three doctors.

The meetings were tape recorded, with the group's permission.[6] The two central-team members also devised a record sheet, which they filled in after each meeting with notes on attendance, seating arrangements, discussion content, verbal flow and silences, and an assessment of the quality of communication and any evidence of group learning in self-awareness.

During the first three meetings the group worked at their task of describing and commenting on their hospital projects, but problems were beginning to develop within the group itself. By the fourth meeting they were able to explore some of them. The meeting began with some stilted discussion on a variety of topics covering previous ground. The group became uneasy, the many silences lengthening until a nurse prominent in previous discussions announced that the group was useless. The convener directed discussion towards an examination of disappointments.

Members immediately responded: the meetings were too short compared with the time some members had to spend travelling. The main trouble was the lack of support from the supporting teams; the group needed enlarging to bring them in. The teams were not ready to discuss feedback problems and the implications of projects yet; most had only got to the data-collecting stage. The 'Tavi-type'[7] group did not work with people in general hospitals. The meetings should be restructured with a presentation by one or two hospital teams and plenty of time for discussion.

The convener offered to arrange a further series of meetings on these lines in the autumn, and the group decided to disband in its present form. The information officer offered to find and circulate published works on feedback and the use of data.[8]

In assessing this second series of meetings, the participant observer commented:

'The meetings were different from what they were expected to be. Few members seemed to realize the group was to be a *self-help, self-teaching group to present feedback problems.* Yet they were told so by letter. It might have been better if the group had been reminded of this at the first meeting and of the fact that it would be non-directive, then we might have been able, all of us, to get on with the task of the group. I certainly feel this was an omission. On the other hand, the meetings responded to the five points mentioned by Revans.[9]

'There can be no doubt that the meetings have been a real part of the Project, measured by these five points. From the beginning the group expected the convener to be directive. If they continue to expect direction in their projects, the success of H.I.C. still seems far away. What is going to happen when there is no central team?'

The writer, as convener to the group, shared these views and also the disappointments of the group members. Certainly they felt it was not a satisfactory learning situation. It was, however, for her. Just as the research assistants of the central team had to temper their beliefs on the proper conduct of research to fit the needs actually expressed by the hospital teams, so she had to modify her beliefs about the structure and conduct of a training group and the use of here-and-now situations for self-learning. Here, the group members helped by saying what they felt was wrong and then going on to work out a new structure that they felt would be more useful. This was the first time the hospital teams had, and took, the opportunity to decide the form and conduct of inter-team meetings, instead of being presented with a central-team plan in the belief that it was what the teams wanted or ought to have. The doers had the opportunity to comment on and influence the organization of what they did, the very process that the H.I.C. Project was trying to achieve in the hospitals. The central team was now showing that it was trying to do what it was urging others to do. This was the one achievement of the second series of meetings: the demonstration to the hospital teams that the central team could receive feedback and modify its own behaviour accordingly. In other words, the central team was beginning to learn. (For another account of the effects of the second series of meetings see note 6, Chapter 16.)

### THIRD SERIES: NOVEMBER 1966–DECEMBER 1967

The needs voiced by hospital-team members attending the second series were incorporated in the design of the next series of seven whole-day meetings held every two months at the Hospital Centre. In addition to the common purpose of all the series, this had two specific aims known and agreed by the members:

(a) to exchange ideas on methods and problems of feeding back project material in the hospitals and, thereby, the problems of including the ideas of H.I.C. in hospital administration;
(b) to give team members experience in group discussion, including decision-making by group methods, in the hope that this might help them when holding similar discussions with their own staff.

The third series came to be known as 'feedback meetings' and were open to all members of hospital, central, and evaluation teams, and to senior staff at the Hospital Centre, with the writer as convener. Personal invitations were sent each time to every member instead of team invitations to the administrative members of supporting teams.

#### *Setting, Structure, and Atmosphere*

Chairs for exactly the number of members attending were arranged in a double or treble circle around a small table. No seats were reserved but members presenting material for discussion usually sat with the convener in the inner circle.

The meetings had a built-in feedback system that ensured that the structure and conduct of the meetings followed the stated current needs of the members and that every member had a chance to influence the development. For example, members changed the programme order after the first meeting, which had comprised three morning presentations, two discussion groups, and a report-back in the afternoon. They wanted to discuss each presentation immediately after listening to it and felt the small groups had broken the exchange of ideas begun in the morning and had led to repetitive discussion after the report-back. They also decided two presentations would give ample material for discussion.

No name badges were used for the first two meetings, because the convener believed that everyone knew each other by then. The students and two new hospital-team members at the second meeting felt they did not belong to the 'in-group' and said so, suggesting that name badges and a list of those attending would be helpful.

Though recordings had been made of the second series of meetings and members had agreed to it, they never knew, or asked, what the central team did with the tapes. The convener believed this may have contributed towards their dependent expectations that the central team 'knew best'. Perhaps it was a mere reflection of this dependence. In the new series, edited transcripts were circulated to people who had attended so that they could look again at how the discussion had developed and at their own part in it. At the second meeting, the convener asked if members wanted non-attenders to receive copies. Most had no objections and some had already shown their copies to colleagues, but others were dubious, and two 'horrified' at the idea. So members decided that the transcripts would continue to be sent only to those who had attended the meeting.

In the second series also, the record sheets filled in by central-team members had never been fed back to the group. Indeed, the group never knew its performance was being assessed. For the third series, a new record sheet,[10] devised by a research assistant, an evaluation-team member, and the convener, attempted firstly to evaluate the usefulness of the meeting to members and, secondly, to help those unaccustomed to group work to learn what to look for when running their own discussion groups. Each member could record his opinion of the meeting and of his own part in it. The collective opinions were circulated so that each member could see how far his opinions matched those of the group as a whole. Over the five meetings assessed,[11] some trends could be seen:

(i) Members tended to rate the meeting as a whole, that is the contribution of all other members, higher than their own contribution.

(ii) Members attending for the first time, rated the first seven questions (on the quality of communication and use of resources in the group) higher than did the 'regulars'.

(iii) Some differences were noted between those who filled in their sheets immediately after the meeting and those who took them home and returned them by mail. The latter tended to be more definite in their opinions, rating all the questions higher or lower than the former.

Attendance was restricted to hospital, central, and evaluation teams, and Hospital Centre staff. The first 'outsider' was the students' tutor whose request to attend was passed to and welcomed by the hospital teams. By the third meeting, new members co-opted for a particular project, or replacing members who had left the hospitals, were being brought along (see *Table 7-1*).

TABLE 7-1 *Attendance at the Third Series of Inter-team Meetings*

A. Attendance at each meeting by hospital teams

Hospital teams

| *Meeting* | *Edg.* | *Hill.* | *Lew.* | *Lond.* | *May.* | *N. Mid.* | *Q.M.* | *St N.* | *Sev.* | *W. Mid.* | *St E.* | *Total* |
|---|---|---|---|---|---|---|---|---|---|---|---|---|
| 1st | 0 | 1 | 3 | 2 | 3 | 0 | 1 | 3 | 2 | 1 | — | 16 |
| 2nd | 4 | 1 | 0 | 2 | 3 | 0 | 1 | 4 | 6 | 3 | — | 24 |
| 3rd | 3 | 1 | 3 | 0 | 4 | 0 | 4 | 3 | 4 | 3 | — | 25 |
| 4th | 0 | 1 | 1 | 1 | 3 | 0 | 3 | 2 | 6 | 2 | — | 19 |
| 5th | 0 | 1 | 0 | 2 | 3 | 2 | 2 | 2 | 6 | 1 | — | 19 |
| 6th | 0 | 5 | 3 | 1 | 5 | 0 | 1 | 2 | 1 | 0 | 4 | 22 |
| 7th | 3 | 3 | 2 | 0 | 3 | 0 | 1 | 1 | 4 | 4 | 6 | 27 |

B. Attendance at each meeting by Project members

Project members

| *Meeting* | *SA* | *SN* | *SM* | *OA* | *ON* | *OM* | *OHS* | *CT* | *EV* | *Other* | *Total* |
|---|---|---|---|---|---|---|---|---|---|---|---|
| 1st | 0 | 1 | 0 | 6 | 6 | 3 | 0 | 6 | 1 | 0 | 23 |
| 2nd | 0 | 3 | 1 | 7 | 5 | 7 | 1 | 9 | 1 | 0 | 34 |
| 3rd | 2 | 4 | 1 | 6 | 4 | 5 | 3 | 6 | 1 | 1 | 33 |
| 4th | 0 | 3 | 0 | 6 | 5 | 3 | 2 | 7 | 1 | 1 | 28 |
| 5th | 0 | 1 | 1 | 5 | 6 | 3 | 3 | 8 | 1 | 2 | 30 |
| 6th | 1 | 2 | 0 | 5 | 5 | 3 | 6 | 9 | 3 | 0 | 34 |
| 7th | 0 | 3 | 1 | 3 | 7 | 5 | 8 | 9 | 3 | 0 | 39 |

C. Total number of attendances by Project members

Project members

| | | | | | | | NEW | | | | | |
|---|---|---|---|---|---|---|---|---|---|---|---|---|
| *Attendance* | *SA* | *SN* | *SM* | *OA* | *ON* | *OM* | *OA* | *ON* | *OM* | *OHS* | *Other* | *Total* |
| 7 meetings | 0 | 0 | 0 | 1 | 1 | 1 | 0 | 0 | 0 | 0 | 0 | 3 |
| 6 meetings | 0 | 0 | 0 | 0 | 0 | 1 | 0 | 0 | 0 | 0 | 0 | 1 |
| 5 meetings | 0 | 0 | 0 | 1 | 1 | 0 | 0 | 0 | 1 | 0 | 0 | 3 |
| 4 meetings | 0 | 1 | 0 | 2 | 2 | 1 | 0 | 2 | 1 | 0 | 0 | 9 |
| 3 meetings | 0 | 0 | 0 | 2 | 1 | 0 | 1 | 1 | 0 | 0 | 0 | 5 |
| 2 meetings | 0 | 3 | 1 | 1 | 3 | 1 | 4 | 1 | 0 | 0 | 0 | 14 |
| 1 meeting | 3 | 4 | 1 | 3 | 1 | 2 | 2 | 3 | 1 | 9 | 3 | 32 |

Key: SA, SN, SM=supporting-team administrator, nurse, doctor
OA, ON, OM=operational-team administrator, nurse, doctor
OHS=other hospital staff; CT=central team; EV=evaluation team

Some members described what they felt about this (from the transcript of second meeting):

ADMINISTRATOR (WEST MIDDLESEX). I first felt we must try and keep the unity we got at Hastings. Now, I've completely reversed my opinion and I think the inclusion of outsiders is a good idea.

ADMINISTRATOR (LEWISHAM). It would be enlightening. They'll probably say things we don't expect.

ADMINISTRATOR (ST MARY'S). They might need some support. They shouldn't come just on their own.

ADMINISTRATOR (ST NICHOLAS). This may be the coming pattern. We have almost a new team now.

Later, one team brought two technical-college staff who had been advising on their project, others brought ward sisters and departmental heads who had been interviewed or whose work was being affected by their projects. By the sixth meeting, the new members were themselves giving presentations.

*Convener's Role*

The convener began a meeting with introductions of new members or those attending for the first time, and a brief outline of the programme. She then handed the meeting over to the presenters. She made no attempt to direct the discussions but followed whatever line members wanted to take, drawing out points that she, as a member of the group, felt needed airing or were of particular interest to her. During the last half hour she became more directive, asking for information on which to base the next meeting's programme, and how members felt about the day. Any subsequent feedback from any source outside and after a meeting was directed back into the next meeting. The convener's role generally was to try to develop an atmosphere that would enable hospital-team members to follow at their own pace and in their own way the two specific purposes of this third series, particularly the second purpose of giving team members experience in group discussion.

She avoided the spontaneous groupings around the bar or the dining tables which continued discussion about the presentations outside the meeting. Whenever the convener was drawn into an 'off-group' of this kind, she was careful to feed the discussion back to the meeting, and to tell her fellow discussants that she would do so. This caused some consternation at first among those members of the hospital and central teams who, for the most part, were accustomed to the semi-secret discussion, manipulative preparation, and decision-making that goes on outside formal committees, but who had no experience of the open, continuous, and consistent feedback system of the kind cultivated in the therapeutic communities and similar non-authoritarian organizations.

The one time the central team as a whole tried to influence the meeting without discussing it first with hospital members, it was without effect. The presenting teams had become accustomed to planning their talk as they wished. Some central-team members became worried about the seeming lack of continuity in discussion, both in the course of one meeting and from one meeting to the next, and believed the presenting team should base its talk on, and the discussion should be directed to follow, Revans's 'Aims and Intentions'. The convener complied with the central team's decision reluctantly, as she believed the change from an undirected approach might damage the developing freedom of exchange and that the central team was falling back into its old habits of telling the teams what to do. In the event, the attempt to influence the meeting seemed to have no effect. The teams continued to present their material as they wished, though Revans's guidelines were usually implicit in their presentations and occasional references were made to what they understood Revans to mean.

*Content*

The presentations were mostly progress reports of current projects that had reached or gone beyond the report stage, given by whoever emerged as the leader or most active member of the hospital team. Occasionally, the results of data collection would be described. An operational team used one meeting to feed results back to its supporting team and the discussion took the form of a demonstration of the role of supporting-team members in deciding on action. At the last two meetings, the newer members, supported by students, gave presentations.

The content of discussion depended on the current preoccupations of those attending. It usually began with questions to the presenting team to clarify or elaborate points in the presentation, then broadened to cover hospital organization, beliefs and expectations of staff, problems of reporting back and taking action, and feelings about the H.I.C. Project as a whole. Some interesting trends emerged.

When a meeting contained three or four members attending for the first time, particularly if they were supporting-team members, discussion tended to become a general helpless grumble about problems endemic in hospital life, such as staff shortage, inadequate training of juniors, lack of money, medical staff's lack of interest in non-medical management, and so on. When the meeting contained mostly regular members, discussion seemed more able to focus on the material presented. As the meetings continued, interest seemed to move away from research design, methods of collecting data, and preoccupation with results, towards the problems of preparing staff, reporting back, involving respondents and other participants in discussion of results and decisions on action (for more details on the content of the feedback meetings see Chapter 16). This general shift of interest may have come about because members felt ready to share these more difficult questions with each other in meetings structured like these, and also, perhaps, reflected what was happening in individual hospitals.

The following extracts from transcripts may give some impression of the kind of discussions that went on. They are, however, no more than small stills of something that was life-size, moving, and full of colour at the time.

*1. On the effects of research (from the first meeting)*

ADMINISTRATOR (ST NICHOLAS). Is it a fact, Miss Barnes, that one would expect to find the staff all perfectly happy except for one splinter group who are unhappy about everything? This is probably what we are looking for.

CONVENER. The only thing I've picked up is that a number of hospitals think that one department is 'worse' than all the rest. It often seems to be medical records. Perhaps they reflect a lot of other problems because they are involved with everything and everyone directly concerned with patients.

ADMINISTRATOR (LEWISHAM). This is our experience so far. We are now in the medical records department. If we'd gone straight there and said, 'How do you feel in relation to your department', I think they would have said, 'We're O.K. except for staffing difficulties'. But we were able to discuss with them what other people said about them. They were horrified. They were doing their job to the best of their ability. Until we pointed it out they were just not aware of other people's feelings about them.

ADMINISTRATOR (THE LONDON). Does your report tell them why other people felt this?

ADMINISTRATOR (LEWISHAM). Not unless the interviewee said why. The report is just a repeat of individuals' comments.

ADMINISTRATOR (THE LONDON). Do you think this is valuable? The possibilities are that it will stir up trouble.

ADMINISTRATOR (LEWISHAM). We've sown the seeds of doubt certainly. They are beginning to see there's a bit more to it than just being pleased with their own job.

*2. On preparing staff*

PROF. REVANS. I'm interested in the deputation from the medical records staff (in St Nicholas Hospital). They feel threatened by the expert (a work study man from a local college), do they?

ADMINISTRATOR (ST NICHOLAS). I think we should admit inadequate preparation. We are quickly trying to make good the damage.

STUDENT (CENTRAL TEAM). Yes, because I was officially introduced by you and they were tremendously co-operative with me.

ADMINISTRATOR (ST NICHOLAS). I discovered yesterday that a lot of information wasn't getting to these lower levels, it was being stopped midway.

NURSE (ST NICHOLAS). This has been happening all the way around and since we realized it we've been trying to make sure that the lower levels know. It makes a lot of difference to morale.

ADMINISTRATOR (ST NICHOLAS). I was a bit disconcerted when one of them said yesterday that if they told the work study man what went on it would only lead to trouble and they didn't want that. I assured them we revelled in trouble.

PROF. REVANS. Maybe our idea of bringing in the top doctor, nurse, and administrator was misconceived. We should have had these lower levels and explained to them they too would feel threatened by all this.

ADMINISTRATOR (ST NICHOLAS). I feel it's our failure, but we are learning.

PROF. REVANS. It's interesting that you have known so quickly they feel threatened.

ADMINISTRATOR (ST NICHOLAS). It came to me through what I would call a step chain, the lower level talked to the one above and so on. In a matter of 10-15 minutes it went through about six levels and got to me.

PROF. REVANS. A year ago that might not have happened.

ADMINISTRATOR (ST NICHOLAS). Probably not. It would have stopped half way.

### *3. On report-writing (from second meeting)*

ADMINISTRATOR (MAYDAY). It's very easy to identify someone if you've only studied a small area of the hospital. Someone may have made a strong point which is well known to others in that area.

NURSE (SEVERALLS). I think every team doing research work has got to be prepared to withhold information where they feel it will do damage by being released.

CONVENER. What sort of things ought not to be in a report?

NURSE (SEVERALLS). Say a number of people comment about a person, that he's difficult or too strict. We are going to get this in our survey. And it will be obvious who that person is however we release it.

NURSE (EDGWARE). Can't you put it generally?

NURSE (SEVERALLS). But if it's only said about one person it's unfair to put it in general terms isn't it?

CONVENER. If everyone interviewed says more or less the same thing about the person the chances are that lots of other people say it too. And he could quite well know it anyway.

NURSE (SEVERALLS). But is it fair to give evidence on which this person could be sacked or moved? I'm extremely dubious. This isn't the object of H.I.C. is it, to get rid of people? There are people just waiting to pick up and use this.

### *4. On operational-team problems and communication between central and hospital teams (from fourth meeting)*

ADMINISTRATOR (ST NICHOLAS). The three of us concerned with our investigations at the moment are working together as comrades in arms, not that we weren't friendly before but we didn't work with the same deep interest. One can only suppose that being involved in the thought processes here at the Centre has produced this kind of situation. One hopes it will develop. That's what Prof. Revans hopes, I think. But it's going more slowly than he thought. Perhaps we misunderstood him in the early days and we thought it would be some very rapid process with a magic key that would unlock all doors. In fact it's very slow ...

CONVENER. Do you feel pressurized by these meetings, or by the central team, or Dr Revans? Are you being pushed too hard? I must say you are relieving my doubts by what you are saying. And people are listening to you in absolute silence, so you are probably speaking for a number of others too. And certainly the central team is concerned about this.

NURSE (SEVERALLS). I think the pressure comes from within. We've got all this material and we want to do something with it, but it's so vast we don't feel that just two or three of us can cope. Perhaps we bit off more than we can chew, but we were never advised not to.

ADMINISTRATOR (ST NICHOLAS). I can't quite accept your view. There is a difference between your team and all the others. Your team has held together. Maybe it's the kind of hospital or something else. But all the other teams have disintegrated, it seems to me. In the early days we talked about teams just to get some representatives from the hospitals. A certain number were collected and put through this process. Then, having been boiled up and sieved off, what remains is one person, sometimes two, sometimes three. And when the team gets down to the odd one or two the strain begins. There is pressure from the central team, but you can look on it as encouragement too.

CONVENER. What do other people feel?

NURSE (SEVERALLS). Some of the teams don't appear in great numbers here.

ADMINISTRATOR (ST NICHOLAS). Some don't appear at all ...

ADMINISTRATOR (LEWISHAM). Isn't it a question of our own satisfaction? We feel there isn't much coming back, we aren't disseminating as well as we should?

NURSE (SEVERALLS). No, I don't think so. Surely we appreciate the fact that we don't change anybody's attitude just by having a chat to them once ...

CONVENER. I think this last discussion has touched the real problems we are all having. There isn't any magic. I'm just wondering what the people setting up their first project make of it. The Hillingdon team, for instance.

ADMINISTRATOR (MAYDAY). Surely the golden rule is to define your problem first.

CONVENER. It's nice if it's as clear as that. But you can't always and you have to go back and redefine it.

DOCTOR (MAYDAY). Yes, but you can use the information you have to redefine it.

NURSE (HILLINGDON). I think the mistake is that anyone was given the impression, or got the impression, that there is a magic wand. I know in my team we're not expecting any magic, but at least an effort is being made to get people rethinking.

ADMINISTRATOR (ST NICHOLAS). I think what's really bothering us is thinking out techniques. You've got to think out what process you are going to use to bring about the changes you want.

CONVENER. The chances are you are going to get better at it. This is the first time.

ADMINISTRATOR (ST NICHOLAS). Oh yes, we would all admit we've learned a lot from this.

CONVENER. But thanks for airing all this. You have certainly been helping the central team to define what our role ought to be now.

*5. On advising a new operational team (seventh meeting)*

ADMINISTRATOR (ST EBBA'S). Can I ask for other hospitals' advice? When you did your reports, did you all give them to your hospital management committee? And if so, did you give any additional information with the bare written statement?

NURSE (SEVERALLS). The one survey we produced a report on, the HMC had the same report that went to the wards and departments. It contained some information about why the project was done and recommendations for using the results. I don't know whether they understood any of it though.

NURSE (EDGWARE). We are talking all the time about communication, how one department interacts with another, that people don't know enough about the other departments. This is our main trouble. Why shouldn't everyone concerned have the report? We did a casualty study and every member of the department who contributed had the full report. We didn't cut it in any way. And this goes for the HMC too. They all know what everyone is thinking. This is communication, isn't it?

ADMINISTRATOR (ST EBBA'S). Yes, it is. But how do you interpret the information you are given. How much weight do you put on everything in the report?

NURSE (EDGWARE). Our report was just what people had said. We had a report back session with the staff and said, 'Now have the interviewers interpreted your remarks correctly?' Just to get it straight to start with. The central team did the interviewing and they may not have interpreted correctly. The staff had the opportunity to say if it was right or wrong. This is where we started off. They were all right. They were quite happy. It was all anonymous and no one knew who said what and it went forward to the HMC just as it was. And from this we got a very good response.

ADMINISTRATOR (ST EBBA'S). I agree with what you say and this is what we shall do as far as our own hospital is concerned. It will go back exactly as it is and be discussed at the meetings we have. Nothing will be edited out. The only thing I wonder is if the HMC should see the full report.

NURSE (EDGWARE). But the HMC ought to know what the staff think about the hospital.

DOCTOR (Q. MARY'S AND ST EBBA'S). I think it's a question of timing. The next stage is the ordinary meeting channels and see from there where we go next.

CONVENER. What do the nursing people feel?

NURSE (ST EBBA'S). If we are only going to feed back to the people interviewed it's not going to tackle communication over the whole hospital. It will have to be fed back to all the staff.

CENTRAL-TEAM MEMBER. I don't think it's a question of 'either or', but whether it's necessary to do the first before you do the second. Both are important. We've heard that at top level there is very clear communication but a bit lower down it gets difficult. And if the junior people don't hear about it, you might be creating some disappointment.

ADMINISTRATOR (ST EBBA'S). I don't know. I can't see we serve a very useful purpose in going back to the people who were interviewed on a basis of anonymity before we go to the general staff on it.

CONVENER. What are they expecting, do you suppose?

ADMINISTRATOR (ST EBBA'S). Andrew, you did the interviewing, what do you think?

STUDENT (CENTRAL TEAM). I think they would like to see some form of report-back at some stage. All we are discussing is at which stage, before it goes to the committee and internal meetings or afterwards. But they definitely would like to see something in writing. They've talked to me for perhaps one or two hours and then they went away and had another think about the project, and now they want to know what is going to happen with what everyone said. That is what they are interested in hearing.

ADMINISTRATOR (ST EBBA'S). And you really think they need this?

STUDENT (CENTRAL TEAM). Yes, I do.

ADMINISTRATOR (ST EBBA'S). Right.

*6. On the formal presentations (from seventh meeting)*

The third series of inter-team meetings ran concurrently with eight formal presentations given between January and December 1967 before an invited audience at the London School of Hygiene. The formal presentations were not strictly an inter-team development but an attempt initiated by Revans to involve and interest a selected public in the H.I.C. Project during its operational stage. As such, they became an important part of the Project and a full account is given below. What belongs to the present discussion is the effect they had on the hospital teams.

The formal presentations presented another new situation to the hospital-team members; for some it was even more threatening than the situation in their own hospitals, though others enjoyed the opportunity to try themselves out in a more public setting. Something of what they felt can be gleaned from the following extract.

DOCTOR (WEST MIDDLESEX). Those of us at the Guy's meeting[12] were keen to keep our links with the central team and to go on with these feedback meetings. They are different from the London School of Hygiene ones, and, for those of us who are participating, more valuable, because there is a freer opportunity to exchange ideas.

CONVENER. That's how I visualized them at the beginning, that we could be a bit easier with each other. I think the LSH meetings are a very good discipline though. (Laughter) You really have to think out what to tell somebody who doesn't know anything about us.

CENTRAL-TEAM MEMBER. The LSH meetings have had a certain value in certain cases, in initiating action within the hospital, more so than the Project itself. But one of the dangers of those meetings is that everyone is on the defensive about what they have been doing, much more than perhaps in these meetings. The LSH meetings obviously haven't achieved what they originally intended to, that it was to be a learning experience for both sides. It often becomes a battle of personalities about particular issues or professional groups taking up a stand. This is my own very personal interpretation of some of those meetings.

DOCTOR (MAYDAY). Yes. You stand there and you have to defend your work.

CONVENER. Is that how it feels?

DOCTOR (MAYDAY). Yes.

CENTRAL-TEAM MEMBER. I don't think it is seen in this light.

DOCTOR (WEST MIDDLESEX). It's the same at scientific meetings. You give a paper and there is a discussion period which is really an excuse for a free-for-all attack. This is a habit of thought we are trained in and I don't know how doctors can get out of it. It may be better for administrators and nurses.

CONVENER. No. You find the same thing at meetings of nurses. Not only is everybody getting at you if you are giving the paper, they are also getting at each other. Whereas, this may be my wishful thinking, but what I think we've done in these meetings here is to work through that defensive barrier to the point where we can talk to each other.

NURSE (SEVERALLS). Here you've got a group of amateurs who are fairly familiar with each other. There you've got a group of amateurs and professionals who are not familiar with each other.

CONVENER. I don't know what you call 'amateurs', Derek.

NURSE (SEVERALLS). I mean us. We're not sociologists are we? We had professors and all sorts when we presented at the LSH. (Laughter)

CONVENER. Yes, but professors are amateurs when it comes to doing anything about research findings.

NURSE (SEVERALLS). They don't think so, do they?

CONVENER. That's their problem, not ours.

NURSE (SEVERALLS). But you know about groups. Those LSH meetings. It's a most incompatible group, isn't it?

DOCTOR (WEST MIDDLESEX). But it's a good way of presenting to the Ministry. It may decide how much money you get next year! (Laughter)

At this seventh and last meeting, members decided to meet again to work out how best to use the remaining months after they had completed their reports. The follow-up meeting was held at the Hospital Centre in March 1968, and about fifteen members, mainly the regular attenders, turned up. No agenda was prepared, and general discussion developed over a wide front, reviewing experiences of the last two and a half years and exploring possibilities for the remainder of the year. The discussion narrowed towards considering a combined project on some problem common to all hospitals.

Two suggestions were: (1) a study of the problems of integrating different kinds of staff in the wards, and (2) a study of hospital-community communication as experienced between hospital staff and patients' visitors. Though both these were common problem areas and would have yielded useful information, they were rejected for the following reasons:

(i) not all the hospital teams would regard them as the most pressing problems of communication,

(ii) some teams had already embarked on new projects and others had plenty of work to do on their current projects,

(iii) neither of the suggested projects would necessarily have any link with previous work done in individual hospitals,

(iv) they would involve another big round of project design and collection of data, with no guarantee of the results being used.

Each hospital team knew best what was possible and necessary in its own hospital and the group decided, therefore, that a combined venture involving all teams could be directed towards answering the question everyone had difficulties with:

'What do you do when you have got the report, and how do you do it?'

This was seen not as a new project, but a further exploration of the most difficult stage in the H.I.C. Project, which might help everyone to understand better what had been attempted and how far it had been carried through.

It was, in essence, to be a natural development of the third series. The meetings would continue throughout the remainder of 1968, with the same informal structure, concentrating entirely on the problems of understanding data, sharing knowledge, and taking action, and not on problems of setting up, designing, and collecting data. The group decided that the Lewisham team (who had begun a project before any other team in late 1965 and whose members, significantly, were not present at this meeting!) should give the first presentation.

The central team agreed to think out some questions on which hospital teams could base their presentations. These were:

1. Who sees and has opportunity to comment on the report?
2. Who is involved in interpreting data, making recommendations and decisions for action, and taking action?
3. How much are all those involved at any stage in the project learning about the problems being studied and how far is this learning being shared and continued?
4. What is the role of the hospital team as a whole, and of its separate members, and what is the nature of communication between them?
5. What are the issues and problems arising from the above and how are they being solved?

Only twelve members attended the next meeting about two months later,[13] four of whom were new members who had never attended meetings before. The two Lewisham members, neither of whom was in the original team, presented a progress report of their most recent project, hardly different in nature from that given during the earlier series, though in subsequent discussion they and the group as a whole tried to explore the problems of feedback and kept off the more practical issues of research arrangements and report writing.

Discussion petered out towards mid-afternoon, and the group decided to meet again in September, after a gap of four months. In the event, no further meetings were held, the hospital teams being reluctant by then either to present material for discussion or to attend.

The atmosphere of the meeting seemed to reflect the fact that the operational stage of the H.I.C. Project in its existing form was ending. By this time, many team members had already broken off contact with the central team, though few had so far stated they wished to do so, and only two hospitals (Edgware and Lewisham) were known to be still engaged in projects. The problem of facing the end of the H.I.C. Project seemed to be as difficult as had been the problem of beginning it.

## FORMAL PRESENTATIONS (JANUARY – DECEMBER 1967)

Six weeks after the third series of inter-team meetings began, the first of the formal presentations was given at the London School of Hygiene and Tropical Medicine (see also item R192 in Chapter 15 and 16). Formal presentation was to be one way of exchanging ideas between the ten hospitals and research workers, senior staff of other hospitals, teachers and students of management, regional board officers, and members of professional organizations. Some notes by Revans explaining the purpose were circulated to those invited.[14]

Eight meetings were held in the early evening over the year, the date depending on when a hospital team felt ready or could be persuaded to perform. Occasionally the date for a formal presentation came near the date for an inter-team meeting and some teams gave this as a reason for not presenting their project or not attending. They would have already 'said their piece' or would hear the same material again. Others used an inter-team meeting as a rehearsal for the formal occasion.

The lecture theatre could hold about two hundred people in serried benches before a broad high table, with lectern at the side, which separated the audience from the speakers by about nine feet. By the third meeting, the chairman and speakers moved in front, on the same level as the first row of the audience about three feet away. On one occasion, the meeting was held in a larger theatre, described by one member as 'a Roman circus'.

The audience was invited and, for the most part, selected by the central team.[15] No list of those invited was sent to the presenting teams beforehand, but they and the other teams were invited to bring along anyone they wished.

The number invited grew steadily with each meeting but appears to have borne no relation to the number attending. Except for the first two meetings, the average number attending was about a quarter of those invited. Few operational-team members and even fewer supporting-team members attended, unless they were giving presentations. Even so, they and other staff from the hospital usually made up about a quarter of the audience, with the central and evaluation teams making up another quarter. Much less than half the invited social scientists attended, but more of them attended more than one meeting than any other group. Regional board officers made up about a tenth of the audience and most came to one meeting only.

The meetings lasted about an hour and a half, with a half-hour for assembly in the basement canteen. The various groups of people attending tended to remain in separate groups during the assembly period, as did new central-team members and students, though the students would occasionally join the hospital team they were working with. The more senior members of the central team, the only ones who would collectively know everyone, would move around attempting to introduce strangers, including, often, the chairman and speakers for the evening. On only one occasion did these last meet for a full briefing session beforehand.

The presentation usually lasted for an hour, leaving half an hour for discussion, and, as in the inter-team meetings, the speakers were usually those who had appeared as the initiators or leaders of a project, though not necessarily those who had been most active.[16]

With only a third of the time left for discussion, and with such a wide range of separate interests in the audience, there was little opportunity for detailed examination. When this was attempted, it was usually about some unclear or poorly documented point upon which people could have untested opinions. For example, after the West Middlesex team's presentation of their nine projects, the greater part of the discussion was taken up with varied advice from the audience on how to counsel student nurses; and Queen Mary's team's presentation attracted some heated opinions on whether or not playing with sick children could be called nursing.

It must be remembered, however, that these were formal presentations before about fifty people, most of whom were strangers to one another. Close discussion of the kind necessary for learning was impossible. Much depended on the chairman's skill in developing a cool dialogue between the researchers and other outsiders and the hospital teams, and in avoiding the devastating competitive debate on which some academics seem to thrive. Most of the questions came from the social scientists, with the central team a close second. Of members of the hospital teams, the nurses contributed most.[17] Audience interest centred mainly on the team's future plans and on general issues of hospital organization, though a good number also took up questions about the effect of the projects on the hospital and on feedback.[18]

To get some idea of the effect of the formal presentations on speakers and audience, the writer collected some reflections from seven people about a year afterwards. Four, who had given presentations, were interviewed; the other three were regular members of the audience (one had also been a chairman) who provided written comments. The four presenters were asked generally what it had felt like and specifically about the preparation, timing, programme, quality of discussion, and the value of the meetings to themselves.

*(a) St Nicholas team member*

The team had had no rehearsal beforehand but had held one meeting to decide who should say what. They also had no prior contact with the chairman and saw her for only a few minutes before the meeting. Neither had the team needed, or expected, help or advice from the central team. 'You've got to do it on your own, then it's your thing.'

The member felt his team had done fairly well but the audience had been so mixed it was difficult to know where to aim the presentation. He felt the experience of presenting to a 'mildly hostile, critical' audience who, he believed, had more knowledge than the team, had been a useful exercise. Most of the questions came from the 'academics' and he found himself 'slipping into their jargon sometimes'.

The atmosphere was generally 'alien and potentially threatening'. At the same time, he saw the other hospital teams' silence as sympathetic support and also felt protected by the chairman's sensitive and kindly manner.

He believed the aims of the formal presentations were to give the Project wider publicity and to justify the money spent. He felt his team must do well and not let down the central team, particularly Revans. He also assumed the meetings were intended to draw together research workers and hospital staff but felt that neither group spontaneously attempted this. Any contact seemed to be made through the central team before the meeting.

(*b*) *Severalls team member*

He was well used to public speaking and had not rehearsed beforehand. The presentation was made too early for him to 'get H.I.C. concepts across'. The main Severalls project was only just entering the analysis phase and he could only talk about preliminary arrangements and the pilot studies. 'Don't think the audience was any the wiser about H.I.C. when I'd finished, but you people asked us to do it then, so we did.'

The team (the member interviewed was the only one to present the material, but others joined in answering questions afterwards) met the chairman for the first time on the platform, but this did not matter much. Not knowing the audience beforehand was more of an advantage than not. 'If I'd known who was there, I would have been much more anxious.'

Two kinds of questions came up; the researchers 'wanted to pick holes in our methodology', and the hospital people 'wanted to tell us how to solve our problems'. He saw the discussion as a battle between 'research amateurs and professionals'. But he felt supported by the central team 'even though none of you said much', and felt confident that he could answer most of the questions.

Having to speak publicly helped him to clarify his own thoughts, and some questions influenced the way the team looked at results later. Another value to the hospital was that a number of other staff who had not heard much about the project until that meeting came with the team. At the beginning of the H.I.C. Project the hospital had a divided nursing staff with two chief nurses. The 'male side' had been less well informed than the 'female side' because the chief male nurse had only become a member of the team after the training courses and had not been invited to the early H.I.C. planning conferences at the Centre. 'We got across more to them that evening than we'd ever done before.'

(*c*) *A team member from the London and a central-team student*

Both felt fairly pleased with their papers though the student had had to rush through his because time was short. (This was the only meeting in which two presentations were given, and, as it was the first meeting, Revans had also given an introductory talk.)

Discussion was divided between researchers and hospital people and, as at the meeting when Severalls performed, the two groups seemed unable to join in mutual discussion. The London Hospital team member also felt the hospital people 'got sidetracked onto solutions'. At the time, he had been disconcerted by one question from a social scientist about how the team intended to use the present project as a baseline for future study. 'If you see him again, please tell him we are still working on this one!'

The student, Kenneth Eason, found the questions about his role interesting because of their relevance to the questioners' own roles as outsiders doing research in hospitals. He also found the question, 'What happens to your work when you leave the hospital?', made the hospital team think about how far they were really committed to the project he was working on.

(*d*) *Department of Health nursing officer* (*research*) – *Marjorie Simpson* (*written comments*)

'The purpose of the formal presentations was clearly in accord with the aims of the Project. How far was the purpose achieved?

'The research aspects of this Project readily lend themselves to confused thought. The teams, including the central team, were engaged in a massive research project to see if what Revans was trying to do could, in fact, be achieved by the means he prescribed and, if so, in what terms his success could be measured. The evaluation of the Project, being undertaken by an independent research team, was never examined in the formal sessions; nor was it intended that it should be. In fact, these sessions formed part of the raw material for the evaluation.

'Research was not the primary object of the H.I.C. Project (see also Chapter 11). Hence, the central team were saying that at the formal presentations discussion was guided towards studying the projects undertaken as instruments for the better understanding of communication problems in hospitals as a whole.[19] Revans said of the meetings, "We need to meet in the same spirit that any group of research workers in any science would meet, listen to a professional presentation of an experiment and then discuss it as objectively as possible." Now, learning to do research has something in common with learning to fence. In pitting oneself against more experienced exponents of the art, one seeks to develop and improve one's skills. Circumstances forced Revans to limit the normal thrust and parry of research discussion by his special rules. For example, the internal content of the experiment, sampling, and questionnaire design were specifically excluded from discussion. Small wonder that the audience is reported to have been often at cross purposes among themselves and that attendance declined over time.

'The meetings, then, were not intended to improve the quality of the research reports nor to help the hospital teams to improve their skills as research workers.

'This leaves unresolved a nagging doubt as to the wisdom of encouraging administrators to act on findings obtained through techniques that cannot stand up to critical examination, and raises the question of the appropriateness of highly skilled administrators using time to carry out projects on an amateur basis. Time and again, speakers pleaded lack of time to do the work involved without neglecting their normal duties. Was carrying out a research project the only possible means of sparking off improved communication? Were there special virtues in their undertaking together something difficult and new to all of them which outweighed the disadvantages? The meetings highlighted these questions as research workers and the hospital teams strove to communicate with each other, but it was outside their scope to proffer answers.

'It would be easy to see in these public presentations an effort to pass on to other people with similar interests something of what had been learned during the Project, and to indicate some of the growing points for further action. Such use of the meetings was specifically excluded by Revans. This stage of the work, he said, "is not intended for the enlightenment of the audience, except incidentally". The audience was brought in to teach rather than to learn. Like all good teachers, they probably got from the sessions as much as or more than they gave.

'As teachers, however, the members of the audience were perhaps underprepared. The objectives of the formal presentations had been set out for them. The hospital team were to present "professional accounts of how these attempts at management therapy have actually worked out", and the guidelines for presentation were laid down. Yet the questions and comments from the audience were ragged, and very rarely were points fully developed and worked out. A great deal depended upon the chairman's skill. One wonders, if these sessions were primarily to help the hospital teams to learn more, whether it would not have been better for one chairman, preferably Revans, to conduct all the meetings, deliberately deciding beforehand the points each project contributed to an understanding of the problems of communication and seeing that these were brought out, enlarged on, and illustrated, perhaps using a small team of speakers from the audience. Indeed, from the hospital teams' point of view, discussing their projects with a small band of experienced administrators and teachers might have been a more profitable learning experience, but this would have cut out the opportunities for others in the hospital and allied fields to learn from the discussion, and that would have been a pity. The hospital teams will have opinions on how much they learned. To the observer, it seemed that the discussion on the use of findings, on feedback and its problems and on implementing change must have borne fruit.

'What came over most clearly was that this adventure had followed the traditional pattern of blood, sweat, and tears. Something of the comradeship of shared adventures came through too, and rifts, if indeed they had occurred, were not apparent, though not all teams survived intact as working units to the end. The first object of the Project had been to develop skills in working together and probably these presentations to an outside audience showed them to best advantage. Many teams had expended much thought and effort on their feedback procedures. Very properly, they were moving gently in the actual implementation of change. Sometimes the audience urged them to move faster, forgetting that all were speaking before the end of the Project and that radical changes in the overall structure of management are not made on the basis of a single, or even of several, small-scale inquiries. There was evidence of many ideas germinating; the harvest will not be reaped in the lifetime of this Project, and much of the seed may wither for lack of nourishment, but there seemed to be evidence that some would grow and flourish.

'The meetings were a good idea, fully in accord with the objectives of the Project. The *nature* of the Project prevented their being used to improve the quality of the research reports. As a learning process, if similar work were undertaken again, it would be worthwhile to structure the meetings more strictly, deliberately using the presentations to bring out and to bring home to the teams the underlying principles illustrated by the reports. In spite of this, it seems probable that the teams were helped by having to meet definite deadlines with their reports, and that they also learned about the difficult problems of introducing change in hospitals. Unintended side effects were almost certainly a degree of learning amongst the audience and a scattering of ideas, which may well develop without acknowledgement or indeed recollection of their origin.'

(*e*) *University lecturer – G. F. Rehin* (*written comments*)

'I was invited to attend the formal presentations through a fortuitous friendship with one of the members of the central team. I was interested in the H.I.C. Project and familiar with Revans's studies. I attended mainly to learn, with no expectation that I might be asked to write an appraisal. Such notes as I took were largely directed to asking questions at the meetings and I am relying almost wholly on memory in writing this account. My judgements may appear distorted both to those deeply involved in them and to those who have access to transcripts and other written records. I read the notes prepared by Revans and circulated before the formal presentations, which contain pertinent questions for any appraisal.

'The meetings were rather too formal, somewhat stiff in atmosphere and impersonal, both during the preliminary cup of tea and in the lecture theatre. Strangers were not introduced. Chairmen were not well informed in advance and, it sometimes seemed, not well acquainted with the aims of the Project as a whole. Microphones and tape recorder were much in evidence and obtrusive. The situation was threatening to the teams, particularly to the presenting teams, many of whom were ill at ease, their relations among themselves at times uncomfortable. They must have felt more under scrutiny than in a "learning situation" of mutual exchange. Much anxiety seemed to underly the meetings, among the presenting team and among the central team. As a consequence, well-meaning chairmen often allowed presenters and audience to escape into prolonged discussion of methods of surveys, peripheral issues, or the "internal content of the experiments". I was often reminded of Revans's pointed formulation of the problem within the hospital: the regenerative process of anxiety, uncertainty, communication blockage (Revans, 1964b, p. 91).

'Much was communicated, and expected information provided, but it was rare for matters to be deeply probed. The presentations were rather mechanical recitations of surveys performed, imperfections revealed, and administrative adjustments made. The audience, particularly those from other teams, frequently closed ranks with the presenting team by turning the discussion into shop talk. Irrelevant questions about methods of surveys would be asked; examples of how imperfections were solved at other hospitals would be given. Much of the discussion involved topics related to communication or human relations within hospitals – for example, the matron's meetings with junior nurses, administrators' conferences with senior officers – but the level of the discussion was often superficial.

'The presentation tended at times to over-emphasize survey methods, particularly the collection and processing of data rather than their analysis, and the focus of most presentations was upon raw information, the significance of which was rarely explored sociologically, or psychologically, or in relation to any theory of hospital administration. Raw data were treated either as evidence of the smooth operation of the hospital or, less often, of minor friction. The predominant impression is that project teams regarded their surveys as discrete monitoring exercises rather than as segments of a continuous learning process.

'While the atmosphere of the meetings and the anxiety engendered undoubtedly account for some of the inadequacies, a more grievous fault, appearing in many sessions and running through all the strata of the H.I.C. Project, was the lack of bedrock foundation, of an underlying conceptual model of the hospital as a "community" or as a social system upon which a significant learning experience could be built. Instead, the model of the hospital that too many participants accepted was that of a rather simple, somewhat mechanical system, which worked according to a rule book. From the accounts presented, it seemed that friction or dissatisfaction disclosed by the surveys was examined at a superficial level to discover what rule had been violated, or the truth or falsity of an implied fact. If the former, action was taken to re-emphasize the rule, to use authority to secure conformity. Implied facts were usually regarded as false, but if true they were often considered to be illegitimate grounds for complaint. Thus it appeared that team members never asked *why* rules were broken or probed beyond the surface of a complaint to find its causes. It was as if the hospital were a machine; when it misfunctioned some minor adjustment was made, and when it squeaked, it was oiled. Deviant behaviour and low morale were rarely read as signs of a deeper systemic pathology.

'One presentation, for example, included a survey of outpatient clinics in which clerical staff had complained that registrars were altering clinic times to suit themselves. Action was taken to remedy this. The medical committee was informed and they reaffirmed the rule that clinic timetables could only be altered by consultants. The junior doctors were told. A situation was revealed of which any hospital administrator ought to have been aware without a "survey", and action was taken to "correct a fault". When I raised the question of *why* registrars had been deviant, implying that this might have been in some way functional for them, I was rather abruptly told off by a team member, a medical consultant, who, in effect, said, "You don't understand hospitals; it is the consultant's prerogative to run clinics and to command registrars." No further discussion of this point was possible.

'Teams were not prepared to probe deeply into the organization itself, into the attitudes of those in authority or, indeed, into their own attitudes. This unpreparedness carried over into the meetings, most of the audience being unwilling to probe the presenting team in relevant ways or to discuss issues raised by interested outsiders. Both the hospital teams and the audience could have been better prepared by the central team before each meeting, somewhere, somehow, initially, for few seemed able to make that necessary but painful confrontation with their own entrenched attitudes and rigidified organization, and with the connection between them.

'Another example will illustrate one of the issues on internal feedback put by Revans in his guiding document and usually raised at the meetings. On one occasion, a differential feedback was described – senior staff received a full report and had opportunities to discuss it; junior staff, in particular enrolled nurses, received one foolscap sheet only. Further inquiries from the audience revealed that enrolled nurses were regarded as both incapable of assimilating more information and unlikely to have any great interest in the project. The team members appeared unable to perceive their own attitudes when they were pointed out to them. There were many occasions when team members displayed hierarchical and authoritarian attitudes. Anxieties had not been worked through to the point where such attitudes could be openly discussed and, therefore, little learning had taken place.

'There is no doubt in my mind that the communication barriers and seeming lack of learning manifest at these meetings were partly the result of a need for defence against the threat of public scrutiny. In more private meetings, I am certain, painful self-examination took place and much was learned by individuals. From the evidence presented formally, however, I would doubt that much in the way of "management therapy" took place. Yet there was goodwill and much open and frank discussion, however superficial, and an evident willingness by many to continue with projects of this sort. I suggest three lessons are to be learned from the experience of these meetings:

1. Formal presentations such as these are not good learning situations.
2. The central team must prepare the inter-team learning situations, whatever their shape, by some process analogous to group therapy, enabling participants to work through their anxiety so that communication can occur.

3. Conceptual analysis that is sociologically and psychologically informed is needed to provide the content of communication.

'I suspect that these lessons are also applicable to individual hospitals and to the whole H.I.C. Project.'

*(f) Deputy senior administrative medical officer – Dr Stephen Mackenzie (written comments)*

'It was not always clear that the hospital had understood the implications of what it was trying to do.

'Some projects seemed to be concerned with matters of internal organization rather than problems of communication, and therefore were more likely to be amenable to organization and method, or simple work study, surveys and solutions, instead of the complicated procedures necessitated by the H.I.C. Project.

'The reluctance of senior medical staff to become involved was particularly noticeable. Some hospital teams were not supported at the presentations by medical members.

'Some hospitals tackled projects that had seemed straightforward at first sight but later proved to be more complex, demanding deeper analysis over a wider field. This imposed a much larger task, needing more time and more workers than had originally been thought likely, and caused some loss of control and impetus.

'Little awareness was apparent that people in key posts would inevitably be subject to change of duties or be promoted to other hospitals, and that unless a project (or a critical part of it) was designed to overcome this defect it might peter out.

'A proper feeling of humility was evident. One had the impression that people were ready to receive criticism of their selection of projects as well as their approach and methods.

'On the whole, constructive criticism came from the audience. But not all other criticism was skilfully rebutted by the team when it could have been – they were perhaps too overawed by the formal nature of their surroundings. Follow-up action was sparsely presented, mainly because the teams had not reached that stage, sometimes perhaps because projects had "run out of steam". Some were not properly communication projects. One came away with the impression that carrying out the projects had done a lot of good in getting people to look at what they did (and said) from someone else's point of view. This aspect and its benefits were almost universally remarked on by participating teams, and, I am sure, applied also to those like myself who merely attended to observe the proceedings.'

## CONCLUSIONS

The inter-team meetings were attempts at helping hospital teams to understand something of the implications of their projects for themselves, for their staff and for the hospital's formal and informal communication system as a whole, through sharing information on each other's projects. An attempt was also made to introduce some type of group- and self-learning within the current situations in which the hospital teams found themselves.

This type of learning can be synthetically produced, as in the so-called 'sensitivity training' or 'T-group', in which a small number of self-selected people, usually strangers at the start, meet regularly for a definite length of time (usually an hour and a half a week) over a period of months, for the purpose of studying the collective experience, feelings, and behaviour occurring in the session at the time – the 'here and now situation' as it is called. The group has a consultant, with psychoanalytic and group training, whose role is to help the group in its study. It is similar in many ways to group psychotherapy, the main differences being that members of a psychotherapeutic group are, and believe themselves to be, psychiatric patients in need of treatment, and the psychiatrist, who hopefully also has psychoanalytic training is chiefly concerned with examining and interpreting transference phenomena. Both T-groups and psychotherapeutic groups are methods of group learning directed towards helping members to become more aware of themselves and how they affect and are affected by each other. Most people who have been members of a T-group feel the experience has helped them personally, and, provided they are able to learn from it, they stand a good chance of making some adjustment in personal attitudes and behaviour. But the experience may not help much, may indeed be a disadvantage, in practical work, because colleagues have usually not shared the same experience, and the structure of the organization in which the work is done remains the same.

A more useful way of providing this experience for those involved in the H.I.C. Project seemed to be to try to use the social situation that develops naturally among a group of people sharing the same task, particularly a novel task, by cultivating it into a learning situation similar to that provided by the network of staff meetings in a therapeutic community (Main, 1946; Weddell, 1955; Skellern, 1953; Jones, 1962). Given time, regularity, and skilled help, students and newcomers in the therapeutic community can begin to develop an ability to examine their interaction, particularly their conflicts, not as a self-indulgent introspective exercise, but as part of their normal job of understanding the current situation and their roles in it in order to help patients. This in itself eases personal communication, and facilitates organizational change and the redefinition of role relationships, because communication blockages and distortions become easier to spot, examine, and clear.

We were not, however, able to get far with this learning process during the H.I.C. Project for the following reasons:

1. Lack of resources in the central team, particularly during the initial training courses and later at the times when individual teams might have been ready for such help, for example, during the stages of staff preparation and discussion of results. (In the event, only one hospital team, Severalls, requested help, and there the staff were already well ahead in the use of groups.)
2. The alien nature of such use of meetings in the world of the general hospital.
3. Irregularity and inconsistency of inter-team meetings, including irregular attendance.
4. Lack of explicit notice at the beginning that study of personal communication would be an integral part of the H.I.C. Project.

Having experimented in the structure and direction of inter-team meetings, and learned from each series how to restructure the next, there seems no doubt that the third series was the most useful to the hospital teams. The series would probably not have developed the way it did, had it begun during the early days of the Project, given the situation as it was at that time. The 'learning process', in the sense outlined in preceding paragraphs, was not nurtured during the initial training courses. Afterwards, the teams were too preoccupied with research methods and the practicalities of setting up their projects to concern themselves with self-learning about communication. Even towards the end, though some members felt they were learning more about their performance in a group setting, there was little evidence that they were making use of their knowledge in their own hospitals.

All this is written with the benefit of hindsight. It is unlikely that this form of learning could have been incorporated into the Project at the beginning. It can only develop at the speed and to the depth acceptable to those involved. The development is always slow, subject as it is to unconscious resistances, even in groups of young people with unformed attitudes and light responsibilities. With older people holding heavy responsibilities, the product of years of training and working in an institution noted for its authoritarian and bureaucratic rigidities, the pace of learning is likely to be even slower – if, indeed, it can begin at all. The important point is, not that the teams could only travel slowly towards self-learning, but that some individual members had so firmly resisted institutional conditioning that they could allow themselves to use the opportunity to explore and redefine old methods, procedures, and their own attitudes.

The formal presentations held even more limitations for the hospital teams. Self-learning cannot occur except in conditions where people feel safe enough with each other to explore at their own pace. The public scrutiny was too much of a threat for the presenters not to behave defensively. They rarely felt safe, either with each other or with the audience, or confident in the material they presented. The meetings were too irregularly placed and attended for any 'in-group' feeling to develop within the gathering as a whole. But the formal presentations were of much interest to outsiders, and many commented after a meeting that they were surprised and intrigued by what they had heard. The presentations also demanded more participation by supporting-team members than any other venture initiated by the central team.

Administratively, the formal presentations were inefficiently arranged. The central team had to organize each meeting separately and was often left to persuade reluctant and unready teams to present their projects in order to keep the meetings going. Many of those invited had their diaries booked months in advance and could not attend because of insufficient notice.

This preamble leads to the following recommendations:

1. In any future project of this nature, the learning process would need to be *developed and cultivated deliberately* in the initial training courses. On return to their own hospitals, the teams could then continue the process in their own team meetings.

2. Having experienced the learning process themselves, and growing more confident in the method, the teams could then begin to use it in their group discussions with staff, particularly during the preparatory and feedback stages of a project. Supervision of these groups could be undertaken by the central team in the form of reviews and analyses of discussions. This could be done by assigning the central team's discussion assistants to individual hospital teams – it implies, however, the need for more central-team members with skills in handling groups.

3. Inter-team meetings like those in the third series could then begin much earlier and develop into continuation training sessions for the teams as well as working discussions to review each others' projects. One or two outsiders with special knowledge and interest in this field could be invited when the teams felt ready to meet them.

4. Formal presentations could be a way of rounding off the project, as a series of weekly or fortnightly conferences during the last few months. The whole programme could be worked out with the hospital teams, giving them time to prepare a more cohesive story for the wider hospital and research public, and the central team time to arrange briefing sessions with the chairmen and to circulate notices some months beforehand and so enable outsiders to book dates well in advance.

NOTES

[1] See Chapter 1, Introduction.

[2] Edgware, Hillingdon, The London, North Middlesex, St Nicholas, Severalls, West Middlesex.

[3] At that time, Mrs Shirley Williams.

[4] Lewisham, Mayday, Queen Mary's.

[5] It must be noted that except for contact between individual central-team members and a hospital team working on a project in a hospital, all exchanges between the central team and the hospitals were conducted by letter or telephone through the administrative members of supporting teams at this time.

[6] See Appendix 7A for Notes on second series.

[7] Reference to study groups run by the Tavistock Institute of Human Relations, London.

[8] Abstracts of two reports were circulated: 'Integrating the Individual and the Organization' by Chris Argyris, and 'An Evaluation of a Program for the Utilization of Survey Findings' by Floyd Mann and Howard Baumgartel. Apart from some disparaging remarks about the Americanization of English, and one team's request for more copies, no one mentioned these papers at any time throughout the Project.

[9] See Chapter 1, Introduction.

[10] See Appendix 7B.

[11] The first two meetings were not assessed, because the convener felt members needed time to settle into the new series before being exposed to further self-examination.

[12] On 17 October, 1967, when representatives of the hospital teams met the advisory committee in Guy's Hospital for a confidential discussion on the future of the Project (see also Chapter 5, p. 94).

[13] From Edgware, Lewisham, Mayday, Severalls, and West Middlesex.

[14] See Appendix 7C, Notes by Revans on Formal Presentations.

[15] See Appendix 7D, Audience Composition and Participation.

[16] See Appendix 7D, Table 7D-iv.

[17] See Appendix 7D, Table 7D-v.

[18] See Appendix 7D, Table 7D-vi.

[19] Third newsletter, May-June 1967, circulated to all Project members.

PART THREE

# *The Hospital Viewpoint - Two Examples*

# *Introduction*

## *HILARY LEIGH*

In the preceding chapters we have discussed, mainly from the viewpoint of the central team, how the Project was conceived and how it subsequently evolved. In this part of the book some of the chief participants from two of the hospitals describe how they experienced the Project and the kind of activities they undertook.

We wanted to include reports from all the hospital teams in this volume but, for a number of reasons,[1] it was eventually decided that the hospital reports justified a separate publication. Thus for a full account of the hospital-team members' own views and the activities they undertook the reader is strongly recommended to consult Chapters 2 to 11 of the companion volume to this book, *Hospitals: Communications, Choice, and Change*, edited by R. W. Revans (in press). In addition some hospital-team members have published accounts of specific activities and subsequent developments elsewhere (Watson, 1966; Zucker and Smith, 1967; Webster, 1967; Perkins and Roker, 1967; Dean *et al.*, 1967; Arie and Fairey, 1969; Coghill, 1969; Stewart, 1969; Fairey *et al.*, 1970).

On the recommendation of the Project's advisory committee the hospitals were encouraged to write up their experiences with minimal guidance from the central team.[2] A brief reminder of the aims and intentions of the Project (see Chapter 1) was sent to all the teams, together with an indication of the desired length of contributions.

Subsequently, when requested, central-team members visited most hospitals to discuss the information that had been circulated. About half the teams said they had found some difficulty in using this information, especially the section describing the kind of learning the members might have experienced through carrying out team projects in their hospitals.

Selecting the contributions that form the next two chapters[3] was not an easy task and many good reasons can be put forward for including contributions from other hospitals. These reports are not intended to be representative; they are two examples that emphasize the practical implications of hospital project work both for hospital functioning and for the senior staff who made up the hospital teams. The authors describe a wide range of specific projects in very different settings and illustrate situations some of which were common to other hospitals. Chapter 8, the Severalls report, is written by a senior nurse and contains additional comments by the physician superintendent. The West Middlesex report, Chapter 9, is written by a consultant physician.

## NOTES

[1] The two main reasons were as follows. (a) It was felt that there were two different potential readerships who might be interested in the Project. For example, applied researchers would want full details of the origins, objectives, methods, outcomes, and evaluation of the Project. Practising managers, on the other hand, would be concerned to hear more about the experiences and conclusions of those participants whose jobs and institutions were centrally involved. (b) The sheer size of book required. If an attempt were made to meet the needs of both audiences in one volume, the cost would be prohibitive.

[2] Initially the editors drew up a list of questions, which it was hoped the hospital authors would use in writing up their experiences. By this method it might have been possible to obtain comparative data on various aspects of the Project from all the hospitals. However, after discussions with the advisory committee it was decided that these questions might inhibit the hospital authors, for example, in writing about topics not included among the questions.

[3] We discussed the possibility of including in this volume a selection of material taken from all the hospital reports. When this suggestion was put to some hospital-team members it became evident that the idea was unlikely to be acceptable. Thus we decided to include two complete reports.

# 8 *Severalls Hospital report*

*D. J. DEAN*

SEVERALLS HOSPITAL
TEAM MEMBERS

| | |
|---|---|
| R. BARTON | Physician superintendent |
| RUTH CLARKE* | Matron |
| J. K. CORBETT† | Director of nursing (replaced Ruth Clarke) |
| D. J. DEAN** | Senior assistant to director of nursing (until 1968) |
| D. J. P. ELLIS† | Psychiatric registrar (replaced J. A. Whitehead) |
| R. FOX* | Consultant psychiatrist |
| ST J. V. HALL | Principal tutor |
| D. J. HOOTON† | Group secretary (replaced C. A. Merrick) |
| L. MANNERS | Deputy director of nursing |
| C. A. MERRICK* | Group secretary |
| E. J. RANDALL† | Deputy matron |
| J. P. WATSON** | Hospital secretary |
| J. A. WHITEHEAD** | Consultant psychiatrist |

This large psychiatric hospital is divided into six clinically autonomous units, each under the control of a consultant psychiatrist. Each unit has approximately five wards accommodating male and female patients. The hospital has a physician superintendent and, until November 1967, had two heads of nursing – a matron and a chief male nurse. Supplies, laundry, occupational therapy, industrial therapy, physiotherapy, pathology, and pharmacy are centralized.

## THE TEAM

By early 1968 only three of the original six team members remained: the nurse member (matron) of the supporting team, and the medical member and nurse member of the operational team had left. One of the remaining three had been promoted. Other members of the hospital staff joined the team at various stages. At one point the team consisted of ten members, the

* Attended appreciation course, 1965.
** Attended one-month course, 1965.
† Attended two-day course, 1967.

majority of whom were nurses. The team was assisted by two social psychology students for approximately six months each, one from Brunel University and the other from Loughborough University.

At first the team was uncertain about the aims of the H.I.C. Project. Professor Revans had given a talk at the hospital's annual study symposium early in 1964. At least two members of the original six were present and were very interested in the talk, which outlined the effects of poor communication in hospitals. Without doubt this had some influence on our decision to participate.

The administrator at that time (1964) left the hospital and his successor was not involved in the original decision to join the Project. Both medical members had some knowledge of research methods and could envisage something of what the future had in store. The nurse members had little idea. The physician superintendent was unable to become one of the supporting-team members because of his numerous other commitments but he gave continuous support and advice throughout, attending a number of early meetings and later introducing the hospital newsletter through which our results were publicised.

On return from the training course at Hastings, the team met the hospital management committee to explain something of what they had learned and to discuss future plans.

Of the three projects undertaken, one involved nurses, another patients, and a third members of the hospital management committee and senior hospital officers.

## PROJECTS UNDERTAKEN

### NURSES' ATTITUDE SURVEY

While still at the training course, team members had discussed possible areas for investigation and had agreed that the nursing staff might be a suitable group because of its great influence on the effectiveness of the hospital. During the course, another hospital team carried out an exercise survey at the hospital which, though not scientifically foolproof, pointed to areas worthy of further investigation. We, as a team, also had preconceived ideas of existing nursing problems.

The team members realized that it was not their own problems alone that needed investigating and correcting. What seemed more important were the problems that the nurses met during the course of their duties. These problems affected the standard of care that the patients were receiving. It would be of little value investigating problems that the nurses themselves were unaware of, so a series of group discussions were organized. Two central-team members each took two groups of nurses selected at random from the hospital. Each group was composed of different grades of staff – sisters and charge nurses, staff nurses and state enrolled nurses, student nurses, and nursing assistants. The groups held two meetings at which they discussed problems encountered in their work in the hospital and in their off-duty time. Then they each selected a spokesman who reported back to the H.I.C. team. The two central-team members commented on the openness of the discussions, and it was suggested that the nurses at Severalls were more familiar with group situations, and therefore less inhibited than the central team had expected.

From the groups' reports six areas were selected for further investigations:

> communication, the unit system, nurses' roles and responsibilities, patients' activities and dependence, training, and staff deployment.

We decided to use a structured questionnaire. A questionnaire of this sort is easier to administer to large groups of people, and we wanted to include all nurses in our sample. We felt that if we did the survey this way, and included everyone, then the feedback of results would have greater meaning, and be more effective. We also thought that a structured questionnaire would be simpler to analyse than a series of interviews.

During the next seven months, the team concentrated on constructing the questionnaire, for they realized this would have to be carefully done. A misleading set of results from a suspect questionnaire could render the hospital a great disservice.

Initially about fifty pairs of statements were drawn up. The statements in each pair were designed to elicit strongly contrasting responses. Two pilot surveys were carried out in two similar hospitals, and in both hospitals about eighty nurses completed the provisional questionnaire and a further twenty were interviewed.

The data were analysed to see which pairs of statements had elicited opposing responses, and the interview material was used to assess whether or not the statements were understood in the way they were intended. A revised questionnaire was produced based on the results of the first pilot run, and the second pilot carried out in a similar way. Then, statements that had failed to elicit contrasting responses from 70 per cent of the population, and any that were still ambiguous, were discarded. The ten pairs of statements that appeared to be the most reliable were included in the final version of the questionnaire as a lie-scale. Only one statement from each of the remaining pairs was selected for inclusion in the final document. This consisted of 79 statements, 55 of which required a response ranging from 'strongly agree' to 'strongly disagree'. The remaining 24 were questions of varying types. (See Appendix 8A.)

During the later stages of construction the team members realized that the analysis would be extremely time-consuming. All of us were still performing our usual jobs and had very little spare time, so we decided to approach the computer department at Essex University for help. The manager agreed that if the team coded the questionnaires his department would transfer the data to punch cards and the information we required would be provided by the computer. After discussions with him about the final design of the document, the survey was carried out in early November, 1966.

While the questionnaire was being constructed, the impending survey was publicized at intervals in the hospital newsletter and again a week before it took place.

Six centres, one in each unit, were set up and supervised by central-team members who were unknown to the nursing staff. The nursing head of each unit was responsible for asking his staff to attend the centre and fill in the questionnaire. After two days most of the nurses had complied. After two weeks, a further opportunity was arranged for anyone who had been absent. In the end, 369 (94·4 per cent) participated. Of the remainder, six refused and the rest were absent throughout the period. Fifteen questionnaires were found to be unusable. The team undertook the coding and forwarded the material to the computer department.

At this time a small crisis occurred. During a meeting a staff member was asked by another member to account for one of the 'results' of the survey. This was before coding had been completed. We felt there must have been some misinterpretation of a conversation one of the coders had had with the medical staff. Whatever the cause, we feared the incident could give rise to some resentment against the project. We decided immediately to write a letter thanking people for their co-operation and stressing that no conclusions would be drawn until the results were received from Essex University. Every nurse and doctor received an individual copy. As far as we know, there were no further incidents of this sort.

Inevitably there was a time lag between the survey and the results. Occasionally, accounts of progress were published in the newsletter in order to maintain interest. We decided not to compile a complete report because this would take more time and risk further loss of interest.

In February 1967, some results became available. Before releasing any of them the ten pairs of statements were examined in the ten per cent sample of the questionnaire, in order to confirm that the results obtained from the respondents at Severalls were reliable. In fact, approximately 75 per cent of the sample of paired statements gained opposite responses, which seemed to us to be a reassuring test of the accuracy of the lie-scale. During March, a gradual release of results through the hospital newsletter was begun. We hoped these would stimulate discussion at the various regular staff meetings. The team's intention was not to introduce changes but to help the staff recognize the need for change themselves and to introduce whatever measures they felt necessary. This method, we felt, was more likely to prove effective and enduring. In addition to visible changes that might come about, there were a number of statements indicating nurses' attitudes to various aspects of their work. It was hoped that involvement in discussion would lead to changes or modifications in attitude in some instances (see Evaluation below). However, the hope that publication of results would be enough to stimulate discussion was not realized. Additional steps were necessary.

Each clinical unit has a nursing head, either an assistant matron or an assistant chief male nurse. These senior nurses have a great influence on the running of their units and the greater involvement of these senior nurses in the project seemed to be one way of increasing interest at ward level. In consequence, they were invited to a weekly meeting, run by the administrative member of the operational team and attended by other team members and the student who worked with us, where they were provided with a more detailed breakdown of results. These results and their implications were discussed in detail and the senior nurses were encouraged to report back and continue discussion in their units. In some instances, this happened.

Many results showed that the lower grades of nurses reflected the opinions of their ward sisters and charge nurses. The teams would have liked detailed discussions with all grades but this was impracticable. However, we attempted to involve the nurses responsible for running the wards. All the sisters and charge nurses were invited to join one of eight groups, each led by a member of the team. The groups met every week for a period of twelve weeks, the team members reporting back to each other at a meeting held after the group discussions. All the groups began by discussing communications at ward level, but later pursued problems of particular interest to the individual group. After four months, three groups disbanded and the remaining five elected to continue. Many topics were taken up and again the group leaders tried to encourage the group members to tackle their own problems.

During December 1967, the team felt that it might be helpful to meet the unit nursing officers at one of their weekly meetings in order to discuss progress and future developments. Although this intention was publicized, less than half the nursing officers attended. The meeting was encouraging in that each nursing officer described action he or she had taken following publication of the results. The meeting appeared to be in agreement with continuing the project in the coming year. It was also decided to hold a similar meeting the following week and to send written invitations to those not present.

Almost every nursing officer attended this second meeting. There was, however, noticeably much less enthusiasm about the project and its future. After discussion had gone on for about an hour, one of the H.I.C. team members suggested a vote to be taken on whether or not to continue the project. By a show of hands it was evident that most of the nursing officers did not wish it to continue.

At the same time it was also decided to discontinue the feedback of results. Some team members were very disappointed by this decision. Their hopes that activities might be resumed early in 1968 were not realized.

## PATIENTS' ATTITUDE SURVEY

Soon after the team began the nursing survey the medical member was given three months' relief from normal duties by the appointment of a locum psychiatrist. To take full advantage of this opportunity the team decided to find out what patients felt about their stay in hospital.

To avoid projecting only our own ideas, twenty free interviews were carried out with patients on the day of discharge from hospital. From these interviews we drew up a semi-structured interview schedule covering the following areas:

| | |
|---|---|
| food | integration of patients and staff |
| accommodation | personal property |
| entertainment | occupational / industrial therapy |
| boredom | cleanliness |
| washing facilities | nurses' uniforms and badges |
| lavatories | transfer to other wards |
| privacy | reception into hospital |
| doctors | progress in hospital |
| nurses | opportunity to see doctor |
| other staff | distribution of medicines |
| freedom | expectations of hospital |
| information | ward administration |
| regimentation | care on discharge |
| relatives' problems | |

All wards were asked to notify the team when any of their patients were to be discharged. One of the team members then made arrangements to interview the patient at a suitable time and place. Depending on the responsiveness of the patient, interviews varied in length from half an hour to two hours. We aimed to interview every patient discharged up to a total of one hundred. In fact about six patients were not interviewed, either because they were anxious to leave or because there was no interviewer available. Using a set introduction, the team members and the student psychologist from Brunel University carried out about twenty-five interviews each, with patients from fourteen wards, two-thirds of them from the male and female admission wards. There were twice as many women as men discharged during the period covered.

During the course of the survey the team felt that a number of patients were trying to please the interviewers by giving favourable answers, and for this reason, a few test questions were introduced. From the replies to these questions it was felt that some respondents were overpraising the hospital and that the total responses were perhaps too reassuring.

At the end of an interview the patient was asked if he or she would mind being interviewed again at a later date. We felt we might get different responses four weeks after discharge. Twenty follow-up interviews were carried out, but we found little difference in response. In the analysis, comments were classified as 'favourable' or 'unfavourable' and expressed as a percentage of the total responses.

The results and some suggestions for dealing with some of the problems revealed, together with a brief description of method, were incorporated in a report, which was circulated to the HMC, all medical staff, senior nursing staff, and heads of departments, with a note from the physician superintendent advising people to read it.

### HOSPITAL MANAGEMENT COMMITTEE AND SENIOR OFFICERS' SURVEY

While planning the nurses' survey and talking about it at meetings, we found that some staff were sceptical about the value of such a survey to the nurses and the hospital. In particular, there were doubts about how far the hospital management committee and senior officers understood the background to it and how far they would be willing to implement any recommendations, especially if they went against a previously agreed policy.

We felt it would be a good idea to get a consensus of opinion from members of the hospital management committee and from group and administrative officers who were particularly connected with the hospital, not so much on the results of the survey (which, incidentally, were not then available) but on what they considered their role to be. The chairman of the hospital's executive subcommittee was approached by a central-team member and agreed to ask for volunteers. Five committee members and six senior officers agreed to be interviewed.

A short standard interview schedule was devised with eleven general, open-ended questions that gave a chance for the respondent to expand his or her answer. A central-team member did the interviewing and wrote a summary of the collective views. Each respondent also received a full report of his or her own interview. However at that time the group was undergoing a change of chairman and secretary. The new group secretary became a member of the hospital H.I.C. team, and the new chairman had taken part in the survey. One report back meeting was held to discuss the summary of collective views and the respondents felt it might be useful to continue discussion after the newly appointed members had settled in their posts. However, for various practical reasons, it was not possible to hold further discussions.

## EVALUATION

No experiment is complete without an attempt to evaluate the outcome. Although the feedback of the results of the nurses' survey was not formally completed it is possible to comment on how the Project affected the hospital, though it was not possible to make a scientific evaluation. Two questions are worth consideration.

(a) What effect has the Project had on the individuals closely involved?
(b) What effect has the Project had on the hospital as a whole?

During 1966 and 1967 the team increased in size, so that ten people became actively involved. It must be remembered that the team members were key figures in the hospital. What value can one place on their experience over the Project period? Working on the Project demanded a great deal of co-operation. We had numerous open and friendly discussions, at least two each week, in which a greater understanding of each other's work led to a more co-operative approach, not only to the exercise in hand, but to many problems outside it. There were instances where meetings had been arranged to discuss hospital problems that two or three years earlier might have been dealt with by a directive in the form of a letter or circular. In early 1968 at a meeting of five team members, it was acknowledged by everyone that our attitudes to dealing with problems had changed. In addition to understanding each other more, we felt we had a better understanding of the problems of other people in the hospital with whom we had had little contact previously.

The effect on the hospital is more difficult to assess, even in such general terms. Much of our effort was directed towards changing the attitudes of some people to different aspects of their work. The amount of success in this area is difficult to estimate. The important question of whether any change will last cannot be assessed until time has passed. It may be possible at some future date to run the nurses' survey again with a sample of the population. An analysis would then indicate more accurately what change, for better or worse, has occurred.

Feedback on the nurses' survey, which was carried out through a series of group discussions, brought together groups of people who had rarely met each other previously, for example, sisters and charge nurses, assistant matrons and assistant chief male nurses. At first some of these gatherings were tense. People were reluctant to discuss sensitive problems. Gradually discussion became more open as the members of the group got to know each other better. In consequence, there was a noticeable improvement in staff relationships, especially at a senior level.

Some problems diminished as more people became aware of the facts. Some discussions led to practical improvements when those involved took it upon themselves to take action which they felt appropriate. The action varied. Further discussions leading to practical measures and better co-operation with other staff were typical. Of importance is the fact that this was action initiated by the people who were involved in the problem and not action imposed by others; an indication that they learnt from their discussion experience. As such, the changes were more likely to be lasting.

We must, however, also refer to some of our shortcomings. During the discussions with the sisters and charge nurses, the lack of involvement of the medical staff became evident. Though we had two doctors in the team, interest in the project did not appear to have spread to their colleagues. For obvious reasons this has been a disadvantage. Nurses look to the medical staff for leadership, especially at meetings. We believe that if we could have involved the medical staff more, the discussions would have been more productive.

The curtailment of feedback from the nurses' survey was a disappointment. Undoubtedly, the value of the project was reduced by the fact that we had not published many of the findings and an enormous amount of material was not utilized at all, or even discussed.

## OTHER CONSIDERATIONS

### TIME AND COMMITMENT

Throughout the H.I.C. Project period each team member had normal duties to carry out. Many members felt they had little time to spare for Project work. Admittedly, a careful assessment of problems is advisable if correct solutions are to be found and should be a normal part of every administrator's work. Nevertheless, to introduce other staff members to the ideas behind H.I.C. meant an increase in the work load of the team members initially involved. In some cases, other aspects of the work of some team members had to be neglected in order to further the aims of the Project. Had there not been one or two team members who were convinced of the value of this kind of work, little would have been achieved. Without doubt the commitment of the team members had a major influence on the subsequent success in carrying out projects and introducing changes. The initial choice of team members in such a Project is of paramount importance.

### STUDENTS

The two university students, each of whom spent approximately six months at the hospital, profited from their experience and they in turn contributed a great deal to our efforts. As far as possible they were involved in all team decisions, attended all meetings, and participated in the practical aspects of the projects. Without them our efforts would have progressed more slowly. They assisted greatly in such tasks as analysis of questionnaires and interviews, and tabulation and presentation of results. This relieved the team members of tasks that they would have found difficult to undertake.

### MEETINGS

Some hospitals had to create channels of communication in order to further the aims of their projects. Our hospital, like many psychiatric hospitals, has for a long time been aware of the value of good communication channels, and a comprehensive system of meetings has developed over the years.

Medical and senior nursing staff have regular gatherings; each unit has regular meetings of all staff, and many wards have weekly meetings also. These meetings provided a medium for discussion of survey results and, with the staff already accustomed to discussion, made it easier to set up new groups. In addition, the hospital publishes a weekly newsletter through which the entire population, including patients, could be kept informed of developments and findings.

### SIZE OF PROJECTS

All three projects were extensive. Did we bite off more than we could chew? Would it have been wiser to complete one project before commencing another? The construction of each survey occupied a great deal of time and, because of inexperience, we failed to realize that the feedback process would demand even more time. In addition, the medical member of the team felt that his three months' relief from everyday duties should be fully used and it was during this period that most of the patients' survey was completed. The time would have been more useful if it had been one or two days of each week spread over a longer period. Though the patients' survey provided extremely useful information, we would not have embarked on it at the time if the medical member had not been released from normal duties for three months. More use could have been made of the results if the team had been able to take an active part in the feedback at ward level.

### REPORTING

It is customary to write a report on findings for presentation to those involved. Three months elapsed before the analysis of the nurses' survey was ready. To compile a report on the amount of material we had would have taken many weeks and it would probably have been too big and complicated to be absorbed by most of the people affected, even if they had read it. We believe our decision to release a little information at intervals was correct. Not only was the information used, but feedback began while participants were still interested in the findings.

### QUESTIONNAIRES OR INTERVIEWS?

At an early stage, we decided to use a questionnaire, reasoning that analysis of questionnaires would be simpler than the analysis of the same number of interviews. However, at the time it was not fully realized how much work would be involved in constructing the questionnaire. It has been said that the reliability of the methods used in gathering information for further action is not of great importance. Our nurses' survey feedback involved a group of senior nursing staff extremely knowledgeable about their work, including some who were not anxious to be involved in change. At the beginning, many attempts were made to discredit findings on the basis of faulty technique. The careful preparation of the research tool made it possible to answer these attempts to delay progress. If logical, reliable explanations had not been forthcoming, we believe that many people essential to the furthering of the aims of the project would have lost interest at a very early stage.

We also feel that the involvement of almost every nurse in completing the questionnaire increased the interest in the project as a whole. It would not have been possible to interview every nurse on such a variety of topics.

### ATTITUDES

Our results indicated that the attitudes and opinions of the nurses in the ward and those of the nurses in charge of wards are closely connected. Without doubt, the attitudes of the nursing administration, in turn, have some effect on those of ward sisters and charge nurses. We attempted not only to alter procedures and attitudes at ward level, but also to involve the senior nurses more closely, hoping for some modification or change in the upper levels of the nursing hierarchy. These nurses were involved in at least thirty meetings, lasting an hour or more, to discuss different aspects of their work. These meetings became increasingly uninhibited and healthy. At two meetings held with H.I.C. team members to disuss the whole Project with especial reference to the senior nurses' involvement, many nurses spontaneously said that the meetings had helped them to reflect on their own ideas and attitudes. Some gave examples of how they had attempted to overcome problems in their particular areas, indicating that some changes had occurred. How far attitudes changed throughout the hospital could be assessed by repeating the survey at some future date.

### COMPUTER FACILITIES

Our task would have been more difficult and less worthwhile had we not had the assistance of the local university's computer department. The different combinations of results that it was possible to obtain from the nurses' survey would never have been forthcoming if the team had had the task of tabulation. Although a few hospitals have computers for their own use it would be encouraging if there was an established computer centre for the use of all health service workers.

### CENTRAL TEAM

Probably every team perceived the role of the central team differently and consequently used the available resources in different ways. Our relationship with the central team centred on:

(a) technical assistance with particular problems;
(b) organized events directed towards hospital-team members in order to impart knowledge and further the aims of H.I.C.

(a) During the month's training course we were completely dependent on the central team. As time passed, our team became progressively more autonomous.

In the early stages, we needed expert help and guidance, especially when we were constructing the questionnaire. However, even at that stage, we participated fully and learnt a great deal from our experience. Those of us in the team at that time would have little difficulty in constructing a similar questionnaire in the future if the need arose. At no time did we expect the central team to advance any stage of our projects without our participating. Without doubt, this has been an important contribution to what we have learnt and to our own feelings of involvement. In addition, it ensured that we were able to answer the many probing inquiries we received throughout the feedback stage. The interdependent nature of the relationship between hospital-team member and expert has been mutually valuable. The expert from outside needed the knowledge of the hospital the team possessed. In turn, the team needed the knowledge of social science methods the experts possessed. Whatever the final valuation of the Project as a whole, there is little doubt among our team that this has been a useful combination, which could be employed in a variety of situations.

It was reassuring at times to find that the central-team members were not always able to answer our enquiries and that they too had been learning along with us.

(b) Perhaps the best measure of our opinions of organized events was the extent to which we attended them. The distance from London made our presence at such events difficult, especially at evening gatherings, such as those at the London School of Hygiene, from which we felt team members gained little. Certainly we heard details of other projects, but the inquiries from the floor that followed added little to the knowledge that could be usefully employed by ourselves. Much of the discussion was too technical and irrelevant.

In contrast, the feedback meetings held at the Hospital Centre were always worthwhile. The informality and familiarity among the 'amateurs' facilitated fairly uninhibited discussions from which a great deal of useful information could be gleaned. Perhaps this accounts for the fact that there were rarely less than three members of our team present on these occasions.

One other aspect of the central team's role has been of great importance to all teams. This was the pressure exerted on hospital teams to report back on their activities and progress. Without this added stimulus many of us would have done very little, especially in the early stages. We still remember that after the training course at Hastings we were expected, within a couple of months, to state our intentions for the future. How many teams would have had *any* future had we been allowed to proceed at our leisure?

## PERMANENT DEVELOPMENTS

Developments consequent to our surveys are difficult to enumerate. It is hoped that there have been adjustments both to the organization and to attitudes, together with improvements in interpersonal relationships. None of these can be measured effectively but they are as important as developments mentioned below, if not more so. Indeed, if success has been achieved in the areas mentioned, more permanent developments should appear as time passes. A number of recommendations from the patients' survey have been considered in detail in some wards and units and have resulted in changes. Many nursing officers have discussed different aspects of the surveys with their staff and this has resulted in a reappraisal of the roles and responsibilities of nurses in some situations. It is impossible in this short account to give details. Two important developments which have occurred are:

(a) A post-graduate course has commenced following requests from the registered mental nurses for further education. All qualified nurses are entitled to apply for the course, which consists of one study day per week over a period of a year.
(b) There appeared to be a lack of understanding among nurses of the role of the social workers in the hospital. Following discussion between senior nurses and social workers every student nurse now spends three days during her initial training with one of the social workers.

## CONCLUSIONS

For nearly three years our hospital team attempted to improve the effectiveness of the hospital by using techniques not usually employed in hospitals. It is our belief that the hospital derived benefit from the experiment. Without doubt, the team members learnt a great deal from their experiences, acquiring knowledge not only of techniques, but of the detailed organization and working of the hospital.

We had difficulties and we made mistakes. Not all of those associated with the Project felt able to contribute or to become involved to any great extent. Much of the work load fell on one or two members together with a university student. In order that the efforts of people involved in such a project can be successful, it is essential that they not only feel themselves to be a team, but are seen as a team by the hospital as a whole. For this reason the initial stages of preparation are of crucial importance.

If this form of management is to succeed, the hospital managers must be fully conversant with the ideas behind H.I.C. and be involved fully in any projects which are undertaken.

## ADDITIONAL COMMENTS FROM RUSSELL BARTON, THE PHYSICIAN SUPERINTENDENT

Just as it is the keener and better-informed staff, who realize how much they do not know, who attend professional meetings, so it is the more efficient and flexible institutions that accept investigations such as the Hospital Internal Communications Project.

The pattern of administration and communication at Severalls Hospital was radically altered in 1961 when the hospital was divided up into firms or units. No prescribed pattern was laid down, each unit being free to formulate its own policy. This is a continuing process and thus no set pattern of administration exists for examination.

The communication projects at the hospital became self-limiting because of frictions and obstructions arising at peer level. From time to time interesting examples of manipulation of situations occurred.

The conclusions drawn were not always patently derived from the facts obtained, and before using these results for planning, one must appreciate that there were no controls and there was some confusion (in spite of repeated explanations) about how far these questionnaires were a democratic exercise designed to make decisions in the hospitals, and how far they were for purposes of research to evaluate what was happening in the hospital.

Communication occurs in two principal forms:

*Propositional* in which facts and propositions are transmitted and
*Emotional* (attitudinal) in which feelings and attitudes are transmitted.

In my view it is the use of communications for emotional purposes that requires the spotlight of scientific investigation. The phenomena of propaganda, rumour, enlistment, usurpation, loyalties, and obstructions and so forth, are the mainsprings of a hospital's enthusiasms and discontents.

Because these questions of morale do not lend themselves easily to dispassionate investigation, analysis, and quantification there has been a tendency to deal with the tangible and concrete, often with diligent futility because the fundamental problems are so difficult to comprehend – 'what you cannot count does not count'.

I hope the Hospital Internal Communications Project will highlight for readers the importance of *people time* – the way people's opinions are listened to and lead with or ignored; the way their feelings are ruffled or respected; thus producing the enthusiastic and willing worker or resulting in the sour dead-beat.

*Object time*, on the other hand, is time that is spent dealing with things, and although accountants, carpentersc, and committees can deal with material things easily, they concern a separate dimension of hospital function and, when the chips are down, the least important one.

If the simple platitude that minds matter and people count is again emphasized and if a more reasonable approach to the happiness and well-being of staff and patients is observed, then this study will be most worthwhile and my own support for it well rewarded.

# 9 *West Middlesex Hospital report*

*N. F. COGHILL*

WEST MIDDLESEX HOSPITAL PARTICIPANTS

| | |
|---|---|
| D. E. BOLT* | Consultant surgeon |
| MARGARET BUNYAN† | Assistant matron (replaced Lucy Pulsford) |
| J. H. CARTER†** | Deputy hospital secretary |
| N. F. COGHILL | Consultant physician and physician for sick staff |
| SANDRA DREIER | Departmental sister, acting personnel officer |
| C. H. DUNN | Senior consultant anaesthetist |
| A. M. EVANS* | Hospital secretary |
| F. P. HALDANE | Consultant psychiatrist |
| JOANNE LAIDMAN | Matron (replaced Dorothy Warren) |
| DOROTHY MURDOCK | Theatre superintendent |
| D. J. PARRY** | Senior registrar |
| LUCY PULSFORD | Assistant matron |
| C. A. STEEL | Group domestic manager |
| E. M. STEFFANS | Hospital secretary (replaced A. M. Evans) |
| J. S. STEWART† | Consultant physician (replaced D. J. Parry) |
| AUDREY THOMAS | Deputy matron |
| MONICA VEALE | Acting matron |
| DOROTHY WARREN | Acting matron (replaced Monica Veale) |
| ELIZABETH ZUCKER | Head medical social worker |

Ours is a large district general hospital of 934 beds. It grew out of the Poor Law system, and from 1935 to 1948 was one of the county hospitals. The hospital caters for a population of about 400,000 and provides a comprehensive range of services to the community. There are large out-patient, accident, and emergency departments. There are sixty consultants on the staff, all those in the major specialties being whole-time or nearly whole-time. During the time of our studies, a new 240-bed medical department was opened.

We came into the H.I.C. Project rather late, in July 1965, because of two

* Attended appreciation course, 1965.
** Attended one-month course, 1965.
† Attended two-day course, 1967.

simultaneous contacts, one through a chance meeting of the hospital secretary with the central-team director at the Hospital Centre, and one through Professor R. W. Revans with whom one of the physicians was already in correspondence. We were asked to join when another hospital withdrew. The medical committee and hospital management committee readily agreed.

## PROJECTS UNDERTAKEN

1. Pilot survey of a paediatric and a medical ward prior to moving to a new building.
2. Opinion survey or domestic services.
3. Project 'paper chase'.
4. Inquiry into the use of operating theatres.
5. Study of medical social work.
6. Student-nurse wastage and nurse counselling.
7. Observations on a medical unit.
8. Study of patients' anxieties in relation to clinical ward rounds.
9. Messenger services.
10. Survey of consultants' attitudes.
11. General improvements in communications.

### 1. PILOT STUDY OF A PAEDIATRIC AND A MEDICAL WARD PRIOR TO MOVING TO A NEW BUILDING, JANUARY–MARCH 1966

These two wards were to be transferred to a new medical block. It was thought that it would be valuable as our first project to obtain knowledge of detailed activities performed in the existing wards, because this would be helpful in planning operational procedures in the new block, as well as highlighting present deficiencies. A total of sixty-four free interviews were carried out by the hospital team with ward staff of all categories on these two wards to determine their attitudes to ward problems. The team at first experienced difficulty in explaining the purpose of the project, but staff were soon forthcoming and co-operative and welcomed the opportunity of expressing their views. They were invited to comment on their work in the ward, the difficulties encountered, their understanding of their roles, and feelings and relationships towards the ward team and others in the hospital. Because of the exigencies of other work the interviews were spread over eight weeks; on reflection we think they should have been concentrated within one week.

This pilot study illuminated the pressures on staff, the complexity of patient care at ward level, and the misunderstandings of roles and relationships between people working in the wards. It was decided that the hospital team, with the aid of students and members of the central team, should concentrate on the three problems which seemed most pressing; the domestic services, the X-ray services (not investigated), and the number of paper forms in use.

2. DOMESTIC SERVICES

The comments of the ward staff during the pilot study about domestic services revealed a problem of a complexity that had not been fully appreciated, although management had realized that the standard of work was low, and unit costs, in relation to other hospitals, high.

With a view to improving

(a) the standard of work done by domestic staff,
(b) the facilities available to the domestic staff,
(c) inter-staff relationships,

the attitudes of the following groups of staff towards the domestic services were surveyed, using semi-structured questionnaires at interview:

fifteen ward sisters and one charge nurse,
fifteen staff nurses and forty student nurses,
fourteen non-nursing heads of departments, three home sisters,
five maternity sisters, and three theatre sisters.

All the staff needed reassurance that the questionnaire was confidential and that their names would not be divulged. The student nurses were apprehensive about the domestics knowing their views.

The following information was obtained from these interviews:

1. On the whole, the domestics were not considered part of the ward team.

2. Nursing staff tended to ignore the domestics, even the permanent ones, on their wards, and there was no personal concern for their feelings as fellow-workers.

3. There was a general feeling that too many coloured domestics were employed; this had created the impression that all coloured domestics were poor workers and a certain amount of colour prejudice seemed to have developed.

4. In the wards where the sister did not clarify her managerial responsibility, the domestics became antagonistic.

5. There seemed to be some reluctance on the part of some of the more senior nursing staff to direct and supervise. In many cases this seemed to be due to lack of interest, in other cases to unwillingness, and, in a few, to fear. Some did not consider that such supervision was one of their duties.

6. There was little communication between the sisters, superintendents, and management.

7. The post of domestic superintendent did not appear to have much status.

The superintendents (assistants to the domestic manager) seemed to have a feeling of inferiority, perhaps due to inexperience, both about the nature of their work and in dealing with people. They were rather young, and probably found it difficult to deal with older women. 'Lack of supervision' of the domestics was a constant criticism. Since the superintendents were inexperienced, the domestic was sometimes left to make her own work routine on the ward. (It must be said here that because the hospital spreads over a considerable area, the work of the superintendents was made much more difficult. For some time they had been understaffed in forewomen, who would normally support them in their work of supervision.)

8. No one knew who was responsible for what, and how much authority any one person had. The superintendents were sometimes afraid of the sisters, and some sisters ignored the superintendents. The student nurses were sometimes afraid of the domestics and there was noticeable antagonism between them.

9. Very few of the nursing staff knew the difference between the various status levels of domestic management, nor did many of them know who was ultimately responsible for the domestic staff. One of the superintendents' complaints was that they were frequently wrongly called 'supervisors', a rank that does not exist in the hospital.

10. The perception of the causes of the domestics' discontent was sharpest among the student nurses and the non-nursing heads of departments. This did not prevent the student nurses from being among the domestics' severest critics, probably because student nurses working under pressure became very frustrated when domestics refused to help in tense situations in the ward.

From this information we felt the following points should be considered:

(i) All sisters and staff nurses should attend a course in management to prepare them better for responsibility (many of the sisters have now attended courses).
(ii) Superintendents should be more carefully selected and prepared for the job. Longer courses, in both practical and management skills, seemed advisable.
(iii) Job satisfaction among domestics would be helped by possibilities of promotion as a reward for good work. Domestics should be able to reach supervision grade after a course in management.
(iv) Better working conditions, changing rooms, and uniforms would give a sense of pride in what appears to be a 'dead-end' job.
(v) There should be better selection of domestic staff.
(vi) A good induction course would help as a form of initial training.

We also decided to ask the central team to interview the domestic staff. They interviewed thirteen ward orderlies and twenty-six domestic assistants, a twenty per cent sample of the total domestic staff.

Beforehand, the domestic manager gave the selected respondents an introductory talk and a letter from the interviewer for the purpose of reassuring them that the interview in no way represented a threat to their continued employment, that it was not a test of aptitude or ability, and that all responses would be presented anonymously in any report. Since they believed in the domestic manager's integrity, there was no difficulty in interviewing them.

They gave us the following information:

1. The main source of recruitment was by word of mouth from relatives or friends.

2. Domestic workers decided to apply for hospital work because they felt they were providing a service.

3. The main reasons for job dissatisfaction were lack of a cloakroom, poor facilities for meals, and lack of joint consultation. Most said that the place to hang personal belongings, wash, and change after work was dirty or inadequate or non-existent.

4. Many seemed uncertain as to why or how long they wanted to continue working at the hospital.

5. Half wanted to wear a proficiency badge, and half did not.

6. Many domestics seemed to think that the nursing staff were in charge of them and only a few thought it should be the domestic manager.

7. The superintendents and the sisters did not always agree on the work to be done and if there was a difference the domestics followed the sisters' orders. The sisters caused them the most difficulty in their work, with the superintendents next.

8. Most of them said they had received no training when they came and that a more experienced worker had shown them what to do. Usually they were not shown round the ward or department in which they were to work and they were introduced only to other domestic workers.

9. Most of them disliked their uniforms intensely.

10. The most contact they had in the hospital was with other members of the domestic staff.

11. The domestic manager was seen as a person to whom they could take problems and difficulties, and most of them said they would do so.

Much of this information confirmed the points for consideration drawn from the nurses' interviews. We felt that:

(i) In order to improve the type of applicant coming forward for vacancies more money must be spent on appropriate advertising.

(ii) Facilities for domestic staff must be improved.

(iii) Domestic staff should understand clearly to whom they were responsible.

(iv) Domestic staff must have a proper training.

(v) Job satisfaction should be improved by better conditions, and better uniforms, and above all by helping them to play a role in the ward team, with other members of the team showing appreciation for their work.

Early in October 1967, a new staff member, a trained personnel officer, joined the nursing administration. She worked with the domestic manager, assistant matrons, and domestic superintendents in devising a plan to solve some of the problems in the domestic situation. In one half of the hospital, the sisters filled in a blank job description of the domestics' and orderlies' work with the times when various jobs were to be done. A meeting of all the sisters was held to explain how the plan was intended to improve communication at all levels. It was decided:

(a) To discuss job descriptions made out according to the sisters' needs, so that relief workers would not find it so difficult to adapt to work on different wards.

(b) To ask the sisters to contact the assistant matron about difficulties with domestic staff so that the senior nursing staff had a clear picture of the problems at ward level. (This plan is still being carried out and has so far improved communications to a limited extent. We hope to put it into operation in the other half of the hospital also.)

(c) To institute more regular communication between sisters, superintendents, and assistant matrons in order to improve understanding of each others' difficulties.

(d) To ask the sisters to release their domestics for meetings with the domestic manager at which problems and new methods could be discussed.

(e) To foster meetings of domestics (which are proving worthwhile and helping to raise morale).

(f) To ask the domestic manager to devise a new training scheme for domestics to be put quickly into operation.

(g) To ask the domestic manager to issue new uniforms to the domestics (which are proving to be popular).

Many of these suggestions are in operation, and co-operation between domestic and nursing staff has improved. Much remains to be done, however.[1]

### 3. PROJECT 'PAPER CHASE'[2]

This was mainly an 'organization and methods' inquiry carried out, at our request, by a student central-team member. The hospital was found to be using 790 different forms of 139 different sizes, costing about £4,000 a year. Approximately three million were used each year. Many were similar, others were redundant or ineffectual. Some departments kept half a year's stock of forms. In addition there was evidence that people's attitudes to available forms to some extent governed their use. The survey showed a weakness in our methods of dealing with form design, control of manufacture, purchase, distribution and storage, and the authorizing and the use of forms. The medical committee has already accepted the need for a general reappraisal of medical record forms.

4. INQUIRY INTO THE USE OF OPERATING THEATRES (see Appendix 9A)

This study was undertaken on the initiative of a consultant surgeon.

One of the major problems facing the hospital was the continuous pressure on beds, and we wanted to study the factors influencing emergency admissions and their effects on the working of the hospital as a whole. As a first stage it was decided to examine emergency surgical admissions. This investigation was deferred until a crisis, arising from a shortage of trained nursing staff in the operating theatres, had been resolved.

For some years the theatres had been under considerable strain and there was a steady wastage of staff, particularly trained nursing staff. By the autumn of 1965, this had reached such a level as to make the continuous full use of the theatres impossible, and action was clearly essential to prevent a complete breakdown. It was realised that the difficulties were due, in part, to a very heavy workload being carried by staff working in theatres unsuited to modern requirements. But it was well known that the least satisfactory theatre, from the standpoint of general facilities, suffered much less from staff wastage than did the other four theatres. It was therefore felt that influences other than physical conditions were contributing to staff wastage. In view of this a committee with representatives of the management committee, the hospital administration, and the surgical, anaesthetic, and nursing staffs, was set up to investigate the matter and seek solutions.

To help in establishing the facts, members of the central team were invited to collect information on how the theatres were used, and to make a study of the working conditions of various groups of theatre staff, and to report on the factors that tended to make the normally heavy strains of the theatre work intolerable for the nurses and technical staff. The whole matter was regarded as one of great urgency because at that time work had had to be reduced by thirty per cent to avert complete closure of the theatres.

During the course of the investigation, many members of the theatre teams were interviewed, individually and in confidence. When the report on the problems was complete, a meeting of all the theatre staff and all theatre users was held to discuss the results. Frank speaking was encouraged and the opinions collected made an important contribution to a general understanding of the steps needed to put the matter right. Some changes that have been made will be mentioned briefly to illustrate the character of the problems that had gone unnoticed for a long time.

*Nursing Staff*

An attempt was made to reduce frequent movement of staff between theatres by building up separate teams for each of the five theatres. Shift working was substituted for broken duties. More adequate facilities for rest and refreshment while on theatre duty were created, and a variety of traditional restrictions that had ceased to serve a useful purpose were eliminated. A better scheme of training for new theatre staff was set up.

*Technicians*

A new work rota was devised and put into operation. The duties of the technicians inside and outside the theatres were redefined to eliminate uncertainties about responsibilities. A clearer line of authority was made for supervising technicians, theatre sisters, and the chief technician. More adequate facilities for training recruits to this service were provided. A common-room specially for theatre technicians was provided.

*Porters*

This group proved to be the most difficult to help without introducing a scheme of working that would prove extravagant in manpower. The problem is still under study but the porters have derived some benefit from the fuller recognition of their problems, and as a consequence, of their status as members of the theatre team. Following this study a charge-hand porter was appointed to facilitate the organization of the portering services for the theatres.

Some problems revealed by the study proved too complex to be dealt with in the context of an emergency programme to avert a major theatre crisis, and it was planned that some of these, such as the widely varying pattern of the workload, should be the subject of further and more detailed study. The limited programme, however, proved its worth in that the crisis was averted for a time. The theatres became nearly fully manned and worked at full capacity. The general efficiency of individual theatres was greatly increased. The working atmosphere also improved enormously.

Unfortunately, in September 1967, it was necessary to curtail again the surgical facilities of the hospital when several of the trained nursing staff of certain theatres left, chiefly for domestic reasons, and no replacements were available. This merely re-emphasized the need for a more detailed and searching study of the theatre situation, and possibly a review of the recommendations that were previously made, to assess whether they were flexible enough to meet the demands of a fluctuating staff structure and workload, which will always be the situation in the operating theatres of any hospital.

## 5. STUDY OF MEDICAL SOCIAL WORK

In March 1966, a seminar was held to discuss Marjorie Moon's report, 'The First Two Years' (Moon, 1966), of an investigation of the experiences of newly trained medical social workers. Medical, nursing, and administrative staff, medical social workers, and a member of the hospital management committee attended. The meeting took place just after the publication of Ministry Circular H.M. (66) 13, on the future development of hospital social work services. The discussion showed that neither the medical social workers nor the medical staff fully understood or appreciated their respective roles and interrelationships. It was clear that there was a need to examine the work of the department.

With the help of the central team, the social work department rationalized its work and organization in the light of its reduced staff. It realized the need to redefine its functions and staff deployment in order to streamline the work both inside and outside the hospital. For example, much work that could be done by clerks was turned over to them entirely. Discussions have been held with local authorities on the possibility of joint appointments and one such appointment has been agreed.

A second seminar was held in October 1966 to discuss the findings with senior hospital staff and representatives from other hospitals.[3]

## 6. STUDENT-NURSE WASTAGE AND NURSE COUNSELLING

In 1966 the acting matron asked the senior medical registrar (member of the H.I.C. team) to interview all student nurses who tendered their resignations. Eight were seen, some several times. Much information was obtained about the wide variety of reasons given for leaving (see Appendix 9B). Seven of these eight girls subsequently left before completing their training, some at the time of interview, and some later.

At the inception of the H.I.C. Project we were undergoing a testing time over certain nursing problems, and like everyone else we were short of nurses. This provided a powerful stimulus to ameliorate the lot of the junior nurses, a first move, we believed, in reducing nurse wastage. We thought we might lessen the number of student nurses leaving before completing their training by encouraging more mature attitudes to, for example, authority, their work, and more personally, their own emotional development. Anxieties caused by our suggestions for nurse counselling were formidable at senior staff (medical and nursing) and at management committee levels, and took many months to overcome.

As a result of a suggestion made by the consultant physician in charge of the care of sick staff members, a small group of consultants and the hospital secretary began to meet in March 1966 to discuss the principle of counselling for student and pupil nurses, and what might be practicable. The acting matron came to some of our meetings and was informed of all our ideas, which were discussed with her. The possibility was raised of discussion groups for the nurses. Unstructured, 'non-directive' groups seemed impracticable for a number of reasons, not least the amount of time they take for the participants; and they do not suit everyone. We thought it would be worth trying a combined system of a few group meetings and individual counselling. Each intake of student nurses would be divided into groups of eight to twelve and a counsellor allotted to each intake. Each group would meet about a month after the start of the introductory course, and again about two months later (i.e. after the nurses had been on the wards for about a month). It was thought that the first meeting of such groups would be introductory but that at subsequent meetings the nurses would do most of the talking.

The counsellors would be available for individual discussion and advice during the full period of the nurses' studentship. Group meetings would enable the counsellor and the group members to get to know each other and matters of interest could be discussed. The counsellor would be available alone for discussion of problems that a nurse might not wish to bring up in a meeting, or that might arise when there was no meeting. It would not be the intention to interfere in any way with existing channels used by student or pupil nurses to communicate with matron or any of her staff including the sister tutors, home sisters, or ward sisters, or with the doctor or sister concerned with the nurses' health; nor with existing arrangements for counselling through the nursing administration or hospital chaplains.

There would be a panel of counsellors drawn from members of the medical staff, senior administrative staff, and medical social workers, and also from outside the hospital if possible. The panel might contain people who were interested but who might not, for various reasons, immediately act as counsellors. The approach would have to be a tentative and empirical one. After the first two meetings of every group all the panellists, whether currently acting as counsellors or not, would meet and discuss what had happened in their groups. The matron, the principal tutor, the hospital secretary, and a member of the central team should be present at all meetings of counsellors. In this way we felt we should all learn a good deal about the problems needing attention, the methods to be employed to bring them to light, and the possible remedies for them.

After the earlier discussions the acting matron agreed to the principle of counselling of nurses in training on condition that the HMC supported her. Therefore the matter was referred to the chairman of the nursing sub-committee. Some members of this committee were strongly in favour, some were as strongly against. The physician to the nurses was invited to explain to the committee in July 1966 what we were aiming at. There was both misinterpretation of our proposals, and fear of their possible results. The matter was referred to the nurses' education committee, due to meet next in October. However, perhaps because of representations over this long delay made to the nursing committee, there was a special joint meeting of the two committees at the end of July. At this meeting it was agreed in principle that there was a need for counsellors for students in the hospitals in the Group, and that the matron and principal tutor of the West Middlesex Hospital, the acting group secretary, the hospital secretary, and the nurses' physician be asked to consider the question of formulating a panel of counsellors for the students at the West Middlesex Hospital as an experiment, and to report upon the manner in which the panel should function.

When, at the beginning of July, the possibility of starting counselling seemed to have been put off till November or December at the earliest, the nurses' physician discussed the matter with the acting matron. For some years he had seen each new nurse individually during her first month at the hospital at the morning surgery. This had served to introduce himself and the health service we offer the nursing staff, to inquire briefly about the home background, and to encourage the nurse to use the facilities freely for any purpose connected with her health. The nurses' physician asked the acting matron if, mainly as an extension of this kind of meeting, and without prejudice to all our other proposals for counselling, she would sanction a meeting of the July intake of student nurses with herself and himself early in August. She agreed but suggested he should be accompanied instead by the senior nurse tutor.

By August 1966, it was possible to make a start on a tentative scheme. The first group of nurses was taken by a consultant physician. The meetings were informal and everyone was usually out of uniform.

In the event little individual counselling was done. One nurse came privately about her troubles to see the physician taking the first group; she was leaving and this was staved off. She said others were equally upset, but although there was talk of them going to see the physician, none did. One nurse left the second group early on, because she was homesick, but she did not see her counsellor. However, the nurses spoke freely in the group meetings of their frustrations, complaints, and difficulties. The topics discussed by the nurses emphasized their preoccupation with the hospital environment; they fell into six main categories:

> lack of social life and activities, defects of communication, personal problems, professional matters, patients, and simple administrative deficiencies.

*Meetings of Counsellors*

Two meetings of counsellors were held, one in October 1966, and another in December 1966. (By October a new, temporary, matron had been appointed.)

The main points reported and agreed on were:

1. Problems of the nursing staff should be considered as a whole—i.e. those of sisters and student nurses together.

2. It was suggested that sisters might receive instruction in teaching tech-

niques to foster a professional teacher-pupil relationship and to facilitate communication and the learning process.

3. The sisters needed to be adequately supported by the ancillary departments in the hospital.

4. Matron had instituted twice-monthly meetings with sisters—a 'business meeting' in which sisters discussed problems in their own work setting, and a 'sisters' forum' in which somebody lectured or showed a film on some topic dealing with hospital life and work.

5. It was agreed that the next intake of student nurses should be taken by someone from outside the hospital, and a list of counsellors was to be drawn up.

In the event, no external counsellor could be found and a consultant psychiatrist took the next intake of student nurses in October 1966.

At the second meeting of counsellors there was general agreement on the following points:

1. These group meetings were taking place possibly too early in the nurses' career.

2. The system adopted was unlikely to result in a nurse bringing personal difficulties to her individual counsellor because the contact between them would be so tenuous, and the fact that the counsellor was a consultant and part of the establishment would inhibit the nurse still further.

3. The supreme requirement for a low nurse wastage was a relaxed, happy atmosphere in the hospital. It was paramount that the nurses should enjoy their training.

4. It was best that arrangements for improving the social life of the hospital should be made from within the department of nursing.

5. There was a need for recognition and resolution of anxieties associated with the nature of nursing work.

6. Machinery was needed to enable contact to be made with the nurse who had personal problems that she could not solve herself and were likely to cause breakdown.

7. The 'hand of friendship' must be the basis of solving 5 and 6 above.

8. Efforts should be made to integrate the sisters to a much greater extent into the life of the hospital.

9. No new intakes of nurses would have group discussions, but the physician and the psychiatrist would continue with the intakes they had taken on.

Three of the nurses had left the first intake: one to have a baby, one to train nearer home because her father was ill, and one just resigned. Another nurse who was not married became pregnant; she was also in need of psychiatric help.

*Subsequent Course of Events*

Altogether seventeen meetings were held; thirteen with nurses, two with sisters, and two with counsellors. There were ten subsequent discussion meetings.

Interesting manifestations were observed in the groups. Young girls in their first year of training discussed in a mature fashion defects and deficiencies in the hospital that affected their lives; and although they felt strongly about some of their complaints, they discussed them with moderation and insight, showing an impressive perception of the hospital structure and of the feelings of their superiors. On the other hand, sisters and consultants, even those taking the nurses' discussion groups, were seen as unapproachable outside the groups. It was evident that during their training many nurses rapidly developed feelings of resignation and hopelessness about the possibility of changing anything, or of obtaining redress, and these feelings were principally responsible for our scheme not being conducive to personal counselling.

We had to consider how sisters might play a greater part in the general life of the hospital, and particularly how they might become involved therapeutically with student nurses' problems, since sisters often seemed unable to help the student nurse in difficulties. At the time of the counselling scheme, most of the pupil and student nurses at our hospital were young girls of just eighteen who had seldom left home before. They were plunged into the maelstrom of anxiety, death, and the struggle for life that is the hospital ward. Even if we were not breaking them down, it might be questioned whether we were doing much more than merely breaking them in.

*Further Meetings*

Owing to frequent changes of matron (we had four in less than two years), and because of shortages and changes in nursing administrative staff, it was some time before it was possible to discuss in detail all the material that had been gathered from the meetings with junior nurses. (At all times the nurses' comments in these groups were, of course, anonymous). However, by October 1967 the new permanent senior matron and deputy matron were 'dug in' and an acting personnel officer had been appointed. In October–December 1967, the personnel officer and the consultant physician who attended the nurses' discussion groups met ten times, usually with the deputy matron present. The matron attended a meeting held by a consultant surgeon's wife and her friends (all ex-nurses) who were interested in befriending the nurses in training.

The matron was determined to provide better social facilities for nurses.

An old hutted ward, temporarily out of use, was made available for a recreation centre. The nurses started to do it up themselves and raised money for this. The Nurses' League gave nearly £500 and the nurses held a Christmas Fair which raised nearly £200. The nurses themselves promoted their own social life in the hospital, and formed committees, societies, and clubs for different activities. Games equipment of various kinds was bought. Most of the defects in the nurses' home were remedied. Television sets, hair driers, and a radiogram were bought. The machinery of the Nurses' Representative Council was renovated. Various other suggestions were examined, such as asking second- or third-year students or pupil nurses to take girls under their wings when they first came to the hospital.

It was evident that many sisters were unhappy about some aspects of life in the hospital. Courses in first-line management for sisters were started at Chiswick Polytechnic. The organizers of these courses made use of material from the reports of the meetings with the junior nurses held by the physician and the psychiatrist, using the nurses' problems in role-playing exercises and discussion groups with the sisters.

In the meetings with the deputy matron and personnel officer, there was discussion of the role of the consultant in helping his ward sister with her problems. Obviously the sister must use the administrative nursing machinery provided for her. However, many ward problems affect doctors as well as nurses, so sisters and consultants must sometimes discuss them together, and offer each other mutual support.

During the introductory course for the January, April, and July intakes of student nurses in 1967, coffee parties were held where a consultant surgeon's wife and three friends (all state registered nurses) met the student nurses informally. By various means it was hoped to foster useful contacts with the young nurses.

As might be expected from the tentative nature of our efforts at counselling, there was no obvious reduction in the wastage of student or pupil nurses. However, as a result of the group meetings with nurses we learnt much about the feelings of young nurses in our large hospital, and gained what were potentially valuable insights into how attitudes may be formed during a nurse's training. The subsequent passage of time has left the impression that although some of us may have a greater understanding of some of the nurses' problems, the treatment of these problems is proving difficult.

At the discussion meetings, the feeling of people concerned with this work has been that a happy hospital is the best guarantee of a nurse completing her training. The practical problem is to achieve this by attention to the difficulties that beset sisters, and to sisters' attitudes to the junior nurses; by providing efficient nursing management; by helping the nurses to organize an adequate social life; and by arranging support for the nurses when they have emotional problems. Some of these are easier to do than others, but a start has been made with all of them.[4]

7. STUDY OF A MEDICAL UNIT

The central-team director spent a week studying one of the medical firms in the autumn of 1966. The following account is taken from his report of the study.

'The two wards in the care of the firm were wooden buildings, built as "temporary" wards in 1938, and had serious disadvantages. There was no day room and all facilities were cramped. However, the wards were due to move to a new building within twelve months. One ward was for males (30 beds) and the other for females (33 beds). It was the object of the observer, during a period of five days, to obtain an overall picture of the work of the firm and to spend some time with each member of it.

'All types of activity except the postgraduate teaching round and the study periods were observed. There were regular opportunities for formal teaching and for clinical conferences, and throughout the activities of the firm consistent efforts were made to record, analyse, and draw deductions from the experience that was gained. The rooms of the physicians contained a library of books, journals, papers, and reprints on gastroenterology and general medicine, a collection of histological microscope slides, and slides for projection.

*Medical Staff*

'The firm was staffed by two full-time consultants, one senior registrar, one registrar, two housemen, and a research registrar. The firm's responsibilities extended beyond the two wards. One of the physicians was the consultant in charge of adult cases of infectious diseases at South Middlesex Hospital which he visited once or twice weekly. He was also in charge of the occupational health service at West Middlesex Hospital. The other physician did a weekly session at Teddington Hospital and half a session at Brentford Hospital.

*Types of Cases Admitted*

'The two wards were described as the Gastroenterology Unit but since the wards had to take in emergency medical admissions from a large catchment area every third day, only about a quarter of the cases could be described as gastroenterological. The remainder covered a variety of medical conditions and a number of cases came in for brief periods to undergo a series of tests.

'There were two other medical units at the hospital and the admission procedure automatically allocated emergencies to the wards which were "on take". In view, however, of the special interest of the firm in gastroenterology some cases of this type were transferred to its wards from other parts of the hospital. Up to sixty per cent of all cases of gastroduodenal haemorrhage were admitted to this unit's beds.

*Ward Rounds*

'Each consultant dealt with one side of a ward during a round which lasted about two hours. The time spent with each of the fourteen or fifteen patients averaged ten minutes, though the time spent on particular cases obviously varied. The consultants were accompanied by one of the registrars, a houseman, and the sister.

'Most patients, on admission, were given about half a dozen tests and in view of the number of questions asked by the consultant about the results and about the earlier medical and social history of the patient, the amount of staff work required of the houseman in preparation for the round was formidable.

'During the round there was considerable discussion about the cases in which the sister, and sometimes one of the nurses, took part. Both the sister and the houseman took notes about treatments and care prescribed. The patients themselves were involved to varying extents. Some were closely examined by the consultant, others were questioned or given information. A good deal of the discussion took place within earshot of the patient, partly no doubt for the convenience of the medical team and partly to enable the patient to ask questions if he wished. Both consultants were keenly aware of the need to take their patients into their confidence, and of the psychological and social factors that might affect their illness. Hence there was a close link in these wards with the medical social workers. In one instance, for example, the medical social worker was requested to visit a patient's employer to find out if his job situation was a source of strain.

'The unit was fortunate in being able to carry out some investigations in a small theatre adjoining its wards. This contained an X-ray machine which enabled such procedures as gastric and intestinal intubation and biopsies to be carried out.

*The Nursing Staff*

'The sister, and also the staff nurse and student nurses, have to be aware of the tests and procedures that are being carried out and to report on the results and the reactions of the patients. Hence, in addition to the normal routines of nursing, they need to be partners in the continuous detective stories that are being played out in the wards. Since, too, the rate of turnover in the wards is greater than in the past the strain on the nursing staff is considerable.

'Both nurses and doctors complained of shortage of nursing staff. These complaints were also due, in part, to the constant pressure of emergency admissions. It was the hospital's policy to put up a proportion of extra beds to cater for emergencies. So habitual had this practice become that there were almost always some extra beds in the ward and it was difficult to know what was the "normal" bed state. One of the sisters, therefore, commented that she usually had to cope with more patients than the number on which her nursing establishment was based. Awareness of these facts had made these physicians and their team very sensitive to the needs and difficulties of the nursing staff.

'Finally, the weekly tutorial for the nurses on the wards was observed. The nurses assembled in the ward and one of the physicians discussed four or five cases with them, among them that of a patient who had had a liver biopsy. Students, particularly those facing examinations, were questioned about procedures and the reasons for them.

*Ward Organization*

'All the medical and nursing developments exerted many pressures on the organization of the ward. The Hospital Internal Communications team at the hospital, however, had started a study of a neighbouring ward and had already discovered a considerable array of problems. Certain points were also noted in the wards under study. One sister regretted that there were not, at present, ward aides in all the medical wards. In wards where increased paper work and even more tests seem inevitable, suitable aides would be invaluable. They might be particularly useful in winter when the pressure on nurses is highest.

'Ward organization generally, and housemen in particular, might also be helped if the admissions system of the hospital were to be examined by an operational research team. Many cases were admitted by the accident and emergency department without reference to an experienced medical registrar. Finally, the task of the houseman and the ward sister was complicated by the fact that, for example, the laboratories closed at 5.30 p.m. Though emergency arrangements existed, admissions and urgent cases could present serious problems at night.

*Housemen*

'An assessment was made of a normal fortnight's work by the house physicians on the two wards. The weekly total hours worked (seventy-seven), plus those on call (twenty-eight), were formidable, and a discussion with one of the housemen underlined their implications. The reputation of the unit was such that a supply of good housemen was always forthcoming and the one interviewed showed his interest and enthusiasm plainly. But the effect of such a régime on his domestic life gave cause for concern. If residential accommodation for young doctors and their wives were available at the hospital the burden of twenty-eight hours on call, on top of a seventy-seven-hour working week, might be just tolerable. When, however, the time required for a long journey to another part of London has to be deducted from the scanty hours off duty there is reason to complain.

'Could hours of duty be reduced? Apart from difficulties of rotas and "cover", housemen in wards such as these have a great deal to do. It was stated that the work of admitting a new patient takes about fifty minutes. After the clinical ward rounds are finished the notes and results of all the patients have to be collated and examined in readiness for the next day. The houseman also has to make personal visits, taking up much time, to the radiological and other departments. It was stated that housemen rarely finished before 10 p.m.

'Finally the houseman is also a trainee with an imperative need to study. His relationship with the patients and his medical superiors was clearly a learning process of great value but the different demands on his time caused some strain. Housemen, in fact, attended the clinical meetings described below but only, it appeared, at the cost of midnight oil.

### *Clinical Meetings and Conferences*

'Five regular teaching meetings took place each week and three of these were observed. In addition there was a weekly meeting over tea to deal with administrative matters attended by all members of the team (including the sisters); and another with the haematologist. The hospital has a good lecture theatre and some thirty doctors from the medical side attended the weekly clinical meeting, which was arranged by the senior medical registrar. An X-ray meeting took place in the radiology department and was attended by three radiologists and the members of the medical unit.

### *Pathology Laboratories*

'The observer interviewed two consultant pathologists who indicated that they were very conscious of the close interaction of their work with the wards. As in most laboratories, the mounting demand for tests was causing acute problems of space and staffing and automation was being developed as fast as possible. Sometimes new methods can cause delays in the wards and one pathologist agreed that a detailed study of the factors that caused or could prevent delays would be very valuable.

### *Clinics*

'The last activity observed was a session by one of the consultants in the out-patients department. Thirteen patients were seen in about three hours and the atmosphere was remarkably relaxed. About half of these patients were returning for check-ups and a very wide range of problems was dealt with. These ranged from the difficulty of communicating effectively with two Indian patients to a long discussion about the best type of university education for a young man whose illness had interrupted his studies. Another patient was referred to the medical social worker for consultation about suitable work in a factory.

### *Concluding Remarks*

'The infinitely complex relationship of the patient, the doctor, the nurse, and the supporting services in a hospital ward merits much deeper study than it has so far received. Medicine, we can safely assume, will become increasingly effective but it will become even more complex. Can we expect to recruit and train for the highly sophisticated skills required, if we cannot reduce existing pressures? And how can we ensure that the whole operation is conducted without wasting scarce resources?

'A start must be made somewhere and this brief survey suggested some possible fields. Reference has been made to the admission system. Which patients have the greatest claims on these highly skilled services? Do they go into the right ward, and do they stay there longer than they need? The obverse is equally important. Do some go out too quickly and what happens to them afterwards?

'There is next the mechanics of the job. Are the forms and facilities that the houseman uses as simple and efficient as they could be? Could some lay assistance or mechanical aids help to reduce the time taken to admit cases or to prepare for rounds? What help could a ward *aide*, housekeeper, or clerk give to the overworked sisters? Could the auxiliaries or orderlies, if properly trained, take some of the work load off the nurses?

'Such a list of problems could be extended almost indefinitely, and it seemed to the observer that in almost every case the initiative should be with the doctor. This is not because the doctor could solve many problems unaided but because of the inevitable reluctance of any other staff to step into the picture without full medical co-operation. The firm studied is conscious of the factors outlined to a remarkable degree but they have not discovered, as yet, the answers to all their problems.'[5]

## 8. STUDY OF PATIENTS' ANXIETIES IN RELATION TO CLINICAL WARD ROUNDS

Partly as a result of the project described above, the consultant physicians asked a central-team member to interview patients on the two wards of the gastroenterology unit.

A brief pilot survey showed (a) the great variation between patients in how much explanation of their illness and treatment they wished to be given; (b) the sense of mounting tension felt by some of the patients who were not seen until the end of the doctors' round; (c) the patients' difficulty in understanding the roles of the different members of the ward team.

The following is a brief representative selection from a large number of patients' comments:

### *Men*

'I would sooner know exactly what is wrong. If they use long medical words I think "My God, what's that?" But if they put it in layman's terms it's better, for example, "You have some fluid on your lung which we are going to drain off".'

'I want to know and don't want to know (about my illness). If it's not nice news then I don't want to.'

'I must say I was puzzled about my X-ray. I went down and it wasn't explained that it was just a normal routine check and so I told them they were X-raying the wrong part of me. It's something to do with my kidneys, you know. I fairly had to squeeze the information about the X-ray out.'

'No, I don't worry about ward rounds, I just want to know when I can go home.'

'I have been conditioned by films; you see people learning their trades, even the comedy ones where they make a joke of it. If I hadn't seen films I might have been worried by the bunch of doctors, I might think "What's the matter with me? Why do I need all these?"'

*Women*

'I do feel that patients who are at the far end of the ward get into an awful state while they are waiting for the doctors to get up to them. They keep asking "What number are they up to now?" They get into a frightful state. They do worry and wonder who exactly all the doctors are.'

'I'm terribly interested. I try to listen in to other people's complaints. I like to hear all I can! Other people's complaints are always shrouded in mystery.'

'Patients do wonder who the doctors are and it would be no use explaining they are a house physician, registrar etc., because they just wouldn't understand that either.'

'I hate being kept in the dark. Some people accept anything and don't ask questions.'

'It isn't a question of discussion with the doctors—I feel doctors are always a little diplomatic and evasive, not necessarily in my case because I think they have been very frank.'

'It is perhaps not always wise to give people the full gen—it may harm them emotionally.'

As a result of the survey this medical unit has made a more conscious effort to assess the extent of each patient's genuine desire for 'explanation'. The formality of the clinical ward rounds has been reduced by varying the order in which patients are seen, and a stencilled information sheet describing the roles of the different members of the unit staff is given to each patient on admission. This leaflet also provides other information of practical day to day use and a supplementary page has been included explaining the significance of the many different nurses' uniforms. This last part will be superseded by the new hospital information leaflet.[6]

## 9. THE MESSENGER SERVICES[7]

A survey of the messenger services and general communication channels was undertaken by David Keay, a postgraduate student from Brunel University. He investigated particularly internal and external mail, and the delivery and collection of medical records, pharmacy preparations, pathology forms and specimens, X-rays, etc.

From this survey it is hoped to rationalize the present organization and thus to save effort and personnel, while providing an improved messenger service. Taking into account the layout of the hospital, a time-table has been evolved that will allow three of the messengers and the post-room porters to cover all parts of the hospital at set times during the day. They will each be responsible for covering a particular area and will operate from a central post-room.

### 10. SURVEY OF CONSULTANTS' ATTITUDES

In the autumn of 1968, as a preliminary exercise for another study, a survey of the para-clinical attitudes of consultants was undertaken at this hospital. Although the exercise was not labelled an H.I.C. project, it was initiated by an H.I.C. team member and the content and results are highly relevant. Full details of this survey are published in Chapter 12 of the companion volume to this book (Revans, in press).

### 11. GENERAL IMPROVEMENTS IN COMMUNICATIONS

A number of steps have been taken during the H.I.C. Project period to improve internal communications by greater consultation among various staff groups. For example, more information is circulated through official channels such as the medical committee, the divisional committees, the monthly meeting of heads of departments, and the sisters' meetings; a monthly diary of events is circulated and it is hoped that this will shortly become a proper news sheet or hospital magazine.

Many of the studies we report have been nurtured in an air of crisis, thereby emphasising the need for more time to be devoted to identifying the problems we face now and will, to an increasing degree face in five to ten years' time. As one measure to meet this need the HMC two years ago asked the senior hospital staff (medical, nursing, and administrative) to formulate a plan of future developments for the hospital. Some forty schemes, in order of priority, have been scheduled for the next three years with a further list of developments needed for the period 1971–1976.

It is felt that the H.I.C. Project has been one not unimportant factor leading to an increasing number of staff of different professional interests and at various levels becoming more attuned not only to problems within their respective departments but to the wider problems facing the hospital. The hospital secretary and other senior officers have been addressing new entrants to the nursing schools, and giving talks at induction courses for newly qualified staff nurses and at the first-line management courses for sisters at Chiswick Polytechnic. One of the physicians gave two talks on 'staff interdependence and relationships', and the psychiatrists gave four lectures on patients', nurses', and doctors' attitudes during Mental Health Week, 1967.

In the past we had often discussed the need for a physicians' committee. When we participated in the H.I.C. Project the time was ripe for the physicians and surgeons to organize their work into respective divisions within the hospital. This evolutionary process was fostered by the presence of the

H.I.C. Project and the self-examination to which it gave rise. The immediate reasons for the formation of the physicians' committee, in October 1966, were the need to increase postgraduate education within the hospital, to rationalize some of the clinical and laboratory procedures in use, and to consider ways of reducing the work load of the junior doctors. Numerous topics have been discussed, many with the service departments. In short, problems that might otherwise never have been tackled at all (some have waited for years!) have not only been discussed, but have been dealt with by appropriate action. All the medical work of the hospital is now organized in divisions (Stewart, 1969). The medical committee has a special subcommittee for studying all kinds of routine procedures in the hospital with the aim of introducing agreed measures of standardization where practicable, and another for introducing economies in the use of drugs, dressings, and surgical equipment. A registrars' committee has been started by the registrars themselves with the encouragement of the senior staff. The object of this committee is to provide a forum for the registrars to discuss ideas for increasing the efficiency of the hospital service and for passing them on to the medical committee.

The study of medical social work brought the realization that the hospital will probably have to work in closer liaison with local authority medical social workers. Partly as a result of this, two physicians worked for a time with our own medical social workers and with Mr Eugene Heimler's team of social workers in the London Borough of Hounslow on a joint research project studying the rehabilitation into their families and work of men who had suffered from cardiac infarction.

Of all the projects we have undertaken the one most completely solved, and that within a reasonably short time, concerned the medical social work department. This was an illuminating tribute to its members as individuals and to their training.

## CONCLUSIONS

*Know then thyself, presume not God to scan,*
*The proper study of mankind is man.*

ALEXANDER POPE

Many of the conclusions will be self-evident, but one fundamental aspect needs emphasizing, namely that without the impact of the H.I.C. Project it is unlikely that the hospital as a complex organization would have been subjected to the same degree of self-analysis.

Industry, transport, and other human institutions do not always run smoothly or productively. This is often due to defects of communication between humans, and these in turn may be due to ignorance of roles and attitudes, and lack of concern for people's feelings.

Hospitals are not exempt from institutional failings; low morale, leading to absenteeism and poor work standards, is all too common. Any difficulties in the management of a concern must stem in part from the activities of human beings as individuals or in groups. Reflecting that awareness and understanding of problems arising from such activities should begin, like charity, at home, any hospital nurse, doctor, administrator, or technician might well consider it his duty to develop an interest in the social pathology of the institution where he works.

Let the staff be concerned first with their own hospital. They might be encouraged in their research by consideration of certain unique properties of hospitals as human enterprises.

People who work in hospitals do so in a milieu that could hardly be more human-oriented; their training and skill is ostensibly directed to the relief of human suffering. Nevertheless doctors' and nurses' preoccupations have hitherto, of necessity, been with curing, controlling, or ameliorating physical and mental disease. Hospitals are anxious places, and, too often unhappy places for some who work in them. To ensure the best use of money, staff, buildings, and equipment, it is necessary for those who work in hospitals to have some knowledge of their social pathology. (It is an interesting current phenomenon that so many young people are more interested in the social workings of man's environment than in its purely physical attributes.)

The great majority of hospital staff who actually work all their lives 'at the bench' (i.e. at the bedside, in the consulting room, in the laboratory, or in an office) also constitute in large part the intellectual elite of the hospital establishment. Such people must be uniquely placed to develop insights into some of the problems that beset humans when they come together to work. What does this mean in practical language? We believe it means understanding others, and themselves, rather better; for some of the difficulties facing nurses, junior doctors, and other staff derive from senior doctors', sisters', and administrators' attitudes and actions.

Like most hospitals, this one has its difficulties of organization, management, and welfare. The H.I.C. Project was seen as a good opportunity to get help with them, and to participate with others in solving some of them (Coghill, 1969).

In a social organism such as a hospital, although things may obviously need changing, local inertia may prevent anything being done. However, internal stresses may set the scene for innovation, and an outside agency can be of great value in providing a stimulus to change at an appropriate moment. (Biologically, change in an organism or group is frequently initiated from outside.) Thus a conjunction of external and internal stimuli provide ideal opportunities. As we see it the H.I.C. Project has been the external stimulus.

It has acted also by showing us new techniques for examining human and mechanical problems, with some advice in their application and in the assessment of results. The techniques are largely of the kind that the people involved in the problems – consultants, nurses and sisters, administrators, cleaners, records staff, catering staff, and so on – can, if necessary with some outside practical help, themselves use to investigate and analyse their problems, learning much in the process. With the Project's help it has been possible to look afresh at the hospital and to see more clearly the defects of the underlying structure.

Attempts to correct all faults by purely mechanistic managerial methods usually fail. Work study, administrative expertise, statistical analysis, operational research, will help with many problems, and cure some. But even in the better hospitals twenty to thirty per cent of nurses leave before completing their training and domestic workers are hard to obtain and retain; the consultant may be felt at one extreme to be uninterested, and at the other overbearing; sisters are discontented; consultants feel the administration is inefficient; there are unhappy relations with governing bodies, and so on.

The concept of administration as something that an administrator does to the administered – as a manipulative act – is outmoded. Just as the best discipline is self-discipline, so the best administration is self-administration (Hunter, 1967a; Hunter, 1967b). This means that consultants and sisters and others must share the burden of management with the administrative staff, and in turn that means they must be managers for a part of their time. Such partial involvement by scientists and others in managerial tasks is becoming increasingly common in industry. In fact consultants and sisters have been managers for years. After all, we speak of the 'management of the case', meaning the total care of the patient. The most important conclusion of the investigation into the discontents of the domestic workers was that the tendency of sisters to opt out of managerial responsibility for some of the activities in a ward, and concentrate on purely nursing tasks, is fatal to efficient domestic work. Unless the domestic worker can be integrated into the ward team, and only the sister and her nurses can do that, she will continue to be an inefficient worker.

But there are some problems in hospitals that require new techniques for their solution. Some of them have been unrecognized or misinterpreted. For example, the nursing shortage has been seen mainly as a problem of recruitment rather than wastage; discontent among sisters, manifesting itself in a variety of destructive ways, is dismissed as a natural characteristic of battle-axes, rather than seen as due to anxieties, arising from training or connected with their work and life, that remain uninvestigated. The 'brain drain' of young doctors is seen by some as black ingratitude to the hands that fed them; we do not try to find out from the individual doctors what motivated them. Patients in one hospital stay twice as long as in another for the same complaint, a financially and socially costly phenomenon barely recognized, let alone treated. The instances can be multiplied.

We cannot start to solve a problem until we recognize its existence. So the organization must be re-examined with greater intuitive speculation. If nurses leave prematurely, why not ask them their feelings about the hospital, preferably before they resign, and find out what they think is wrong with it? Instead of complaining about the sisters we could try, as Revans did in Lancashire (Revans, 1964b), to understand some of the episodes of hospital life that upset them, and to investigate their feelings about the hospital environment; then we might go on to try to alter the administration so as to help the sisters. It is obvious to anyone who has given any consideration to the matter that some of the difficulties besetting student nurses arise directly from the sisters. But as the boy is father to the man, the student nurse is mother to the sister. When are we going to break this vicious circle?

The medical profession is coming to see that one of the most important causes of the medical 'brain drain' is nothing to do with the National Health Service, but is mainly the lack of a proper career structure and postgraduate programme for young hospital doctors. This becomes plain when one talks to young doctors, or indeed, if one remembers one's own career before becoming a consultant. (It looks as if much the same cause is operative in the 'brain drain' of scientists generally.)

It would be absurd to suggest that all the existing social or managerial investigations and projects carried out by the ten-hospital consortium, and indeed in numerous hospitals up and down the country, were entirely due to the H.I.C. Project. One of the most encouraging aspects of the NHS is the number of ideas being generated in its hospitals for their betterment. (This alone, incidentally, suggests that there is far more resilience in the hospital service than some of its critics evidently believe.)

Nevertheless we believe it is true that the presence of the H.I.C. Project has encouraged in the ten hospitals projects of a greater number and variety than would otherwise have been undertaken. It has done this by offering, firstly, information on methods of sociological investigation (technical expertise), secondly, practical help with advice and extra pairs of hands, and, thirdly, support (feedback and other meetings and discussions, and its mere presence). These supports, arising from the comradeship of a common venture, are valuable in exploring relatively new areas doubly valuable when the scope of investigation and therapy involves the feelings, attitudes, and emotions of human beings, and trebly so when those humans are ourselves and our own medical, nursing, and administrative colleagues.

What, to us, has made the H.I.C. Project so useful is that by its presence it has often made possible the objective investigation of hospital activities and attitudes that, undertaken purely internally, might have proved explosive and destructive. By being outside the 'ring' as it were, and by supplying methods and some outside helpers, it has provided the means of investigating delicate hospital situations previously guarded by walls of protective anxiety. For example, we were sustained in our efforts to overcome the difficulties of starting the nurses' discussion groups by the background presence of the H.I.C. Project, and we felt the climate of opinion arising from its presence and activities was a help in overcoming reluctance about this and other schemes. The Project made our own suggestions more respectable and acceptable to colleagues and authority.

## THE FUTURE

We believe that this work should continue. We are as yet only on the threshold of recognizing and understanding some of the problems, pressures, and complexities that make up a hospital organization. Certainly we who work in hospitals must be prepared to expose ourselves to self-analysis, to share our problems with others, and to participate in a programme of re-education aimed at overcoming the many organizational defects that exist and the out-of-date attitudes and prejudices held by many hospital staff. We hope, as the present project comes to an end, that the following will happen:

(a) A central bureau for dissemination of advice and information will be set up, possibly by the Department of Health or the King's Fund or the Nuffield Trust. Perhaps this organization could focus on one, or maybe two, problems common to all hospitals, for example nurse wastage, or patient turnover, which they might all join in investigating and treating, perhaps working on different aspects of a subject. This would not exclude a hospital from pursuing any other problems it wished. Discussion between hospitals is important in this kind of work for offering support and disseminating information. So we would suggest that meetings of project members from participating hospitals should take place at least several times a year, perhaps on a regional basis.

(b) The educational and training needs in this area of activity will be met through special courses arranged at recognized hospital educational centres, e.g. in London (King's Fund College of Hospital Management), Leeds, and Manchester.

(c) Local links will be established between hospital groups, universities, and technical colleges: in this context it is hoped that the links already established between ourselves, Brunel University (particularly for the secondment of students), and the Chiswick Polytechnic can be continued and strengthened.

## NOTES

[1] A fuller report of this study may be obtained from the Hospital Secretary, West Middlesex Hospital, Isleworth, Middlesex.

[2] For full details of this project see Goldschmidt (1968).

[3] For full details of this project see Zucker and Smith (1967).

[4, 5, 6] More detailed reports of these studies may be obtained from the hospital.

[7] This project is not included in the central-team or evaluation analyses of hospital projects because

(a) the study was undertaken as a result of direct negotiation between the hospital and Brunel University and was not discussed in H.I.C. meetings or with central staff,

(b) the study findings were not available for consideration by the hospital administration until after the writing-up stage of the Project had begun.

PART FOUR

# *Evaluation Report*

*GEORGE F. WIELAND*

# 10 *Introduction to the evaluation*

My first information about the H.I.C. Project came in 1965. A colleague at the University of Michigan took part in one of the three-day appreciation courses and reported that there was a need for a social scientist who could help with the Project work and the measurement of its effects. At the time I was interested in learning more about action research and changing organizations, to supplement my background in the more usual academic kinds of research. I wanted to learn more about 'action' as well as 'understanding'. The H.I.C. Project seemed to be very suitable, particularly since the relatively large number (ten) of organizations involved in the project would facilitate the kinds of comparative analyses that I had found to be powerful research procedures.

A fellowship proposal to the U.S. Public Health Service highlighted the unique character of a ten-organization change project, and it detailed four major activities: (1) learning about action for organizational improvement, (2) learning about evaluating or assessing changes by using survey methods. (3) learning about action research, or research by changing and manipulating variables, and, at a lower priority, (4) learning about differences in hospitals in the U.K. compared with those in the U.S.

The fellowship funds were awarded in March 1966, and I took up my fellowship post in London during May of that year. The latter part of May and most of June were used primarily for acclimatization and orientation, and in late June, some notes on a tentative plan for evaluation were submitted to the advisory committee of the H.I.C. Project. The idea of an 'independent' evaluator was agreed upon and the work leading up to this report began.

Discussions with advisory committee members established the desirability of a comprehensive, detailed measurement of Project outcomes, particularly turnover of staff and length of patients' stay in addition to 'communications', and an application was made for Ministry of Health funds to provide further help. A research assistant was hired to do this work, and a separate budget was provided for the various expenses involved in the independent evaluation. Thus I, as an evaluator, became part of an evaluation 'team', and was to continue so to the end of the Project some three years later.

I have described the formal beginning of the evaluation, but the real beginning is much earlier. I have indicated elsewhere (Wieland, 1968a) my views on the inevitability of, and even need for, a 'non-independent' evaluation. Interaction between evaluator and those being evaluated must occur, and in the process each is bound to affect the other. By being aware of this process, the evaluator may mitigate its detrimental effects on the 'objectivity' of the evaluation, and even make positive use of such interaction. Thus, the evaluation may be said to have begun at least upon the arrival of the potential evaluator and his initial interactions with the staff of H.I.C.

However, there are even earlier influences on the evaluation, which may have potentially detrimental effects that cannot be treated in such a cursory fashion. The earlier influences are found in the background and experiences of the evaluator, and in his resulting values and ways of viewing the world. These are the lenses through which the facts of the H.I.C. Project are seen and evaluated. They determine what the evaluator chooses to study and how he goes about it. But the most important point is that these determinants of the evaluation are often unrecognized. To recognize them is to acknowledge the weaknesses – and perhaps the strengths – of the evaluation, and ultimately to obtain a more objective and more valid view of the activities being evaluated.

I joined the H.I.C. Project with the view that it was an organizational change project, like others being undertaken in the U.S. at the time. Of course, precisely what was to be changed, and the methods to be used, differed in varying degree from other projects. From contact with research done by colleagues at the University of Michigan, I arrived with a number of views of what is and what is not important in the study of organizational functioning and organizational change. First of all, effectiveness, i.e. in the case of hospitals the quality of medical and nursing care provided – is what an organization is all about, not 'morale' or some other factor. There are other reasons – connected with individuals and their psychological satisfactions – for studying staff morale and turnover, but in terms of organizational effectiveness, turnover and morale are side issues (see Chapter 13 for further details). However, while patient-care is a most important aspect of hospitals, earlier work at Michigan demonstrated to me the great difficulty involved in its measurement (Georgopoulos and Mann, 1962). To collect valid data would first require considerable developmental work.

An alternative to measuring end-products of organizational functioning is to examine the immediately preceding factors in the set of determinants. The so-called 'human-relations' approach at Michigan and elsewhere provides a number of leads based essentially on the relations between organizational members or groups (see, e.g., Likert, 1961, on 'supportive relations' and Georgopoulos and Mann, 1962, on 'co-ordination'). Particularly important, to my thinking, is the work of Tannenbaum (1966) on the relationship between 'high total control', or mutal influence systems, and organizational effectiveness. In fact, when asked to speak to others about 'communications' I have invariably pointed out that, in my view, 'communication' or providing information is not really important – what matters for an effective organization is whether the recipient of a communication listens and acts on the information, i.e. whether he is 'influenced'.

Other work at Michigan by Katz and Kahn (1966) has highlighted the problem of 'levels' in organizational change. Attempts at changing individuals – sending them to sensitivity training groups, for example – are not likely to change organizations without still further change efforts. Organizations are likely to be changed only if organization-level phenomena are changed directly – or changed indirectly by some linkage between individual, group, and organizational phenomena.

These, then, are some of the most important views, or 'biases', that I brought to my role of evaluator in the H.I.C. Project. While this evaluation report does not test any theories of organizations, a knowledge of the intellectual background of the writer is still useful, because the reader can better understand and himself 'evaluate' the evaluation. Given these biases, what is an evaluator likely to look at, and what is he likely to overlook or distort? How will he design the evaluation and measure what he is 'looking at', and how are his conclusions liable to be biased or unwarranted from the evidence provided?

The evaluation proved to be a much more difficult undertaking than expected, and ultimately over three years were devoted to it. The data described here were for the most part collected while the author was the recipient of a United States Public Health Service Postdoctoral Fellowship (No. 2F2MH29181-01) at Guy's Hospital Medical School. Financial support was provided by a research grant from the Ministry of Health to Guy's Hospital Medical School, while office space and facilities were provided by The Hospital Centre of the King's Fund.

Grateful appreciation is expressed to Project hospital staff who gave generously of their time and to Professor Revans and the central team of the H.I.C. Project, who not only made the evaluation possible, but consistently encouraged it. The Project advisory committee provided equal encouragement, as well as patient understanding when difficulties were encountered. The individuals who have helped in the assessment and evaluation of the H.I.C. Project are many. Mr Alan Ogborne, Mrs Elizabeth Stenning, Mrs Patricia Day, and Mr Roger Watts all worked diligently as research assistants on the evaluation. Special thanks go to Mrs Gillian Cowan and Mrs Marion Anderson, who did most of the interviewing and questionnaire distribution, to Mrs Angela Archer who served ably both in typing and in coding responses for computer analysis, to Mr Ang-Lip Lim for a competent job of programming, and to Mrs Kathleen Chapman who patiently and skilfully carried out both clerical and secretarial tasks. Professor R. W. Revans, Mr Duncan N. Smith, Dr Nelson Coghill, Dr James Stewart, Professor Mayer Zald, Mr Ernest Weston, and Mrs Sharon Wieland read portions of the evaluation report and provided useful comments, and they were able to point out to me some of my errors and oversights. Special thanks go to Mr Jasper Woodcock for his editorial assistance.

# 11 The H.I.C. Project and the evaluation design

In the first half of this chapter we shall provide an evaluation-team view of the aims of the H.I.C. Project. The second half of the chapter describes the evaluation design used to assess the achievements of H.I.C.

No single definite research proposal setting out fixed and detailed objectives for the H.I.C. Project exists. They must be extracted from a series of notes and guidelines written during the Project, from reports on planning conferences, from Project progress reports, etc. But if we take these sources and expand them with earlier work by Revans and his associates, a relatively extensive and detailed picture emerges.

The main theme of the Project is, of course, 'communication'. Revans (1964b) has presented a view of the hospital characterized by cycles of anxiety, communication blockage, and malfunctioning, leading to more anxiety, communication blockage, etc. Communication or lack of it is a major problem in hospitals:

> '... some of the problems facing the Hospital Service today can be traced to difficulties of communication within the hospitals themselves and between people in different departments and specialties and at different levels in the organisation' (The Hospital Centre, 1966b).

The H.I.C. Project is basically an attempt to improve hospitals in a practical sense. The aim was to attack, and solve, some of their problems and to improve their efficiency. The letter of invitation sent to the hospitals spoke of 'a new method of solving problems'. Communications problems are basic, and it was expected that their solution would improve the 'morale' of staff (i.e. reduce turnover) and improve the efficiency of patient-care as measured by length of stay:

> 'Our evidence suggests that the effectiveness of hospital communications is likely to exert a major influence upon two important characteristics of the hospital, namely, the speed with which it can treat its patients and the attachment it can command from its staff' (Revans, 1967, p. 32).

> '... people are ... looking for ... intelligibility. People want to understand what is going on around them ... In the course of his research Revans has found that those hospital systems that arrange employees intelligently, assigning functions in a manner understandable to the workers, not only

retain staff longer but discharge patients more quickly' (Milbank, 1966, p. 246).

Problems, however, were not to be limited to communications problems. If the problems were of concern to staff and their solution would improve work effectiveness, then their solution could be a part of the H.I.C. Project:

'Existing senior staffs should be helped to identify problems creating anxiety within their own hospitals' (Revans, 1964a).

In addition to the solution of communications problems, and the solution of other kinds of problems, the Project had an educational aim. Those individuals involved in studying problems would learn how to 'see' problems; they would become more 'aware' of problems and in this sense become better communicators. They would also become more aware of their own behaviour, and they would presumably change their behaviour so as to communicate better their intentions and desires to others in the hospital:

'Since, it seems, that the principal defect of many hospitals is a lack of awareness of their internal problems, education in this sense is of great importance. The Project aims to provide it' (The Hospital Centre, 1966a).

'If communications are blocked because senior staff do not appreciate their continuous teaching function and subordinates are thereby prevented from learning and adjusting, only some process that improves the perception of the seniors can effectively free them. This is essentially the objective of education as it is implied in this paper. The first need of management education in Britain today is to heighten the awareness of managers of the effects they have upon their subordinates' (Revans, 1964a).

This emphasis on changing people and their behaviour is clearly detailed in 'The Aims and Intentions of the Project' (see item 6 of the Aims) and flows directly from earlier work by Revans. A survey of Lancashire factories (Revans, 1965a) showed that the attentiveness of management was one of the most important factors associated with worker satisfaction. Revans concluded, 'our task is to help managers learn the art of listening'.

Furthermore, the aim of improving communications of the H.I.C. Project is not restricted to relations between superior and subordinate:

'[H.I.C. is] ... an attempt to treat the whole hospital and improve its efficiency by encouraging members of the medical, nursing and administrative staff to work together in diagnosing, examining and remedying their own hospital problems ... and the fostering of friendly and helpful relations between one hospital and a neighbouring one, to the extent of calling in staff from one to locate a stumbling block in the other, and to advise on methods of its removal or circumvention' (Craig, 1966).

Turning now to the primary means or activities to be used by H.I.C. in meeting the above aims, we find that:

'The two initial steps to be taken were identification of the problems by senior hospital staff, which would be analysed by detached and qualified observers, trained in management problems, and working outside the hospital. The hospital staff would then undergo training in social research and conduct "attitude surveys", preferably in other hospitals. The problems uncovered would then be analysed and solved by the methods of group therapy' (*British Medical Journal*, 1964).

'... those in charge (of hospitals) may be helped to overcome such problems by methods developed by research workers in the social and administrative sciences' (Revans, 1968).

'The hospitals themselves, personified by their administrators, their doctors and their nurses, must actively join these studies, and members of these professions must learn to conduct surveys, to interpret their findings, to seek the structure of the problems so revealed and to build the programmes of participation by which these problems may be ameliorated' (Revans, 1964b, p. 98).

'It is therefore necessary to experiment with continued exercises in self-teaching. Since it is essential that those in the working situation shall also learn their own part in it, these exercises must involve a responding group ...' (Revans, 1967, p. 70).

These quotations do not, by any means, exhaust the available statements on how problem-solving, communications, and management educational aims were to be achieved.[1] However, it seems fair to say that the emphasis was to be on attitude surveys done by hospital staff themselves. Attitude surveys were the main focus of the month-long courses given by the H.I.C., and help in doing surveys was generally the kind of help provided by the central team when their help was requested. However, the ideal was that hospital staff were to do as much of the work as possible themselves. These two features, attitude surveys and self-help, are the key aspects of the H.I.C. Project that go far to explaining what actually happened in the Project and also what came of it. The combination of these two features is also quite unusual in organizational change studies, and consequently the Revans Project provides an interesting supplement and contrast to the work of others in the field.

Let us turn now to the problem of evaluating the H.I.C. Project.[2] The ideal evaluation design is that of the classical controlled experiment. One assembles a representative sample of cases from the general population to which one will generalize the findings. These cases are then assigned randomly (or, at second best, by matching) to the experimental or control treatments. One measures both groups of cases before and after treatments. The only way in which the two groups differ is the presence or absence of experimental treatment, and change in the experimental cases over and above that in the control cases consequently indicates the effect of the experimental treatment.

Such an ideal design encounters many problems when it comes to implementation. Control groups require some of the participating hospitals to submit to measurement procedures without sharing in the benefits of the changes made in the experimental hospitals, and co-operation of this kind may be difficult to obtain (see, e.g., Houghton, 1968). Control groups also double the costs and effort required in measurement procedures. Before-and-after measurement is, of course, also twice as costly as a single measurement, but a more serious obstacle to its use is the problem of what to measure in the 'before' measurement, when the specific aims and directions of the change activities often are yet to be defined.

These are some of the problems in using an experimental design to evaluate change efforts. But despite these problems, the experimental design commends itself to the evaluator because of its precision in demonstrating the degree of change free from any contaminating influences, and its precision in linking the effects with the change efforts, free from any alternative explanations or relationships. Unfortunately, in evaluating the H.I.C. Project, no such design was feasible. This was true for two reasons: (1) it was decided that the evaluation would be independent of the change activities, thereby preventing the evaluator from having control over who gets the experimental treatments, a very necessary requirement; and (2) the evaluation activities did not begin until after the H.I.C. Project had already started in earnest, thus preventing the evaluator from measuring 'before' as well as 'after', another vital aspect of experimental design.

We shall strive in the evaluation to attain the standard of an experimental design. For some of the work – in the use of regional average figures for length of patients' stay – we shall approach this ideal using a 'quasi-experimental design' (Campbell and Stanley, 1963). However, for the most part, the evaluation design used here will be a 'survey-correlational' design.[3] A survey, in its simplest form, consists of a collection of data at one point in time. However, some data may pertain to earlier times as well as those concurrent with the survey. For the evaluation, we have collected current information on the criteria or outcomes of the change programme as well as information on the earlier change activities – i.e. what was done that might have produced the outcomes.

The experimental design facilitates evaluation since comparisons can be made between 'before' and 'after' states and between 'experimental' and 'control' groups. Thus one knows just how much better or worse the treated subjects have become. In the survey design used here, less straightforward procedures for comparison must be used. First of all, one may take results at 'face value' – do they seem 'good' or 'bad' in themselves? Comparison groups are really implicit in this; for in judging something as it is, one considers likely alternatives, either similar subjects or the treated subject itself, at an earlier point in time. For example, if three-quarters of the staff of a hospital say on the average that they are 'satisfied' with their work, we consider whether this is typical of staffs in similar hospitals, or whether it is typical of this particular hospital staff over the course of the past year or so. But if actual figures are not available for comparison, such evaluations are not very reliable or objective.

If we must use the survey design, then the most reliable and objective alternative to the experimental design described above must be an 'internal' comparison or evaluation. For the most part, our comparisons will in fact be of this nature (see Chapters 14-18). By 'internal', we mean that answers to one question in the survey will be compared with those to another in the same survey – questions regarding different kinds of outcomes, or questions for different H.I.C. activities, etc.

The most basic problem in any evaluation is to decide on the criteria, those things which are to be judged or weighed in determining a project's success. Above, we have cited as examples from Revans's writings: the provision of information or 'intelligibility', improvements in communicating, listening, and being aware; the solving of various hospital problems and the improvement of the work of project participants; and finally the reduction of staff turnover and length of patients' stay. These criteria seem to be, to varying degrees, the goals or intentions of those planning and carrying out the Project.

In addition to what is consciously intended, however, there may be other outcomes of value to various project activities. Increasing the influence of project participants upon the functioning of their hospitals is one such possible outcome. Giving project participants skills by which to study their hospitals and to set right various problems may lead to their having a greater influence over the activities they are studying. Furthermore, there is considerable research evidence showing that increasing the influence of various echelons in organizations leads to more effective organizations (Tannenbaum, 1966).

A very useful way to look at the above criteria is as points in a sequence or chain of events, from the planning of a project, to the implementation of project activities, to immediate and subsequent outcomes (see, e.g., Suchman, 1967). No single point in the chain provides sufficient data for an evaluation (see, e.g., *Figure 12-1*, in Chapter 12). This is because success at any one point in the chain of events is not always directly related to success at subsequent points. Furthermore, it is particularly unfair to select only some ultimate event in the chain as a criterion, because failure in reaching some extremely high standard is still compatible with success at some earlier point in the chain characterized by more modest expectations. In fact, in a novel, exploratory project such as the H.I.C. Project, even achievement of preliminary sub-goals may be of significance, and the evaluator does well not to overlook these events.

Having decided to look at events at several points along a chain – from project activities to achievement of sub-goals and to the achievement of relatively final outcomes – we need only ask how, or with reference to what, one evaluates the project events. First of all, there is what one might term the 'level' of activities or outcomes. Thus, according to our discussion above about 'internal' comparisons in surveys, we may report that the level of sending communications is higher than the level of receiving communications.[4] Similarly, we may say that 'feedback' meetings are rated more 'useful' than are the meetings at the London School of Hygiene, or vice versa. The level or extent of H.I.C. outcomes (i.e. criteria of H.I.C. success) is described primarily in Chapters 12-14 below. The level or extent of determinants is covered in Chapters 15–18.

The second portion of the evaluation analysis consists of an examination of the relationships between determinants and outcomes.[5] The basic question is, given some differences or variation in outcomes and criteria, what are the determinants of these differences? If some hospital-team members, for example, say there has been an improvement in the amount of information they now have about the functioning of other departments in their hospitals, and other team members say there is no difference, what factors can account for this? Differences in such outcomes are successively related to various suspected determinants in order to specify how, for example, more knowledge about other departments comes about. In short, given differences in outcomes, what difference in initial conditions, initial resources, amount of effort, procedures used, or whatever, account for the outcome?[6] These analyses are found in Chapters 15-18.

The most positive evidence for the 'success' of H.I.C. (i.e. for beneficial outcomes from H.I.C. activity) appears in Chapter 14, coming from questionnaire data on increased information, communication, problem-solving, and action in the hospitals. Chapters 12 and 13, on the effects of the Project on length of stay of patients and turnover of staff, do not, by and large, provide any significant indication of H.I.C. success in changing organization-level phenomena. For this reason some readers may wish to turn first to the more positive H.I.C. outcomes described in Chapter 14, and the determinants of these outcomes described in Chapters 15 to 18. Staff turnover and patients' stay are ultimate criteria of success and require attention on that basis, but the findings here are not wholly encouraging.

## NOTES

[1] If an organizational change project is to make a diagnosis and to fit outcomes to what the client really needs – and what the change-agent can give (compare Lorsche and Lawrence, 1969; Klein, 1969) – then it is likely that the goals of a project initially stated to the client must be incomplete and lacking in clarity.

[2] For an account of some different views on evaluating H.I.C., see Appendix 11A.

[3] There is one sense in which the correlational approach is superior to the experimental approach. The correlational approach, in contrast to the experimental approach to evaluation, focuses on the *process* of change. Instead of the experimental 'black box', where a large number of inputs are made to treatment units and outputs measured, the correlational approach follows inputs to look at immediate consequences, intermediate consequences, etc., as well as ultimate outputs. There are, of course, problems in assessing directions of causation, but the correlational method does begin to cast light on how change comes about. By measuring change-agent and client activities one begins to develop a theory of 'changing', as Bennis (1966) has so aptly put it. One of the aims of the present evaluation is to relate such variations in process to variation in outcome.

[4] See Chapter 14 for more details on interpreting survey data.

[5] Because no probability sampling design is utilized here, statistical significance tests are inappropriate for ascertaining whether relationships are 'real' relationships or not. However, we shall use the standard tests as an aid to interpretation.

[6] Correlations show only association, not causation. However, when one is able to make assumptions about causal directions for some variables, the causal directions for relationships with other variables may be inferred by the magnitude of relationships (Blalock, 1964). We shall use this approach, as well as the more usual one of assigning causal direction on the basis of observational evidence and inference. In the final analysis, however, none of the correlations reported here can be interpreted other than as reflecting association.

# 12 *Patients' stay*

In this chapter we shall take an important criterion of hospital functioning – the average length of patients' stay, and attempt to examine the effects of the H.I.C. Project upon this aspect of the participating hospitals. As we have indicated above, requiring changes in such an ultimate criterion may be unfair and too stringent a test of the success of a project. In fact, the analysis reported in this chapter – changes in the average length of stay of patients in H.I.C. hospitals compared with changes in other similar hospitals – does not demonstrate any improvements as a result of the H.I.C. Project. However, some readers may feel that the analysis was not carried far enough, or that it was not comprehensive enough. For these reasons the analysis is outlined in detail in this chapter, enabling the reader to draw his own conclusions.

Patient characteristics are important in this evaluation not only because patients are the most important measure of hospital output or effectiveness, but also because Revans (1964b, pp. 86-90, 125-127 and 1967, pp. 26-28) has detailed some expectations specifically about the effects of improvement in communications on the length of patients' stay.

Revans (1964b, pp. 13-21, 105-106) shows that the length of stay for a number of different medical or surgical conditions appears to vary systematically over hospitals. If a hospital tends to have longer than average stay for one category of patient, then it tends also to have longer than average stay for other categories. Furthermore, Revans shows that the average length of stay for several different kinds of nursing staff is also associated, negatively in this case, with the length of stay of patients. Hospitals with staff who remain at the hospital a long time – staff with presumably high 'morale' – are also hospitals with relatively short stay for patients. Revans suggests that the association between length of stay for patients and length of stay for nursing staff may be attributable to some organizational factor, perhaps 'atmosphere of the ward'.

Further analysis by Revans (1964b, pp. 78-90) has provided some elaboration of this relationship and its possible determinants. Sisters' perceptions of the approachability of their superiors, sisters' attitudes towards the integration of their student nurses, and staff stability and length of medical and surgical patients' stay show a significant pattern of relationship ('concordance') overall. However, the attempt to show a specific relationship between either of the measures of attitudes and either of the measures of patients' stay is not very successful. Only the correlation between sisters' attitudes towards the integration of student nurses and the mean period of stay for medical patients is significant just at the 5 per cent level.

Arguing from the tendencies displayed in his data, Revans sees the information in the organizational system as the crucial organizational factor. Thus, '... the sisters' attitudes to their subordinates will determine the amount of information passed, not only to the physicians but also to the paramedical units upon which the diagnosis and treatment of the medical patient so much depends' and 'it would also affect the solicitude that the student nurse would show to the patients' (Revans, 1964b, p. 83). This seems to suggest that the information and improved communications provided by the H.I.C. Project could have a possible effect on length of patients' stay in at least two ways: (1) the H.I.C. training and the hospital project work of the hospital-team members may have an effect on their own work efficiency – they may become better 'communicators' – and this will then affect the efficiency of their subordinates, and, eventually, patient-care (Links a and b in *Figure 12-1*); (2) the training and projects may also have effects upon the morale of those trained and, directly or indirectly, upon their subordinates, and eventually on patient-care (Links c and d or a, c, and d).

FIGURE 12-1 *Possible sequences for the effects of H.I.C. activity on H.I.C. outcomes*

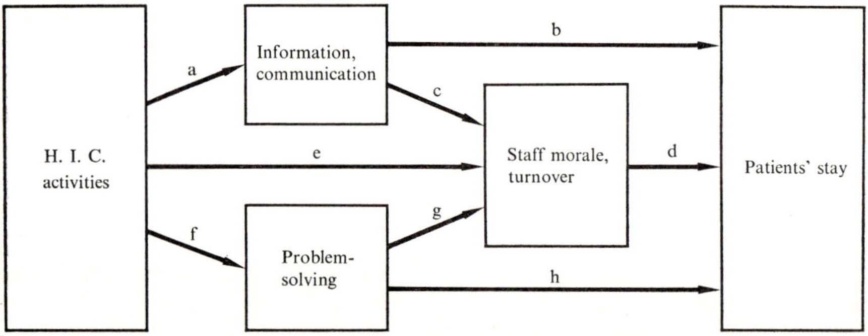


A third way is somewhat similar to the first in that efficiency is improved, but the means are different. Namely, hospital projects may be used to solve hospital problems that have been impairing the efficiency of patient-care (Links f and h, or possibly f, g, and d). These are not so much problems having to do with people and their attitudes towards work, but rather problems having to do with technology – patients getting lost because signposting within the hospital is not clear, records being mixed up because of confusions in report forms, in filing systems, or because of lack of storage space, etc. In other words, the hospital projects can solve problems that have impeded good, efficient patient-care.

The question for the present analysis is not a comparison *between* hospitals in the length of stay for various patients. The H.I.C. hospitals vary considerably in the types of patients they attract and the kind of work done by their staff. The basic question is instead, given the average length of stay of patients in each hospital, what changes have occurred within hospitals over the course of the H.I.C. Project? Has the length of stay for some, or all, categories of patients been reduced and, if so, by how much? In short, the hospital serves as its own control. How is each hospital doing now, compared with some earlier time?

Assuming that all other things remain equal or constant apart from the introduction of the H.I.C. Project, an increase (or decrease) in length of stay from before to after the Project is likely to be due to the effects of the Project. In stronger terms the question is, has the H.I.C. Project made the average length of stay longer or shorter *than it used to be* in that hospital?[1] However, all other things are not equal over time. In the last few years there has been a general tendency throughout England and Wales for the average length of stay to decrease for most categories of patients. This phenomenon should be evident in H.I.C. Project hospitals as well, suggesting that some proportion of the reductions found in H.I.C. hospitals may be due to the 'normal' course of events. New techniques of medicine, nursing, and administration are being continually introduced into hospitals, together with better facilities and better-trained staff, etc.

It is probably an impossible task to measure all these other factors and try to separate their effects on reduction of stay from those of the H.I.C. Project. Instead we shall compare the H.I.C. hospitals with another similar group of hospitals, which are presumably subject to the same 'normal' determinants of reduction in stay. Matching the H.I.C. Project hospitals with other hospitals on some key determinants of reduction in stay is one possible approach. Unfortunately, all of the major determinants of length of stay are not fully known, and consequently the dangers involved in a matching procedure are high (Campbell and Stanley, 1963). An alternative, more practicable, method is to compare H.I.C. hospitals with the average of all hospitals in the region in which they are located. The question at issue thus becomes not merely 'have changes in stay occurred in H.I.C. hospitals?' but rather 'are changes in stay in H.I.C. hospitals greater or less than changes occurring in their regions?'

The data utilized here are obtained from the Department of Health and Social Security Form S.H.3, submitted each year by all hospitals. This is a report of the gross patient statistics for the year, broken down into some thirty different departments, or categories of patients. In each hospital, we have utilized only those categories in which at least 500 discharges (or deaths) occurred in the comparison years. For most of the H.I.C. hospitals, these categories included (a) general medicine, (b)

TABLE 12-1 *Average Length of Patients' Stay for 1964, by Hospitals*[1]

| | Project hospitals | | | | | | | | | |
|---|---|---|---|---|---|---|---|---|---|---|
| *Patient categories* | *A* | *B* | *C* | *D* | *E* | *F* | *G* | *H* | *I* | *J* |
| General medicine | 28·66 (1505) | 23·23 (2571) | 24·58 (2576) | 24·38 (2433) | 23·22 (1547) | 20·00 (2216) | 16·88 (3817) | 18·55 (3511) | 16·52 (2411) | |
| Paediatrics | | 9·54 (385) | 12·29 (585) | 8·20 (276) | | 8·27 (871) | 12·08 (707) | 13·78 (970) | 8·09 (822) | |
| General surgery | 15·61 (1285) | 14·29 (2764) | 14·31 (2858) | 17·38 (2079) | 13·11 (1791) | 12·44 (1943) | 12·30 (3603) | 11·04 (4524) | 11·10 (3987) | 15.90 (500) |
| Traumatic and orthopaedic surgery | 62·00 (318) | 25·13 (628) | 18·57 (354) | 19·00 (1054) | 28·93 (320) | 19·00 (1078) | 16·94 (953) | 11·93 (1605) | | |
| Gynaecology | | 8·68 (1773) | 7·53 (1833) | 8·35 (1772) | 8·73 (1143) | 7·18 (2054) | 12·75 (829) | 8·97 (2837) | 5·53 (1564) | |
| Obstetrics | | 10·14 (2811) | 11·22 (2578) | 9·49 (2672) | | 9·32 (2879) | 11·00 (1294) | 9·30 (3020) | 8·93 (3591) | |

[1] First entry gives mean patients' stay in days; second entry, in parentheses, gives number of discharges during the year, upon which the mean is based. Blank cells in the table mean that those hospitals had no discharges in the particular patient category.

TABLE 12-2 *Average Length of Patients' Stay for 1964 by Regions and Nation*[1]

| | *Regions* | | | | | |
|---|---|---|---|---|---|---|
| *Patient categories* | *North-West Metropolitan Region* | *North-East Metropolitan Region* | *South-East Metropolitan Region* | *South-West Metropolitan Region* | *London Undergraduate Teaching Hospitals* | *England and Wales* |
| General medicine | 19·38 (50,981) | 20·38 (45,419) | 21·29 (37,674) | 19·63 (34,763) | 19·11 (44,966) | 17·88 (609,661) |
| Paediatrics | 10·12 (9,985) | 10·64 (9,748) | 11·49 (6,743) | 10·97 (5,636) | 14·98 (6,242) | 11·34 (132,664) |
| General surgery | 11·29 (71,647) | 11·68 (71,660) | 11·85 (60,545) | 11·92 (51,251) | 12·64 (58,251) | 10·98 (957,419) |
| Traumatic and orthopaedic surgery | 15·80 (22,945) | 20·63 (16,034) | 24·44 (18,095) | 18·78 (17,900) | 19·03 (13,125) | 18·54 (319,920) |
| Gynaecology | 8·39 (32,454) | 9·06 (25,807) | 9·22 (23,109) | 8·95 (21,312) | 9·41 (21,866) | 8·40 (379,827) |
| Obstetrics | 9·36 (47,030) | 9·59 (47,721) | 9·31 (35,630) | 9·59 (32,241) | 10·40 (26,186) | 8·80 (583,641) |

[1] First entry gives mean patients' stay in days; second entry, in parentheses, gives number of discharges during the year, upon which the mean is based.

paediatrics, (c) general surgery, (d) traumatic and orthopaedic surgery, (e) gynaecology, and (f) obstetrics. These categories will be presented in the tables accompanying this chapter. A number of the hospitals also had sufficient patients in (g) geriatrics, (h) ear, nose, and throat (tonsils and adenoids), (i) ear, nose, and throat (other), and (j) urology. Some total scores based on these four categories, together with the six already mentioned, will be presented in the text below.[2]

The next problem in the analysis is to determine the appropriate time periods for comparison. Because the data are only readily available in the form of yearly averages, year-to-year comparisons are used. The H.I.C. Project began in 1965, thus the previous year (1964) may serve as a baseline for comparisons. The H.I.C. Project presumably had no effect on the length of patients' stay during that year.

Probably 1967 is the best year for comparison with 1964, in order to measure Project effects on length of stay. Activities during 1966 may have begun to provide opportunities for changes in patients' stay. During this year, all of the hospitals started projects and, by about the middle of the year, the 'average' hospital had one project report in hand (the earliest was in January 1966, and the latest in January 1967). This, however, is not to say that these project activities had any marked effects during 1966 on hospital staff, other than team members, or on patients. Hospital-team administrative actions based on project findings may have occurred, on the average, from about the middle of the year onward, but more pervasive effects, through feedback of project findings and discussion groups among those studied in the project, would not occur in many of the hospitals until 1967. Consequently, if one considers the full possible array of project effects on changes in length of stay, the year 1967 is the most appropriate.[3]

*Table 12-1* shows the average length of stay for six major categories of patient in the H.I.C. hospitals during 1964. It may be noted that the length of stay for each category of patient varies considerably from hospital to hospital. General medical patients, on the average, stay as long as 28 days in one hospital and as little as 16 days in another. However, the prime focus of our interest is not these differences between hospitals, but rather the changes in the length of stay that are found in the same hospital during the course of the H.I.C. Project.

However, first let us look at the relationship between length of stay in H.I.C. hospitals and national and regional averages. The last, right-hand column of *Table 12-2* gives the national figures (for England and Wales) for patients' stay. Many of the hospital figures in *Table 12-1* show a longer average stay than for the nation as a whole (34 out of 44 departments with 500 discharges or more). The regional averages for the five regions relevant to the H.I.C. hospitals (in *Table 12-2*) are also generally longer than the national averages, so that H.I.C. hospitals may not be abnormal in this respect. In fact the figures in *Table 12-3* show that the average stay in H.I.C. hospitals is just as often shorter than the regional

TABLE 12-3 *Average Length of Patients' Stay for H.I.C. Hospitals Compared with Respective Regions, for 1964*[1]

| | Project hospitals | | | | | | | | | |
|---|---|---|---|---|---|---|---|---|---|---|
| *Patient categories* | *A* | *B* | *C* | *D* | *E* | *F* | *G* | *H* | *I* | *J* |
| General medicine | +9·03 | +3·60 | +5·20 | +3·09 | +1·93 | −0·38 | −2·23 | −0·83 | −2·86 | |
| Paediatrics | | (−1·43) | +2·17 | (−3·29) | | −2·37 | −2·90 | +3·66 | −2·03 | |
| General surgery | +3·69 | +2·37 | +3·02 | +5·53 | +1·26 | +0·76 | −0·34 | −0·25 | −0·19 | +4·22 |
| Traumatic and orthopaedic surgery | (+43·22) | +6·35 | (+2·77) | −5·44 | (+4·49) | −1·63 | −2·09 | −3·87 | | |
| Gynaecology | | −0·27 | −0·86 | −0·87 | −0·49 | −1·88 | +3·34 | +0·58 | −2·86 | |
| Obstetrics | | +0·55 | +1·86 | +0·18 | | −0·27 | +0·60 | −0·06 | −0·43 | |

[1] A positive sign indicates hospital length of stay is more than the regional average; a negative sign, less. Figures refer to patients' stay in days. Blank cells in the table mean that those hospitals had no discharges in the particular patient category for 1964. Parentheses indicate less than 500 discharges for the year.

TABLE 12-4 *Increase or Decrease in Average Length of Patients' Stay, 1964 – 1967*[1]

| *Patient categories* | *Project hospitals* | | | | | | | | | |
|---|---|---|---|---|---|---|---|---|---|---|
| | *A* | *B* | *C* | *D* | *E* | *F* | *G* | *H* | *I* | *J* |
| General medicine | −3·56 | −3·97 | −3·27 | −1·04 | −2·41 | −1·87 | −0·72 | −3·15 | −0·27 | |
| Paediatrics | | (−1·04) | +1·02 | (+1·76) | | −2·84 | −0·82 | −4·07 | −1·31 | |
| General surgery | +1·20 | −0·85 | −2·84 | −4·87 | +5·33 | +1·08 | −0·33 | −0·69 | +0·13 | −7·90 |
| Traumatic and orthopaedic surgery | (−12·89) | −1·74 | (−5·10) | +2·28 | (−9·40) | −3·20 | −1·23 | −1·80 | | |
| Gynaecology | | −1·33 | −1·00 | −0·96 | −0·35 | −0·08 | −4·06 | −1·10 | +0·46 | |
| Obstetrics | | −0·32 | −0·51 | −0·84 | | −0·32 | +0·85 | −1·64 | +0·15 | |

[1] A positive sign indicates an increase, a negative sign a decrease. Figures refer to patients' stay in days. Blank cells in the table mean that those hospitals had no discharges in the particular patient category in either 1964 or 1967 or both. Parentheses indicate less than 500 discharges in one or both years.

TABLE 12-5 *Increase or Decrease in Average Length of Patients' Stay, 1964 – 1967, by Regions and Nation*[1]

| *Patient categories* | *Regions* | | | | | *England and Wales* |
|---|---|---|---|---|---|---|
| | *North West Metropolitan Region* | *North East Metropolitan Region* | *South East Metropolitan Region* | *South West Metropolitan Region* | *London Undergraduate Teaching Hospitals* | |
| General medicine | −1·18 | −1·08 | −1·99 | −1·33 | −1·31 | −1·28 |
| Paediatrics | −1·62 | −1·44 | −1·59 | −1·57 | −3·08 | −1·84 |
| General surgery | −0·79 | −0·78 | −1·25 | −0·92 | −0·44 | −0·68 |
| Traumatic and orthopaedic surgery | −1·50 | −1·23 | −2·24 | −1·98 | −1·13 | −1·34 |
| Gynaecology | −0·69 | −0·96 | −0·92 | −1·35 | −1·11 | −0·80 |
| Obstetrics | −0·46 | −0·69 | −0·51 | −0·69 | −0·70 | −0·70 |

[1] A positive sign indicates an increase, a negative sign a decrease. Figures refer to patients' stay in days.

average as it is longer (23 out of 44 departments show shorter stay in H.I.C. hospitals). H.I.C. hospitals are apparently not atypical of the London metropolitan area, although they would appear to be atypical of the nation as a whole.[4]

*Table 12-4* shows the increase or decrease in average length of stay from 1964 to 1967 for the 6 different kinds of patient categories. Of all 44 departments (with at least 500 discharges or deaths), 35 show decreases in the length of stay in the H.I.C. hospitals, while 9 departments show increases. If other departments with at least 500 discharges are included, such as urology, ENT, etc., the record is much the same – of 49, 37 show decreases in length of stay. However, *Table 12-5* shows that the average length of stay in the regions in which H.I.C. hospitals are located is also decreasing in these patient categories, and it would appear that on the average the extent is generally comparable to the national decrease, and to the decrease in the H.I.C. hospitals.

The precise comparisons are made in *Table 12-6*; this shows the changes in length of patients' stay in H.I.C. hospitals, relative to the changes in their respective regions. In 21 out of 44 departments (about half) there are decreases in length of stay greater than the regional changes. Taking all departments with 500 or more discharges, the length of stay is reduced in 24 out of 49 between 1964 and 1967. Using all ten different kinds of patient category examined, and including departments with less than 500 discharges, we find similar results: reductions in length of stay in 35 out of 75 departments between 1964 and 1967. The comparisons of 1964 with 1965 and of 1964 with 1966 are very similar. In no case is there a statistically significant proportion of departments showing reductions in stay greater than the reductions found in the relevant regions.

The above analyses have considered changes in length of stay in the H.I.C. hospitals simultaneously for all departments with 500 or more discharges annually. While it would be capitalizing on error variance to select arbitrarily certain promising categories of patients for further analysis, Revans has provided some *a priori* arguments on this point in his earlier research. 'Socially dependent' categories are most sensitive to changes in the communication systems of hospitals (Revans, 1964b); included in the present data are two categories of patients that are socially dependent in Revans's terms – 'general medicine' and 'paediatrics'.

Looking at general medical patients, a test of the changes between 1964 and 1967 suggests that the differences found in average length of stay may be significantly greater than the changes in the regional averages (i.e. a Walsh test is significant at $p = \cdot 05$, one-tailed test). However, there is one possible question about this finding, and that is whether the data from one of the nine hospitals should be included in the test. This hospital is said to be 'unique', and comparisons with regional averages may be somewhat questionable. However, more doubtful than the validity of comparisons is the stability of the measures from this hospital, because length of stay of

TABLE 12-6 *Increase or Decrease in Average Length of Patients' Stay, Relative to Regional Change, 1964 – 1967*[1]

| *Patient categories* | *Project hospitals* A | B | C | D | E | F | G | H | I | J |
|---|---|---|---|---|---|---|---|---|---|---|
| General medicine | −2·23 | −2·64 | −2·09 | +0·95 | −0·42 | −0·79 | +0·59 | −1·97 | +0·91 | |
| Paediatrics | | (+0·53) | +2·64 | (+3·35) | | −1·40 | +2·26 | −2·45 | +0·31 | |
| General surgery | +2·12 | +0·07 | −2·05 | −3·62 | +6·58 | +1·86 | +0·11 | +0·10 | +0·92 | −7·12 |
| Traumatic and orthopaedic surgery | (−10·91) | +0·24 | (−3·60) | +4·52 | (−7·16) | −1·97 | −0·10 | −0·30 | | |
| Gynaecology | | +0·02 | −0·31 | −0·04 | +0·57 | +0·88 | −2·95 | −0·41 | +1·15 | |
| Obstetrics | | +0·37 | −0·05 | −0·33 | | +0·37 | +1·55 | −1·18 | +0·61 | |

[1] A positive sign indicates an increase in length of patients' stay relative to the change in the average patients' stay for the region in which the hospital is located. Thus a positive sign may refer to a *larger increase* in length of patients' stay than obtained in the region generally, or to a *smaller decrease* in stay than found in the region. The opposite obtains for negative values. The operation used was to subtract algebraically the regional average change from the hospital average length-of-stay change. Figures refer to patients' stay changes in days. Blank cells in the tables mean that those hospitals had no discharges in the particular patient category in either 1964 or 1967 or both. Parentheses indicate less than 500 discharges in either or both years.

its general medical patients varied markedly, both up and down, in the past few years (from 29 to 31 to 39 to 25 days in 1964, 1965, 1966, and 1967). If the 1964 to 1967 change score for this hospital (a net decrease of 2·32 days, over and above the regional decrease) is excluded, then the decreases in stay in the remaining eight H.I.C. hospitals are not significantly greater than the regional decreases in stay (see *Figure 12-2*). There is no firm

FIGURE 12-2 *Average length of stay 1961 – 1968 for general medical patients in H.I.C. hospitals*

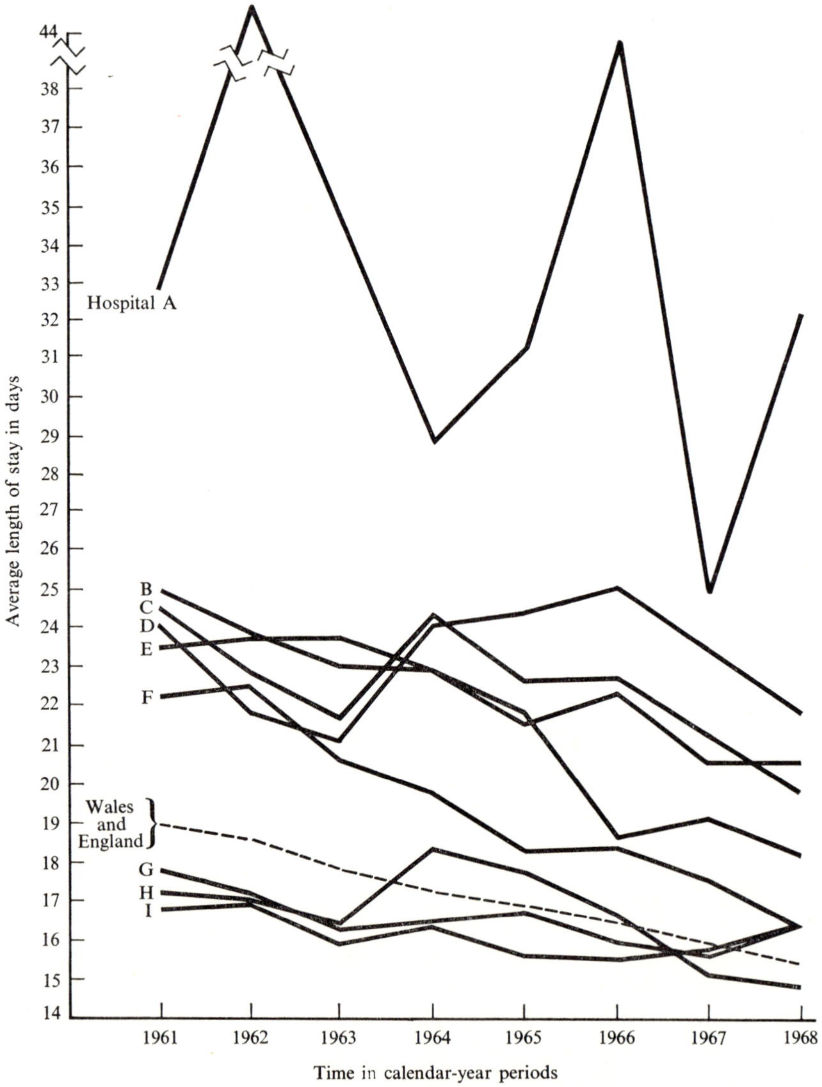

evidence that length of stay for general medicine has decreased as a result of the H.I.C. Project.

An examination of changes in stay in paediatrics and all other departments (utilizing hospital scores based on 500 or more cases per year) shows no other department that is significantly different from the average regional changes (two-tailed tests). Thus, the finding that one category of socially dependent patient (i.e. general medicine) shows decreases over and above regional decreases must be balanced against the lack of similar findings in the one other category with an *a priori* expectation of H.I.C. effects (i.e. paediatrics). Hence no general conclusion about decreases in the stay of 'socially dependent' patients can be reached.

There are a great number of possibilities that may help to explain the absence of significant decreases in length of patients' stay in H.I.C. hospitals, over and above regional decreases. First of all, the H.I.C. Project may have been ineffective. However, we shall show in subsequent chapters that the Project in fact has had some effects, at least on problem-solving and on communications.

Other possibilities rest more directly with the relationships demonstrated by Revans (1964b), and the related expectation for H.I.C. hospitals. The demonstrated relationships are correlations or associations and not necessarily direct causal relationships. It is possible that the association between nursing 'communication' and length of stay is produced by some third factor, such as the attitudes and behaviour of doctors, and that the associated factors are related in a 'spurious' way, being results of a common cause.

Alternatively, nursing 'communications' and morale may be directly related to length of patients' stay, but with the latter being the determinant. Revans suggests that the former determines the latter, but it is just as likely that hospitals that acquire efficient care and short length of patients' stay may subsequently show improvements in nursing 'communication' and 'morale'.[6] If length of patients' stay is the determinant, then improving communications by means of an H.I.C. Project may have little effect on stay.

In summary, Revans provides some data suggesting that organizational characteristics (such as 'communications' or certain attitudes) may be associated with the length of patients' stay and the stability of hospital staff. The H.I.C. Project is an opportunity to test this relationship and the causal assumptions involved. Data on length of patients' stay were gathered from H.I.C. hospitals for the year before change activities began and for the three subsequent years of H.I.C. activity. Most of the categories of patients examined showed reductions in average length of stay, but when these reductions were compared with changes in the hospitals' respective regions, H.I.C. hospitals appeared to be improving at much the same rate as the regions generally. A closer look at length of stay in general medical and in paediatric patients (since Revans views these 'socially dependent' patients as most likely to be affected by improvements in communications) also does not provide any clear evidence of decreases over and above regional decreases in stay.[7]

## NOTES

[1] In examining the length of patients' stay, we assume that a long stay is undesirable, wasteful, and to be avoided. An alternative view of the length of stay is that a shorter stay means that care of poorer quality is being given. However, Revans (1964b, pp. 128-132) provides some data showing that the mortality rates in long-stay and short-stay hospitals are the same. Our assumption is derived from studies of British length-of-stay statistics in relation to those of other nations, showing that British hospitals consistently keep patients in hospital longer (e.g. see Pearson *et al.*, 1968). The basic argument is that care in other countries does not seem to be appreciably worse despite the shorter stay, so that while shorter stay may not be better for the patient, it is at least not worse, and the savings obtained by shorter stay can be used to give better care to the nation as a whole.

[2] It should be noted that the analysis procedure followed at this point uses the patient category, and not the hospital, as the unit of analysis. There is some basis for this since such categories tend to reflect somewhat independent sub-units within the hospital system. Furthermore, since length-of-stay figures for different categories of patients tend to co-vary by hospital (Revans, 1964b), a hospital analysis should not provide widely differing results from the preliminary investigation here, as long as there are not widely varying numbers of categories from hospital to hospital – giving undue weight to some hospitals.

An examination of data (using Kendall's coefficient of concordance) for the six hospitals with all six types of patient categories, does not replicate Revans's findings (*see Table 12-1*). If, however, traumatic and orthopaedic surgery is omitted (because some hospitals have less than 500 cases), and a seventh hospital (which has cases in the five remaining categories) is added to the analysis, a significant coefficient of concordance results. A similar result follows from an analysis omitting both paediatrics and traumatic and orthopaedic surgery (because of low numbers of cases in both categories) and again using data from seven hospitals.

Since there is some evidence that length of stay is a hospital-related variable, one might ask whether *change* in length of stay is also hospital-related? In other words, do hospitals with relatively greater decreases (or increases) in length of stay (relative to regional changes) for one category of patient also show relatively greater decreases (or increases) for other categories? Tests utilizing the coefficient of concordance and the above three permutations of hospitals and categories fail to show a statistically significant relationship. An alternative examination of the possible relationships between absolute changes in length of stay, category by category, also yields no significant overall relationship. That is, the greatest decreases or increases in length of stay, across hospitals, are not necessarily in the same category of patient. Consequently, for simplicity, we examine changes in length of stay by category instead of hospital, even though either procedure would seem permissible.

[2] In addition, 1966 has been compared with 1964 in our analyses, but the results show no greater effects than those between 1964 and 1967.

[4] The former conclusion is rather important in the examination of hospital

changes or reductions in length of stay compared with the regional reductions. If H.I.C. hospital patients' stay is longer or shorter than for the 'average' hospital (as shown by regional figures), statistical regression may create an artificial impression that hospital scores are decreasing or increasing more than regional scores. Fortunately, the relative equality of hospital and regional scores in these data obviates any serious possibility of statistical regression effects on the general trend of changes.

[5] After the analyses for this chapter were completed, the figures for the year 1968 became available. These data for general medical patients are shown in *Figure 12-2*. When an analysis comparing hospitals with their respective regions is performed, no relative improvement in H.I.C. hospitals is demonstrated.

Also shown in *Figure 12-2* are the figures for 1961 to 1963. These figures show that the 1964 averages are abnormally high compared with 1961 to 1963, and, consequently, use of the 1964 base-line probably gives an overestimate of the improvements in length of general medical patients' stay obtained in H.I.C. hospitals between 1964 and 1967.

[6] A similar situation has been found in the study of 'human relations' practices in organizations. For a long time it was thought that certain supervisory practices would lead to higher performance. Recently it has been demonstrated that higher performance can strongly affect the use of human relations practices in supervision (Likert, 1967).

[7] Analyses identical to those in this chapter (but for 1964 to 1968, 1969, or 1970) yield no significant changes either for all departments or for general medicine or paediatrics alone. The only exception is a reduction in length of stay for general medical patients, from 1964 to 1970 ($p = \cdot 027$, one-tailed Walsh test).

# 13 Staff turnover and absenteeism

In this chapter, we continue our examination of the effects of the H.I.C. Project. As in the previous chapter, we shall find no clear-cut evidence for positive (or negative) H.I.C. results. The several analyses here, and in Appendix 13A, are first approximations, and we shall not advise the reader to view the findings of 'no H.I.C. effects' as definitive. The findings must be weighed in the light of the measurement problems encountered and the assumptions made.

The study of staff turnover should have a place in any evaluation of the H.I.C. Project because of the earlier research done by Revans (1964b) and its role in the genesis of the H.I.C. Project. As indicated above (Chapter 12), Revans showed in *Standards for Morale* that communications practices, staff turnover, and length of patients' stay are related to one another. There, and elsewhere (see, e.g., Revans, 1967), Revans argued that an improvement in communications practices in hospitals would lead to a subsequent improvement in staff-turnover rates (see *Figure 12-1*).

There is now additional research evidence that certain communications practices are associated with turnover and that these communications practices, in fact, determine or have a causal effect on staff turnover (Wieland, 1969c). Therefore, one could examine staff turnover in the H.I.C. hospitals for evidence of changes in communications practices induced by H.I.C. activity. This chapter will examine some of the indirect evidence on communications changes. However, it is more practical to examine communications practices directly, as will be done below (see Chapter 14), than to use an imperfect measure of communications such as turnover.

Another ostensible reason for measuring turnover is because of its value as an indicator of morale (or worker satisfaction), and because high morale may be a necessary condition for an effective organization.[1] That is, high morale may produce high-quality, efficient patient-care. However, this also is an inadequate reason for using turnover to evaluate the H.I.C. Project. First of all, the degree of evidence from Revans's earlier work (Revans, 1964b, p. 82) provides no firm support for an assertion that morale affects care. Furthermore, there is research evidence (see Kahn, 1960; Vroom, 1964; Likert, 1967) from a number of other kinds of organizations that suggests that morale is not a direct determination of effectiveness, but is generally only indirectly related to effectiveness. This indirect non-causal relationship occurs because both morale and effectiveness arise from aspects of organizational functioning, such as communications practices. This evidence from other organizations leads us to suggest that turnover may not be a direct determinant of hospital effectiveness or of the quality and efficiency of patient-care.

Because staff turnover is not as direct an indicator of the nature of staff communications practices as are measures of communications themselves, and because staff turnover is probably not a direct determinant of hospital effectiveness, we shall not place a great deal of emphasis on this aspect of assessing the H.I.C. Project. Turnover and associated staff morale or satisfaction can, of course, be of interest as ends in themselves (Wieland, 1969c), and it is in part for this reason that the analyses in this chapter are undertaken. But the indirect nature of the relationships between staff turnover and other important effects of the H.I.C. Project, together with our own observations and subjective impressions of the possible extent of H.I.C. effects on a staff turnover, have led us to place relatively less emphasis on this aspect of the evaluation compared with other aspects found in subsequent chapters. Measures of patient-care are certainly important, and 'communications', also, but in our view, measures of 'morale' are probably somewhat less important in ascertaining and assessing the effects of the H.I.C. Project.

The analysis here utilizes measures of absenteeism, as well as staff turnover, in assessing 'morale' (in the sense of work satisfaction). There is considerable research evidence indicating that turnover and absenteeism are related to each other, and to work satisfaction (Vroom, 1964; Lyons, 1966). The aim of the analysis is to examine absenteeism and turnover among those hospital staff who were most directly affected by the projects or studies carried out by H.I.C. team members. That is to say, we take some of the respondents in hospital project surveys, and their colleagues, and examine the changes in turnover and the absenteeism over the course of the H.I.C. Project. Some comparisons examine the changes between 1964 before H.I.C. started and the end of H.I.C. in 1968. Other comparisons deal with turnover rates during periods of high H.I.C. activity (such as 1966) and rates in earlier years. Finally, still further analyses (reported in full in Appendix 13A) deal with rates during and after those months in which data collection or feedback occurred in hospital projects, compared with some other equivalent time periods.

Turnover and absenteeism rates have been computed on a monthly basis, starting in July 1964 and continuing until July 1968 in most cases. Turnover is measured by the number of staff leaving the hospital, expressed as a percentage of the average number of staff employed during the period examined. In most cases, we compute the turnover rate for a particular grade of staff, such as sisters, rather than the hospital staff as a whole. Staff promoted from one grade to another are not counted as leavers. Years and quarters are the basic units of time utilized in the analyses.

Absenteeism is measured in terms of 'spells' or periods of absence from work. Each absence of one-half day or longer, no matter how many days in length, is counted as one spell of absence. The absence rate, or the average number of spells of absence per staff member, is calculated from the total number of spells for the particular staff category during a given period, divided by the average number of staff employed during that period. For some further analyses, absence rates for short spells of absence only are utilized. It is our expectation that shorter spells of absence – such as three days or less – will tend to reflect poor 'morale' rather than genuine sickness and longer spells of absence the reverse.

For the first set of analyses or comparisons, three increasingly inclusive sets of staff groups are utilized.[2] Comparisons are made year by year from mid-1964 until mid-1968, each year beginning in July and ending in June, and comparisons are also made between years before H.I.C. and years during, or after, the high of H.I.C. activity (i.e. between 1964 and 1967; 1965 and 1967; and 1964 and 1966). For each group, we ask whether turnover (or absence) increases or decreases between the two years compared. Assuming there are no long-term trends in rates of absence or turnover, and assuming all other things are equal, then those comparisons for years spanning or including the H.I.C. Project should show the effects of Project activity. Different groups of staff are the unit of analysis. By chance, in any comparison, half of the groups might show an increase in turnover, and half a decrease in turnover, but if the H.I.C. Project has reduced turnover then a statistically significant proportion of groups should show a decrease in turnover.

The primary comparisons are based on ten groups of nurses with the rank of sister or above, each group comprising at least thirty individuals. The secondary comparisons, including less 'pure' groups, utilize the first ten groups and an additional ten, making a total of twenty groups. These ten additional groups are either more heterogeneous (e.g. casualty department nurses including both the trained and the untrained), or homogeneous but not made up of nurses (e.g. medical records department staff, or porters). The tertiary comparisons involve thirty-one groups of staff, made up of the twenty groups just mentioned, and eleven other groups of smaller sizes with, consequently, more unstable and fluctuating levels of turnover or absenteeism (e.g. X-ray department staff, assistant matrons, etc.).

The eighteen different comparisons of turnover show only one 'suggestive' result. Of 20 groups of staff, 13 show an increase between 1964 and 1965, and 7 show a decrease ($p=0{\cdot}10$, one-tailed, by a binomial test; Siegel, 1956).[3] Unsupported by any other similar findings from comparisons between other pairs of years, this result may be due to chance. If enough comparisons are made, one is bound to be 'significant' by chance, and so we defer any conclusions until further data are examined.

The absence comparisons, however, provide some consistent but rather unexpected results. While the primary comparisons show nothing reaching significance, the secondary comparisons for 1964 to 1966 are suggestive, showing 13 groups with increasing absence rates, and 6 with decreasing rates ($p$=·08). The tertiary comparisons for the same two years, also show an apparent increase in 21 groups and a decrease in 9 groups ($p$=·02). These significant comparisons are quite pertinent, since they relate to the period during which H.I.C. Project effects manifested themselves – they reflect a change from immediately before H.I.C. began (the year beginning mid-1964) to the time when Project activities were at their peak (mid-1966 to mid-1967).

These findings are further supported by analyses of short spells of absence only. The primary comparisons for 1965 to 1967 show a significant pattern of increase ($p$=·01), as do the secondary comparisons for 1964 to 1966 ($p$=·02) and the tertiary comparisons for the same years ($p$=·002). In addition, the increases in the secondary comparisons for 1965 to 1966 are nearly significant ($p$=·06), while the tertiary comparisons are significant ($p$=·01). There is only one set of comparisons that shows a decrease (at $p$=·07), but this is between a year of high H.I.C. activity (1966-67) and a year of somewhat lower activity (mid-1967 to mid-1968). These findings suggest that the H.I.C. Project has had, instead of a beneficial effect on the absence rate, an adverse effect. One could speculate that perhaps the H.I.C. Project has 'stirred up' matters in the hospitals, increased tensions, and thereby increased absence rates.

There is, however, one serious question about the apparent finding of adverse effects from H.I.C. Almost all of the adverse comparisons are based on the year mid-1966 to mid-1967 as the year providing increased absence. If, for some reason other than H.I.C., this year showed an elevated absence rate, then the effects of H.I.C. and effects of the other determinants would be confounded, and no definitive statement of H.I.C. effects would be possible. In fact, the year under question spans a winter of extraordinarily high absence rates in the country as a whole – a severe winter with a high incidence of 'flu (see Johnson, 1968).

It is possible that the apparent adverse effects of H.I.C. on absence rates are due to this atypical winter. Firstly, turnover does not show similar adverse effects, although one might expect some correspondence. Secondly, absence comparisons between the year before H.I.C. (1964-65) and a year of relatively high H.I.C. activity (1967-68) do not show similar adverse effects, as one might expect if H.I.C. was creating tensions in the hospitals. We cannot be sure that the apparent adverse effects on absence during 1966-67 are due to the severe winter rather than H.I.C., but a subsequent data analysis provides a test of the effects of H.I.C. avoiding this confounding influence and showing that H.I.C. did not, in fact, increase absence.[4]

The analysis presented in Appendix 13A examines turnover and absence by quarterly periods, and compares rates before, during, and after the data-collection, reporting, and feedback stages of 17 different projects. Various 'simple' and 'complex' (difference-of-a-difference) analyses, at different calendar periods, provide some control of: (1) historically unique events contemporaneous with H.I.C. activity (e.g. the 'flu' in early 1967), (2) seasonal variation (especially evident in absenteeism), and (3) long-term, secular trends or changes in absenteeism and turnover rates. The analysis provides no evidence of either positive or negative H.I.C. effects. Although there may be some momentary turnover effects immediately before and during project data collections, and a perceptible, but short-term, reduction in absence rates at the time of feedback, the application of the above controls in various comparisons leads to a conclusion of no major long-term H.I.C. effects (positive or negative) on staff turnover and absenteeism.

In summary, the effects of the H.I.C. Project on staff turnover and absenteeism are studied because of the interest of various observers in staff morale. However, too great an emphasis should not be placed on any finding, either positive or negative, since neither staff turnover nor 'morale' are probable direct determinants of hospital effectiveness, as measured in terms of patient-care. Neither is turnover as good an indication of 'communications' as are direct measures of these phenomena. The view here is that studying turnover is valuable primarily to indicate levels and changes in staff satisfactions, which are valued as ends in themselves. This would be an important outcome of H.I.C., but perhaps not as important as some other outcomes, such as improved patient-care, or improved communications practices.

Absence and turnover rates are studied from 1964 to 1968 for a number of large, relatively homogeneous groups of staff, generally sisters, involved in projects or surveys in the hospitals. Year-by-year comparisons suggest an increase of absenteeism from before project activity started (the year starting in mid-1964) to the period of highest project activity in the hospitals (year starting in mid-1966). However, because many of the comparisons are based on one particular year, with an abnormally severe winter and high absence rate, these results are inconclusive. The turnover comparisons seem to show no effects, either beneficial or adverse.

Further analyses (Appendix 13A), using quarterly periods before, during, and after project events as bases for comparisons, control for various distorting factors including historically unique events. No major long-term H.I.C. effects are found. The general conclusion from the analyses in this chapter is: no major long-term H.I.C. effects, positive or negative, on staff turnover and absenteeism can be demonstrated.

## NOTES

[1] We take Revans's 'morale' to refer to an emotional state, not a motivational one, because the indicators of 'morale' used by Revans are turnover and absence (see, e.g., Vroom, 1964).

[2] There are a number of considerations that must be taken into account in selecting the appropriate staff groups for calculations of turnover and absenteeism. The ideal group would be large and homogeneous, with primarily

'voluntary' reasons for leaving or for absence. There would be moderately large rates of turnover or absence with no constriction of variation because the rate was close to zero. Finally, the group should be subject to fairly direct effects from the activities of the H.I.C. Project.

Ward sisters meet a number of these requirements. They are present in large enough numbers in each hospital to give fairly stable graphs of turnover and absence. Sisters are also fairly homogeneous in terms of experience. Unfortunately, however, the turnover and absence rates for sisters (or for any groups fairly high in organizational status) are relatively low in magnitude, and one must contend with a constriction of variation at these low levels. That is to say, if turnover is zero, then participation in H.I.C. activities cannot improve the turnover rate, for it can get no better than it is. The other important shortcoming in selecting sisters for the examination of turnover is that, in our view anyway, much of the turnover seems to be 'involuntary', due to retirement or marriage, for example.

These factors make it no great advantage to choose sisters instead of other groups, such as staff nurses, or students. However, the deciding factor is the relationship of sisters to the H.I.C. Project. Sisters may be expected to be directly affected by participation in H.I.C. Revans in his approach to organizational change emphasizes starting at the top of an organization, and sisters are often direct subordinates of – or one level removed from – the top-level participants in H.I.C. Furthermore, in almost every one of the H.I.C. hospitals, ward sisters have been involved in projects as respondents or recipients of 'feedback'. The H.I.C. emphasis on sisters and on ward studies is, of course, based directly on Revans's earlier research and publications and on the staff groups studied there. For these various reasons, ward sisters are the most commonly used group in the evaluation of staff turnover. Other staff groups used are staff nurses, assistant matrons, casualty department nurses, medical records staff, X-ray department staff, porters, etc.

[3] One-tailed tests are used since we expect H.I.C. to produce a decrease in rates of turnover or absence. A significant result in the opposite direction is embarrassing, but to revert to two-tailed tests here, and later, would be unfair to the H.I.C. Project and would make it relatively more difficult to demonstrate Project effects.

[4] The available data also permit a further analysis, controlled to some extent for long-term trends – or at least for those trends that are straight-line. Such control may be obtained by projecting trends from non-H.I.C. years to years during which H.I.C. Project activity occurred in the group studied. The projected turnover or absence rate (obtained by either extrapolation or interpolation) is compared with the obtained rate, the difference presumably reflecting the effects of H.I.C. Project activity on the group. Turnover data for two years more or less free from hospital project activity, and for an adjacent year during which there was project activity are available for six groups of sisters. To extend the analysis, three smaller groups of trained nurses (sisters and staff nurses) can be added. The results with respect to turnover, using either 6 groups or all 9, are equivocal, but with respect to absence the results are in the direction reported above – namely, the project seems to have affected absence adversely: 4 groups out of 6 show absence rates higher than projected, and 2 lower ($p=0.34$); using all 9 groups, 7 are higher, 2 lower ($p=0.01$).

Unfortunately, there is again a systematic bias in the comparison year during which project activity occurred. In most cases it is the year beginning July 1966, and encompassing the severe winter mentioned above. For this reason, the above results for absence are still somewhat equivocal, and conclusions must be deferred until later in this chapter when analyses controlled for this 'historical' source of error, in addition to the long-term (straight-line), secular trend errors and seasonal variation errors, that have been taken into account here, are reported.

# 14 *Hospital-team members and H.I.C. outcomes*

In this chapter we turn from relatively 'objective' evaluation data to more subjective data – ratings by H.I.C. participants. In addition, the focus is on outcomes that are more immediate than changes in turnover or length of patients' stay. Here, we shall be concerned with changes created by H.I.C. in the hospital-team members and those around them. As we understand the possible effects of the H.I.C. Project, these changes in hospital-team members are probably necessary, but not sufficient, conditions for more widespread organizational changes, such as changes in staff turnover or patients' stay.

In order to discuss the H.I.C. outcomes as hospital-team members see them, we will first have to examine the procedures used to obtain the data – the two surveys of hospital-team members by interview and questionnaire. In presenting the research design and methods, we also introduce the primary source of data for our subsequent examination of the determinants of H.I.C. outcomes. Even though special supplementary research instruments were developed to measure aspects of central-team functioning, project activities by central and hospital teams, and feedback meeting interaction, comparability between determinants of H.I.C. outcomes is obtained basically from the two broad surveys. Consequently, this chapter not only reports what the hospital-team members see as H.I.C. outcomes, but also introduces the reader to the bulk of the data and methods used in the remainder of this evaluation report.

In terms of substantive matters, we shall suggest that information characterizes the outcomes of the H.I.C. Project better than problem-solving – although both are reported to varying degrees by hospital-team members. Responses about work improvement and communications outcomes are on the average not wholly optimistic either, although again there is considerable variation in the reports.

## THE SURVEYS

Two surveys at widely spaced points in time were utilized to provide information on how hospital-team members saw the H.I.C. Project. The population for the 'first questionnaire' was defined as those members of

H.I.C. hospitals who were on the Project mailing list and were considered active hospital-team members by the Project secretary at the time of the survey (the period February to April 1967), a total of 72 individuals. Of these, 31 attended the one-month operational course, 26 the three-day appreciation course, 13 the two-day course, while 2 did not attend any course (43 per cent, 36 per cent, 8 per cent, and 3 per cent, of the survey population, respectively). The numbers in the three different professional categories were as follows: 28 in administration, 21 in medicine, and 23 in nursing (39 per cent, 29 per cent, and 32 per cent, respectively). There were from 6 to 10 team members in each hospital.

After a personal interview session with open-ended items, lasting on average 45 minutes, respondents were given a questionnaire to be returned by post to a private address. There was only one case of non-response (a refusal) to the questionnaire and a 100 per cent response for the interview.[1] Items from this first questionnaire are identified here by the prefix 'F' in the item numbers.

Respondents generally completed their questionnaires at some time during the period April-July 1967. Consequently, the data from the first questionnaire apply to events up to that time, but not afterwards. By the time the questionnaire was administered, H.I.C. courses were long since over, the first wave of students had come and gone, the second series of Project meetings had been completed, the third and fourth series of meetings had started, and the central team had been reorganized. All ten hospitals had completed one hospital project (in the sense of carrying out some 'feedback'), and eight out of the ten hospitals had completed or were completing a second project. This suggests that there was in fact something to assess at the time hospital members were asked to rate the effects of H.I.C. activities in their hospitals.

A second survey of hospital-team members was carried out in December 1968 and January 1969, at the formal end of the H.I.C. Project. The population surveyed included the 72 earlier respondents plus 21 new team members (identified from Project lists or informal contacts in the hospitals). After a short interview comprising three open-ended questions, and a series of precoded rating items on hospital projects, respondents were given the 'second-survey' questionnaire. Some questionnaires were completed on the spot, but most were mailed back. These items are identified by the prefix 'R'.

Excluding from the population those respondents not available because of death, the temporary nature of their assignment to H.I.C., illness, or other 'involuntary' reasons, there is a total of 87 in the population, and of these, only 3 are non-respondents, giving a response rate of 97 per cent for the questionnaire portion of the second survey.[2] The 84 respondents were made up of 35 administrators, 20 doctors, and 29 nurses (42 per cent, 24 per cent, and 34 per cent, respectively). There were 22 who attended the three-day course, 13 the two-day course, 30 the one-month course, and 19 who had not attended any course (26 per cent, 15 per cent, 36 per cent, and 23 per cent, respectively). To the first portion of the second survey, comprising the interview and the questions on projects, there was only one 'voluntary' non-response, giving a response rate of 99 per cent.

Most of the items in both questionnaires were Likert-type items with 5-point scales. Partially to keep the use of questionnaire space and respondents' time to economical levels, items were presented in a tabular format, with the same responses (e.g. 'much', 'some', etc.) applying to each item. A further reason for using a tabular format was that it facilitates comparisons between questions, and diagrammatic presentations of the comparisons. For purposes of analysis a series of similar items with identical response alternatives was extracted from the questionnaires, and the mean response for all respondents was entered on the numerical scale used by the

FIGURE 14-1 *H.I.C. Project Outcomes—Hospital, as Rated by Hospital-team Members*

(A diagram of mean responses superimposed on questionnaire items)

Taking into account *all* of the various H.I.C. projects and activities in this hospital, how much have the H.I.C. project activities involved each of the following? (Circle one number for each line)

| | *H.I.C. activities have involved:* | *Amount involved* *Very much* | *Much* | *Some* | *Little* | *None* |
|---|---|---|---|---|---|---|
| F72 | Giving the hospital H.I.C. team more knowledge about problems that exist in the hospital (3.5)* | 5 | 4 | 3 | 2 | 1 |
| F73 | Giving others in the hospital knowledge about problems that exist in the hospital (3.2) | 5 | 4 | 3 | 2 | 1 |
| F76 | Solving, or reducing, hospital problems (2.8) | 5 | 4 | 3 | 2 | 1 |
| F77 | Telling hospital staff that the top people are concerned about them and their problems (3.3) | 5 | 4 | 3 | 2 | 1 |
| F78 | Helping you and the hospital H.I.C. team to set right a number of problems (2.8) | 5 | 4 | 3 | 2 | 1 |
| F79 | Getting the people studied to work themselves on solving their problems (2.8) | 5 | 4 | 3 | 2 | 1 |

* The mean response for all respondents ($N$=62 to 66) is given at the end of each item.

respondents. For clarity, these mean values are linked by a line, allowing the reader to pick out easily those items given on the average either higher or lower values than other items (see, e.g., *Figure 14-1*).

For single non-tabular items, average responses (usually the mean, occasionally the median or 'middle', score) are reported in the text. Because means are sometimes misleading because of skewed or non-normal distributions or responses, and because the use of means involves assumptions of measurability not completely warranted by the data here, percentage distributions for the responses to items are provided in Appendix 14A.

## THE INTERPRETATION OF THE QUESTIONNAIRE DATA

Special care must be taken in interpreting or evaluating the meaning of the data described here. For the most part, an average rating of 'much', 'some', 'little', or an intermediate value will be reported for the various questionnaire items. For example, *Figure 14-1*, shows that respondents apparently felt 'giving the hospital H.I.C. team more knowledge about problems that exist in the hospital' was a factor with between 'much' and 'some' relevance to H.I.C. activities. On the 5-point scale from (5) 'very much' to (1) 'none', the average rating for all hospital-team members answering the question was 3·5.

To evaluate the meaning of the responses to this item, one must know if 'much' or 'some' are relatively 'good' responses or not. With the present data, the only way this can be done with confidence is to *compare* the responses to this item with those for another item having the same judgements (or words) as responses. In a sense, one ignores whether the average response is 'much' or 'some' or whatever, and instead concentrates on whether the average response for the item in question is greater or less (better or worse) than the average responses for other items. For example, in *Figure 14-1*, it becomes clear that the average response to item F72 is 'higher' or 'better' than for any of the other items in the figure. Comparison with other items shows that 'knowledge' (item F72) is felt to be more characteristic of the H.I.C. Project than, for example, 'problem-solving' (item F76).

This kind of comparison does not say whether the H.I.C. Project has provided more knowledge than some other alternative programme, such as a survey by management consultants. A comparison of H.I.C. with such an alternative would only be feasible if some of the H.I.C. Project participants (or a set of equivalent 'control' hospital staff) had been involved in an alternative programme, and comparable data had been gathered.

Similarly, the data described here cannot be used, at least in any simple, direct fashion, to determine whether the 'knowledge' (or 'problem-solving', etc.) situation in H.I.C. hospitals is now any better than before the H.I.C. Project began. Data collected both then and now, and using the same response alternatives ('some', 'much', etc.), would be necessary for this kind of comparison.

In spite of the inability to make these kinds of comparisons there is still much to be learned from the data presented here. Many comparisons between questions or items are possible. For example, one might ask whether courses are more useful than 'feedback' meetings, or vice versa? Have the administrative or the nursing members of the teams had more influence on H.I.C. activities? These and other questions can be answered by making comparisons between the average response for one item and the average response for another item with the same response alternatives.

To reiterate the main point, conclusions based on the average response (whether 'some', 'much', 'good', 'bad') to any one judgemental question *alone* can be misleading. Ideally, responses to items calling for judgements, such as 'some', should be *compared*, either implicitly or explicitly, to other items producing similar judgements as responses. Evaluations of more or less, or good or bad, can only be made with some comparative reference, and the most appropriate comparison is another item with the same judgemental scale.

## H.I.C. OUTCOMES–KNOWLEDGE, PROBLEM-SOLVING, AND INFLUENCE

In the first questionnaire, two sets of questions were asked to obtain some of the views of hospital-team members on the possible outcomes of the H.I.C. Project. The first set of questions (items F72-F80) was introduced by these words: 'Taking into account *all* of the various H.I.C. projects and activities in this hospital, how much have the H.I.C. project activities involved each of the following?' A list of possible outcomes from the H.I.C. Project (see *Figure 14-1*) followed together with rating scales from 'very much' to 'none'. In answering these questions, the respondent presumably took into account whatever he thought the H.I.C. Project had done in his hospital, whether for him personally or for others. The general perspective of the introductory statement was reinforced in each specific item by the mention of 'hospital' or 'those studied', etc.

*Figure 14-1* shows the mean responses for six items included in this first series of questions. Three items stand out with relatively high means – between 'much' and 'some'. All three of the items (F72, F73, and F77) deal with the provision of knowledge or information.[3]

The average ratings for items concerned with 'problem-solving' (items F76, F78, and F79) are not as high as the ratings of knowledge or information outcomes. There are a number of possible explanations to account for this lower rating. Perhaps the emphasis of H.I.C., as exemplified by courses, etc., is not on problem-solving, but on obtaining knowledge. A review of statements by Revans and others, and a review of the various project activities, however, shows that no such exclusive emphasis was made. One could also argue that, at this relatively early stage of the H.I.C. Project, team members had obtained some knowledge but had not yet had much time for problem-solving. This is probably a valid explanation to some degree, as is the next point. One might view these ratings of problem-solving achievements – 'some' tending in the direction of 'little' as being of possible concern to further users of the H.I.C. Project for improving their organizations. Project activities in the hospitals may make team members more knowledgeable about their situation, including bringing formerly hidden problems to light, but the H.I.C. Project for some reason may not help greatly to solve these problems (see also Chapter 4).[4]

FIGURE 14-2 *H.I.C. Project Outcomes—Personal, as Rated by Hospital-team Members*

(A diagram of mean responses superimposed on questionnaire items)

| How much has the H.I.C. Project affected *you* in the following ways? (Circle one number) | *Very much* | *Much* | *Some* | *Little* | *None* |
|---|---|---|---|---|---|
| F82 Giving you information about the functioning of the hospital generally (3.0)* | 5 | 4 | 3 | 2 | 1 |
| F83 Giving you information about the functioning of close work associates in the hospital (2.5) | 5 | 4 | 3 | 2 | 1 |
| F85 Increasing your influence over the functioning of the hospital generally (2.0) | 5 | 4 | 3 | 2 | 1 |
| F86 Increasing your influence over the work of close associates in the hospital (1.8) | 5 | 4 | 3 | 2 | 1 |
| F87 Providing you with solutions to some specific problems (2.4) | 5 | 4 | 3 | 2 | 1 |

* The mean response for all respondents (*N*=68 to 69) is given at the end of each item.

The second set of H.I.C. Project outcomes (see *Figure 14-2*) is obtained from the following question: 'How much has the H.I.C. Project affected *you* in the following ways?' This second set of outcomes is different from the first set above in that the effect of the H.I.C. Project on the respondent personally – on 'you' – is emphasized.

The two 'information' and 'knowledge' items (F82 and F83) in this set of measures are rated somewhat lower than the information or knowledge items in the first set. Perhaps the difference can be attributed to the fact that these items refer to the individual himself. The respondent may feel that others on the team or others in the hospital (the referents in the first set of outcome items) may have obtained more information than he has himself. An alternative explanation of the lower rating for these information items is that they refer to general information, while the first set of items refers to 'knowledge about problems'. Interview comments indicated to us that the H.I.C. Project might do a great deal to demonstrate the existence of problems, but that it was not quite as effective in providing the general information often needed to solve problems.

One should also note that 'information about the functioning of the hospital generally' is rated more highly than 'information about the functioning of close work associates' (3·0 and 2·5 respectively). Presumably this is because most of the studies or projects were about lower levels in the organization, and intermediaries or direct subordinates of team members were often bypassed.

Again, problem-solving is rated less highly than informational outcomes from the H.I.C. Project (item F87 is rated 2·4, compared to 3·0 for item F82). Seemingly one must infer that hospital-team members were somewhat more pessimistic about problem-solving outcomes than about informational outcomes (see Chapters 4, 5, and 6 for similar views and some recommendations).

Finally, two items (F85 and F86) in this set deal with changes or increases in the influence of team members over general hospital functioning, and over the work of close associates in the hospital. Both of these items are rated relatively low (2·0 and 1·8, respectively) by the respondents. Further details on first survey outcomes may be found in Appendix 14B.

## COMMUNICATIONS OUTCOMES

The three questions shown in *Figures 14-3* and *14-4* may be taken as indicating some basic aspects of 'communication' behaviour changed or improved in the participating individuals and their hospitals by the H.I.C. Project. One question deals with communicating to others, another with receiving communication (listening, etc.), and the third question with knowledge and understanding of others.

Each of the respondents in the second survey was asked to rate all of his hospital-team colleagues on these three characteristics (results only for the six course-defined roles are shown in the diagram). First of all, respondents were asked to rate the 'typical level' of functioning, so that subsequent ratings of 'change' would be facilitated. For example, how much does the administrator, who attended the 3-day course, communicate to others: 'very much', 'much', 'some', 'little', or 'none'? The average scores (when values

FIGURE 14-3 *'Communications' Behaviour and Changes in Hospital-team Members, as Rated by Team Colleagues*

(A diagram of mean responses superimposed on questionnaire items)

How much does each of the following H.I.C. team members typically *communicate to others—share information, provide explanations*? Please indicate first the typical *level* during the past 2 or 3 years, and then how much *change* (from whatever source) has occurred in the past 2 or 3 years:

| *Items* | | *This is the Typical Level:* | *Very much* | *Much* | *Some* | *Little* | *None* | *Amount of Change:* (Due to *all* causes, not only H.I.C.) | *Very much* | *Much* | *Some* | *Little* | *None* |
|---|---|---|---|---|---|---|---|---|---|---|---|---|---|
| R28, R39 | 3-day Admin. | (3.8)* | 5 | 4 | 3 | 2 | 1 | (3.0) | 5 | 4 | 3 | 2 | 1 |
| R29, R40 | 3-day Doctor | (3.0) | 5 | 4 | 3 | 2 | 1 | (3.0) | 5 | 4 | 3 | 2 | 1 |
| R30, R41 | 3-day Nurse | (3.4) | 5 | 4 | 3 | 2 | 1 | (3.4) | 5 | 4 | 3 | 2 | 1 |
| R31, R42 | Month Admin. | (3.6) | 5 | 4 | 3 | 2 | 1 | (3.2) | 5 | 4 | 3 | 2 | 1 |
| R32, R43 | Month Doctor | (2.8) | 5 | 4 | 3 | 2 | 1 | (2.9) | 5 | 4 | 3 | 2 | 1 |
| R33, R44 | Month Nurse | (3.4) | 5 | 4 | 3 | 2 | 1 | (3.5) | 5 | 4 | 3 | 2 | 1 |

How much does each of the following H.I.C. team members typically *receive communications* (listen, seek information from others, and appear receptive and open to new ideas)? Please indicate *level* and then *change* in past 2 or 3 years:

| | | *Typical Level:* | | | | | | *All Change:* | | | | | |
|---|---|---|---|---|---|---|---|---|---|---|---|---|---|
| R50, R61 | 3-day Admin. | (4.0) | 5 | 4 | 3 | 2 | 1 | (3.1) | 5 | 4 | 3 | 2 | 1 |
| R51, R62 | 3-day Doctor | (3.4) | 5 | 4 | 3 | 2 | 1 | (3.0) | 5 | 4 | 3 | 2 | 1 |
| R52, R63 | 3-day Nurse | (3.5) | 5 | 4 | 3 | 2 | 1 | (3.2) | 5 | 4 | 3 | 2 | 1 |
| R53, R64 | Month Admin. | (3.8) | 5 | 4 | 3 | 2 | 1 | (3.2) | 5 | 4 | 3 | 2 | 1 |
| R54, R65 | Month Doctor | (3.2) | 5 | 4 | 3 | 2 | 1 | (3.0) | 5 | 4 | 3 | 2 | 1 |
| R55, R66 | Month Nurse | (3.6) | 5 | 4 | 3 | 2 | 1 | (3.4) | 5 | 4 | 3 | 2 | 1 |

* The mean response for all respondents ($N=33$ to 52) is given to the left of each scale. In addition it should be noted that in the questionnaire, respondents were provided with the names of their hospital colleagues, written in after the titles '3-day admin.', etc.

of 5 to 1 are assigned from 'very much' to 'none') obtained from all those answering these questions are found in the middle of the diagram under the heading 'Typical Level'.

Communicating, listening, and having knowledge and understanding are all generally rated between 'much' and 'some' for most of the different roles in the hospital teams. The 'three-day' administrator, or the supporting-team administrator who attended the three-day appreciation course, tends to be rated 'much' on these three items, and at the other extreme, the

FIGURE 14-4 *Further 'Communications' Behaviour and Changes in Hospital-team Members, as Rated by Team Colleagues*

(A diagram of mean responses superimposed on questionnaire items)

How much does each have *knowledge and understanding of the behaviour of others*—of *what* people are doing and *why*, and *what they think and expect of him*? Please indicate *level* and then *change* in past 2 or 3 years:

| | | This is the Typical Level: | | | | | | Amount of Change: (Due to *all* causes, not only H.I.C.) | | | | | |
|---|---|---|---|---|---|---|---|---|---|---|---|---|---|
| *Items* | | | *Very much* | *Much* | *Some* | *Little* | *None* | | *Very much* | *Much* | *Some* | *Little* | *None* |
| R100, R111 | 3-day Admin. | (4.0)* | 5 | 4 | 3 | 2 | 1 | (3.2) | 5 | 4 | 3 | 2 | 1 |
| R101, R112 | 3-day Doctor | (3.3) | 5 | 4 | 3 | 2 | 1 | (3.2) | 5 | 4 | 3 | 2 | 1 |
| R102, R113 | 3-day Nurse | (3.5) | 5 | 4 | 3 | 2 | 1 | (3.3) | 5 | 4 | 3 | 2 | 1 |
| R103, R114 | Month Admin. | (3.6) | 5 | 4 | 3 | 2 | 1 | (3.2) | 5 | 4 | 3 | 2 | 1 |
| R104, R115 | Month Doctor | (3.4) | 5 | 4 | 3 | 2 | 1 | (2.9) | 5 | 4 | 3 | 2 | 1 |
| R105, R116 | Month Nurse | (3.6) | 5 | 4 | 3 | 2 | 1 | (3.6) | 5 | 4 | 3 | 2 | 1 |

* The mean response for all respondents ($N$=304 to 409) is given to the left of each scale. In addition it should be noted that in the questionnaire, respondents were provided with the names of their hospital colleagues, written in after the titles '3-day admin.', etc.

'month' doctor, or operational-team doctor who attended the month-long training course, tends to be rated 'some'. According to the results diagrammed, administrators in the hospital teams seem to be the 'best' communicators, or at least they are seen as doing more in the way of 'communication'. The medical members of teams are seen by their team colleagues as doing the least 'communicating', with nurse members in between.[5]

The right-hand side of *Figures 14-3* and *14-4* shows the 'amount of change' for the communication behaviour described in the questions. Respondents were asked to rate change 'due to all causes, not only H.I.C.', so one might take these ratings as an over-estimate, or an upper limit, for the changes created by the H.I.C. Project. The rating scale for 'change' was somewhat modified from that used for 'typical level', so that both positive and negative changes could be rated – from 'much increase' to 'some' to 'little' to 'no change' and finally 'decrease' in the particular behaviour. Overall, the ratings seem to indicate 'little' change, although some averages, for some hospital-team members, are between 'some' and 'little' change.

In terms of differences between team members in the amount of change, once again there is a fairly consistent pattern in all three questions. The 'month' or operational-team nurse is rated as having changed or improved in her communication practices most, of the six kinds of team members rated. Next, in extent of change, is the 'three-day' or supporting-team nurse (that is, the matron). After the nurses come the administrators, and finally the doctors, in showing improvements in their communication behaviour over the 'past 2 or 3 years'.

Of the three groups of staff, nurses, then, seem to have improved their communication behaviour most. While the average amount of change does not seem to be very great for most staff (i.e. 'little' change), for nurses it approaches 'some'. Communication changes are generally rated a little lower than some other outcomes such as increases in knowledge or information, although the questions here (with their somewhat different response scales) are not entirely appropriate for a firm conclusion in this direction.

## WORK IMPROVEMENTS

So far we have discussed changes in the communications behaviour of team members produced *presumably* by H.I.C. as well as by other factors. An attempt to compare the relative effects of H.I.C. and other factors would also be desirable. In the last section of the second questionnaire, respondents were asked to rate how much their work 'changed for the better or worse' during the last two or three years, because of participation in various kinds of improvement programmes other than H.I.C. (see *Figure 14-5*). Thus respondents were asked about changes due to courses of various kinds, improvement programmes within their hospital such as management by objectives, having the results of surveys, reading professional journals, etc. Finally, respondents were asked about work changes specifically due to '*participating in the H.I.C. Project*'. Here the question is explicitly about the value of the H.I.C. Project in comparison with these other factors.

*Figure 14-5* shows that courses are generally rated quite highly. 'Courses of all kinds (excluding H.I.C.)' are rated as having changed and improved the respondent's work 'somewhat' (a mean of 4·0). 'Management' courses and 'residential' courses are rated just as high, but 'interdisciplinary' courses rated rather lower.[6]

'Participating in improvement programmes within my hospital (e.g. in "management by objectives")' was rated as improving work as much as courses, namely 'somewhat'. Rated lower were 'having survey or project results from my hospital' and 'reading professional or hospital journals' (rated 3·7 and 3·8, respectively). Apparently of 'little' value in improving work was 'having survey or project results from other hospitals'.

Some other sources of possible work improvement – but not necessarily formalized, planned programmes of improvement – are included in the question for comparison purposes. These are generally rated lower than the activities specifically intended to bring about improvements in work behaviour.

FIGURE 14-5 *Hospital-team Members' Rating of the Effects on their Work of Various Activities, including Participation in the H.I.C. Project*

(A diagram of mean responses superimposed on questionnaire items)

There are many different ways in which hospital personnel may try to improve their work. In the following items, we are trying to learn about the effects of various activities, excluding H.I.C., which may have helped to improve the work.

During the last 2 or 3 years, how much has the quality of your work *changed for the better or worse* (in the widest sense) *because of the following*? (Please ring one answer for each line)

*My work has changed:*

| *Because of:* | | *Much better* | *Somewhat* | *Little* | *No change* | *Worse* | *Not done* |
|---|---|---|---|---|---|---|---|
| R290 | Attending courses of all kinds (excluding H.I.C.) (4.0)* | 5 | 4 | 3 | 2 | 1 | ND |
| R291 | 'Management' courses (4.0) | 5 | 4 | 3 | 2 | 1 | ND |
| R292 | Interdisciplinary courses (3.7) | 5 | 4 | 3 | 2 | 1 | ND |
| R293 | Residential courses (4.0) | 5 | 4 | 3 | 2 | 1 | ND |
| R294 | Participating in improvement programmes within my hospital (e.g. in 'management by objectives') (4.0) | 5 | 4 | 3 | 2 | 1 | ND |
| R295 | Having survey or project results from *my* hospital (3.7) | 5 | 4 | 3 | 2 | 1 | ND |
| R296 | Having survey or project results from *other* hospitals (3.1) | 5 | 4 | 3 | 2 | 1 | ND |
| R297 | Reading professional or hospital journals (3.8) | 5 | 4 | 3 | 2 | 1 | ND |
| R298 | Changes in (the nature of) my duties (3.4) | 5 | 4 | 3 | 2 | 1 | ND |
| R299 | Changes in facilities, equipment, or money (3.4) | 5 | 4 | 3 | 2 | 1 | ND |
| R300 | Changes in patient load or changes in patients (2.7) | 5 | 4 | 3 | 2 | 1 | ND |
| R301 | Changes in staffing (3.2) | 5 | 4 | 3 | 2 | 1 | ND |
| R302 | Changes in the functioning of superiors or peers (3.1) | 5 | 4 | 3 | 2 | 1 | ND |
| R303 | Changes in the functioning of direct subordinates (3.4) | 5 | 4 | 3 | 2 | 1 | ND |
| R304 | Participating in the H.I.C. Project in all its aspects (3.7) | 5 | 4 | 3 | 2 | 1 | ND |

* The mean response for respondents ($N$=40 to 81) is given at the end of each item.

With the above ratings as a comparison, it is interesting to examine the value placed on the H.I.C. Project by participants. 'Participating in the H.I.C. Project in all its aspects' (item R304) is rated about the same or a little less than either courses or participating in improvement programmes. Somewhat surprisingly, participating in the H.I.C. Project is rated only on a par with reading professional or hospital journals. On the positive side, the H.I.C. Project is rated considerably higher, or better, than having survey or project results from other hospitals.[7]

In general, it would appear that H.I.C. is not viewed with enthusiasm by hospital-team members as significantly more effective than most other improvement programmes. If anything, hospital-team members may perceive the more traditional approaches to change and improvement – courses – as very slightly more beneficial for their work than the H.I.C. Project.

Several other items scattered throughout the second survey questionnaire are suitable for use as measures of H.I.C. Project outcomes in the areas of work improvements and actions (see *Figure 14-6*). Items R214 and R215

FIGURE 14-6 *H.I.C. Project Outcomes—Administrative Actions and Work Improvements*

(A diagram of mean responses superimposed on questionnaire items)

| | *Very much* | *Much* | *Some* | *Little* | *None* |
|---|---|---|---|---|---|
| Two items dealing with a hospital project which respondents claimed to have the most knowledge about, in terms of data and reports produced: | | | | | |
| R214 How much *administrative action* on your part resulted? (2.8)* | 5 | 4 | 3 | 2 | 1 |
| R215 How important, or *how worth while* were the actions in the hospital taken as a result of the project? (3.4) | 5 | 4 | 3 | 2 | 1 |
| Three miscellaneous items: | | | | | |
| R236 How much are any changes made in *your work*, because of H.I.C., the 'right' changes (they won't have to be modified later)? (2.7) | 5 | 4 | 3 | 2 | 1 |
| R237 How 'right' are changes made in your *hospital* because of H.I.C.? (3.2) | 5 | 4 | 3 | 2 | 1 |
| R239 How much has the H.I.C. Project, in general, improved your work? (2.8) | 5 | 4 | 3 | 2 | 1 |

* The mean response for all respondents ($N=62$ to 82) is given at the end of each item.

are part of a series of items dealing with hospital project data and use of such data. The two items provide some evidence about the actions resulting from projects and the value of these actions. The results for item R214 corroborate the findings above that problem-solving was not a pervasive result of H.I.C. The average rating here for administrative action does not quite reach the level of 'some'. Even this may be an overestimate of the action taken, for respondents are answering for the one project, of all the projects in their hospital, with which they had the most contact and involvement. Projects with less involved team members may have produced less in the way of actions taken. Finally, however, it appears that when actions were taken, they were relatively 'worth while' (a rating of 'some' to 'much', or 3·4). Item R239, dealing with work improvements, is very similar to item R304, and not surprisingly, despite a change in the kinds of scale alternatives available, the average rating is very similar (2·8 or less than 'some' for R239, and 3·7 or less than 'somewhat' for R304). The remaining two items in *Figure 14-6* are used to examine feelings about the value of changes made because of H.I.C. One item – how 'right' were the changes in the work of the respondent (item R236) – is rated 'some' or a little less, on the average; while the other item (R237), dealing with changes in the hospital, is rated 'some' or a little more.

In general, hospital-team members are not very enthusiastic about the outcomes of the H.I.C. Project – at least in terms of the questions asked here about these outcomes. 'Some' is the usual answer for most items. Evidence will be provided in later chapters showing that there are some aspects of the H.I.C. Project which excite hospital-team members, but generally the outcomes of the H.I.C. Project do not arouse much excitement.

However, so far the discussion has been about average responses to items. The average ratings of 'some' are in fact often comprised of ratings of 'very much' by a few hospital-team members, as well as ratings of 'none' by other team members. To take item R239 for example – 'How much has the H.I.C. Project, in general, improved your work?' – the majority of team members answer the question with 'some' (41 individuals or 54 per cent), but there are 10 individuals (13 per cent) saying 'none', and, more important, there are 7 (9 per cent) who say 'much' and 5 (6 per cent) who say 'very much'.

How is it that some individuals report considerable benefits from H.I.C.? If one can maximize the factors creating this apparent benefit – whether the factors are characteristic of team members themselves, or perhaps of the way they went about participating in H.I.C. – then a subsequent H.I.C. Project, or one similar to it, can be rather more successful than the present one. The remaining sections of this report will be devoted primarily to this task. However, before attacking this problem, we must first examine the intercorrelations among the criteria used as measures so as better to understand their make-up.

## RELATIONSHIPS AMONG DIFFERENT CRITERIA

We have described so far some 20 different criterion measures for the H.I.C. Project. This number has been reduced somewhat by intercorrelation and selection of measures in limited and relatively defined clusters. Furthermore, examination of correlations with various determinants of H.I.C. outcomes provides information on redundant measures. By these procedures, some 16 measures have been selected for use in our analysis of the possible determinants of H.I.C. success. Details on the intercorrelations of most of the outcomes may be found in Appendix 14C. Here we shall summarize the main points and considerations in the examination of outcome intercorrelations.

Most, but not all, of the measures are interrelated; the more of one outcome reported by hospital-team members, the more of other kinds. To some extent these intercorrelations may be determined by 'halo' or response-set relationships 'in the head of the rater'. However, the absence of some relationships between items adjacent in a questionnaire – between items that could be evaluated similarly by respondents, as well as the presence of relationships between similar items despite measurement nearly two years apart – suggests that relationships in the data are based to some degree on valid observations.

In terms of the different patterns of relationships, there is some evidence that the above-termed 'problem-solving' (items F76, F78, F79, and F87) and 'administrative actions' (items R214, and R215) are similar outcomes. These are, in turn, related to another set of variables termed 'work improvements' (items R239 and R304).

In addition, acquiring 'information' about associates or others in the hospital (items F82, F83), and increasing one's 'influence' over these associates or others (items F85, F86), seem to be related to the above set of variables, but especially to making improvements in one's work. Finally, 'knowledge' about problems (item F72) shows some relatively limited relationships with several other variables.

One of the most important criteria for evaluating the H.I.C. Project must be the changes in the 'communication behaviour' of the hospital-team members. However, other H.I.C. measures show few significant correlations with these communications criteria. While this absence of strong relationships may be due in some degree to the nature of the construction of the communication items, other correlations elsewhere in the evaluation study suggest that this is not the full explanation. At this point we shall have to conclude tentatively that communications outcomes are apparently unrelated to many of the other outcomes from H.I.C. such as administrative action, problem-solving, and various kinds of information.

However there is an alternative explanation for the lack of relationship, namely the referent of the communication items – 'all' communication changes, whether due to H.I.C. or not. The absence of correlations could be due to the fact that other determinants are operating to create changes in team members' communication behaviour. In relation to these other determinants, H.I.C. may be a relatively insignificant factor. We turn now to make some comparisons of this nature.

## H. I. C. AND OTHER DETERMINANTS OF COMMUNICATION IMPROVEMENTS

*Table 14-1* shows that in fact many other possible determinants of improved communication (items R290 to R303) do not seem to be related to

TABLE 14-1 *Relationships between Various Determinants of Work Improvement and Changes in Communications Behaviour*

($N = 39$ to 80 individuals)

| | | *Changes in communication behaviour* | | |
|---|---|---|---|---|
| *Work improvements due to* | | *Change-communicate RC100* | *Change-listen RC260* | *Change-understand RC420* |
| R290 | All courses | ·18 | ·14 | ·16 |
| R291 | Management courses | ·14 | ·10 | ·21 |
| R292 | Interdisciplinary courses | ·12 | ·16 | ·30** |
| R293 | Residential courses | ·29* | ·19 | ·24 |
| R294 | Improvement programmes | ·27** | ·12 | ·38** |
| R295 | Survey in own hospital | ·31** | ·12 | ·19 |
| R296 | Surveys in other hospitals | ·06 | −·05 | ·04 |
| R297 | Journals | ·12 | ·02 | ·05 |
| R298 | Changed duties | ·01 | −·08 | ·00 |
| R299 | Changed facilities | −·02 | −·16 | −·07 |
| R300 | Changed patients | ·16 | ·03 | −·05 |
| R301 | Changed staffing | ·21* | ·21* | ·18 |
| R302 | Changed superiors – peers | ·29** | ·24** | ·30** |
| R303 | Changed subordinates | ·24** | ·25** | ·23** |
| R304 | H.I.C. participation | ·23** | ·19 | ·26** |

* Significant at a probability less than 10 per cent, two-tailed test.
** Significant at a probability less than 5 per cent, two-tailed test.

the improvements in communication measured here. More precisely, improvements in work behaviour produced by these various alternative improvement programmes, or changes in the hospital situation, are usually not related to improvements in communication behaviour.

Two significant exceptions do, however, suggest that the measures of improvements in communication behaviour are valid measures. 'Changes in superiors or peers' and 'changes in subordinates' are the two exceptions. The extent to which the respondents report improvements in their work because of these kinds of changes, is related to improvements in communication behaviour as observed by colleagues of the respondents. These correlations are not so extremely high that the alternative non-H.I.C., determinants of change explain or determine all of the variance in communication change, thus preventing any correlation between H.I.C. variables and communication change. Nor are these correlations so low that one can reject the communication change items as invalid and unrelated to any other variables.

The finding that there is little relationship between various H.I.C. criteria and general changes in communication behaviour must then stand. The lack of relationships cannot be explained by the invalidity of the measures of communications change, nor by the contamination of the measures by extraneous, non-H.I.C., determinants.

The general absence of other correlations in *Table 14-1* suggests that most non-H.I.C. kinds of programme to improve work behaviour, or other changes that improve work behaviour, apparently have little concommitant effect on improving communication. This, of course, must be a tentative conclusion, since a more proper way to examine this kind of relationship is to ask respondents to rate directly the improvements in communication because of various activities. Here, the question is about 'work improvements' due to these activities, and these work improvements are then related to communication improvements – a rather indirect approach to the problem, but more economical in terms of the numbers of questions required of respondents.

However, *Table 14-1* provides evidence that there are several kinds of improvement programme that may have an effect on certain kinds of communication behaviour. Namely, work improvements derived from participating in interdisciplinary courses do seem to include, or are related to, changes in the awareness of the behaviour of others. Participation in improvement programmes, such as management by objectives, would seem to have the consequence of improving work behaviour and apparently also changing and improving communication behaviour. Finally, having survey or project results from one's own hospital would also appear to create improvements in communication to others. In other words, if one is trying to improve communication behaviour of these particular kinds, then some of the improvement programmes mentioned above would seem to be likely means of facilitating improved communication.

Looking at the magnitudes of the different correlations with changes in communication behaviour (*Table 14-1*), it would appear that alternative improvement programmes are perhaps marginally more effective or better than H.I.C. in creating communication changes. That is to say, of all the alternative ways of improving awareness of the behaviour of others (item RC420), participating in improvement programmes such as management by objectives might be a better source of communication improvement than participating in the H.I.C. Project (r=·38 and ·26, respectively). Of course, as we mentioned above, these relationships are rather indirectly measured relationships, but the evidence we have available does suggest that a few specific alternative programmes may be more useful than H.I.C., at least for improving communication.[8]

This is not to say that participating in the H.I.C. Project is without effect on communication behaviour. There are some significant correlations between H.I.C.-determined improvements in work behaviour and improvements in communication behaviour. H.I.C. apparently did have some effect on communication. From *Table 14-1*, one would infer that H.I.C. had, perhaps, more effect than some alternative improvement activities but less effect than a few other improvement activities.

In summary, considering all changes in hospital-team members in communicating to others, listening, and understanding others, it would appear that some part has been played by the improvements in their work behaviour produced by H.I.C. Those team members who say that they have improved their work through participating in H.I.C. tend to be those who are also seen by colleagues as improving their communication behaviour. However, some alternative improvement activities may have a comparable and perhaps more direct effect on work behaviour and communication behaviour. If these observations, derived from an exploratory analysis, are valid, then programmes to improve communications behaviour like H.I.C. should emphasize activities such as interdisciplinary courses, management by objectives, and having the results of surveys in one's own hospital.[9]

In conclusion, in this chapter we have described the two surveys of hospital-team members, and the resulting measures of H.I.C. outcomes as seen by these participants in the Project. From the first survey, informational outcomes seem rather more evident, problem-solving less so, and changes in one kind of behaviour or relationship – influence over others – even less. The second survey provides data on hospital and work improvements, as well as communication changes. For the extent of the former outcomes, 'some' is on the average the best descriptive term, while for the latter, 'little' is more appropriate.

Further examination of the magnitude of H.I.C. outcomes is possible by looking at the effects of H.I.C. in improving the work of team members, compared with the effects of alternative improvement activities, such as attending courses. This comparison also shows the effects of H.I.C., as reported by the average hospital-team members, to be relatively modest. However, H.I.C. did have some positive effects – sometimes major – on the work, the problem-solving, and the communications behaviour of some of the team members, and a major part of the remainder of this evaluation report is devoted to examining the possible determinants of these effects.

One of the final sections of this chapter provides evidence about the relationships between various H.I.C. outcomes, including the finding that communications changes are generally unrelated to other H.I.C. outcomes such as problem-solving. The last section reports some evidence for the effects of H.I.C. participation on improvements in communications behaviour, as well as effects of participation in alternative improvement activities, such as courses, on the communications behaviour of the average hospital-team member.

## NOTES

[1] While the response rate to the questionnaire instrument is high, the inclusion of some respondents who had little interest, or had spent little time on the H.I.C. Project, undoubtedly raised the non-response rate for some items that were difficult to understand or not particularly relevant to someone who had loosened his ties with the Project. Many of the items had over a 90 per cent response rate, but some items had less. The percentage of responses for all items reported here and their item-alternatives may be found in Appendix 14A, and the interested reader may learn the non-response rate for any item by reference to these figures.

[2] Most of the non-response in the survey as a whole seems to have been truly 'unavoidable'. There was one death. One respondent changed hospitals, producing an artifact of non-response, since he did respond in the second survey, but was classed as a 'new' respondent. Two former respondents declined to respond because they said that their assignment to the H.I.C. Project was only 'temporary'. An examination of the job situation of one of the respondents at the time and of the statements of the other respondent to our interviewer in the first survey, indicates that these two respondents were, in fact, temporary. One individual was too ill to be interviewed, and another was working abroad and no forwarding address was available. Only three individuals seem classifiable as 'avoidable' or voluntary non-response. All three of these were three-day course (supporting-team) doctors. Unfortunately, since this survey came at the end of the Project, there was only a limited amount of time to try to get the less easily obtainable questionnaires.

[3] The percentage distributions, providing more precise descriptions of the responses are given in Appendix 14A.

[4] Another explanation for the relatively lower ratings for problem-solving compared to knowledge outcomes, is in terms of 'social desirability'. Respondents may feel that it is more acceptable to say that they have improved their knowledge. To say that one has solved problems to 'some' extent, for example, is to say there were, and may still be, problems existing in the organization – a not entirely easy thing to admit for some people. 'Loyalty' to one's own organization seems to be a rather strong norm among hospital people and would make it difficult to admit that problems did exist. These

points, of course, may apply to any of the ratings of 'negative' functioning found in this study.

[5] One may question whether the hospital-team members can validly rate one another on these factors. We shall present some relevant information below – intercorrelations among these variables – showing that there seems to be adequate discrimination between various rating targets, as well as correlations with other criteria, thereby demonstrating some validity for the items.

[6] Some respondents did not clearly understand the term 'interdisciplinary', it was learned during the course of the survey. The relatively low rating compared to other kinds of courses may be due in part to this lack of understanding.

[7] Respondents were instructed not to rate work effects if they had not participated in an activity. They ringed 'ND' for 'not done' instead. Because of this, there are varying numbers of respondents for different items. Since varying response rates together with the biases resulting from different groups of respondents might account for the differing average responses for items, all comparisons were calculated again, using only respondents who answered both of a pair of items. The same differences were obtained.

[8] The relatively larger correlations between alternative programmes and communications, compared with H.I.C. and communications, may be perhaps conservative estimates of the relative advantage of alternative programmes. In rating *all* communications changes, respondents may have thought of the H.I.C. Project scheme as they completed the questionnaire, and an unduly large amount of the variance in 'all' communications improvements may be due to this salience of H.I.C. for the respondents. If true, this would probably unduly inflate correlations between the communications ratings and measures of H.I.C. activity or effects.

[9] The analyses in this and subsequent chapters are for the most part individual-level analyses, using individuals as units of analysis (a notable exception is Chapter 18, which contains analyses with hospital projects as units of analysis). Analyses-of-variance by hospital, by course attended, and by tripartite group, were made for the sample of hospital-team members and were found to yield relatively few items with significant between-group variance (about 20 per cent of the items from the first and second surveys). The analysis-of-variance by course showed the lowest number of significant items (15 per cent, with most of them concerning the actual amount of effort put into hospital project activity such as administering questionnaires). The analysis-of-variance by hospital showed a larger number of significant items (22 per cent, with many of them concerning the amount or usefulness of central-team help). The criteria of H.I.C. effectiveness were generally not significant. The analysis-of-variance by tripartite group also showed a larger number of significant items (22 per cent, with some of them concerning the amount of central-team help received). More importantly, some of the H.I.C. criteria (dealing with problem-solving) were significant. Doctors tend to report fewer problem-solving outcomes than do nurses or administrators. Further data on doctors and problem-solving are presented in Chapter 18 (see especially *Table 18-3*).

In summary, evidence from analyses-of-variance seems to indicate that an individual-level analysis, rather than aggregating by course attendance, hospital, or tripartite group, is most suitable for the variables studied here, including especially the outcomes or criteria of H.I.C. effectiveness.

# 15 *H.I.C. activities*

In this chapter we begin the task of examining the H.I.C. Project in detail to learn about the specific factors and processes by which outcomes are attained. For almost all of the different outcomes examined in Chapter 14 at least a few, and often considerably more, Project participants report a relatively high level of outcomes. The question considered here is, how do these participants differ from other participants reporting relatively unsatisfactory outcomes? Is the extent of increased knowledge (or any other outcome) reported by participants related to the amount of hospital project work they did, or to the amount of contact with central-team members, or some other apparent 'cause'? By means of correlation coefficients, we shall examine the relationships between various aspects and activities of the H.I.C. Project and the possible outcomes of the H.I.C. Project reported above in Chapter 14.

The plan of this and subsequent chapters about the determinants of H.I.C. outcomes will be similar. For each area we shall look at the 'level' or extent of various determinants. For example, time spent on H.I.C. might be a determinant of H.I.C. outcomes, and so we shall first look at the average time spent on H.I.C. (it turns out to be about 2 hours per week). Then, secondly, we shall investigate whether those who spent more hours report more of various outcomes, than those who spent fewer hours. The relationships between determinants and outcomes will be assessed by means of correlation coefficients.

Each chapter, or section of a chapter, is prefaced by a summary of the major relationships found, accompanied by a simplified diagram (e.g. *Figure 15-1*). The reader interested in greater detail may turn to the summaries at the end of each chapter.

In the first section of this chapter, we shall see that those who rate courses as relatively 'useful' seem to have increased the information they had available. However, the 'usefulness' of courses is not related to problem-solving outcomes. Hospital-team members who rate the central team's help and formal meetings as 'useful' are those who report problem-solving outcomes (see *Figure 15-1*).

## H.I.C. PROJECT PROGRAMMES

Presumably the outcomes or achievements of the H.I.C. Project are deter-

FIGURE 15-1 *Project programmes and H.I.C. outcomes**

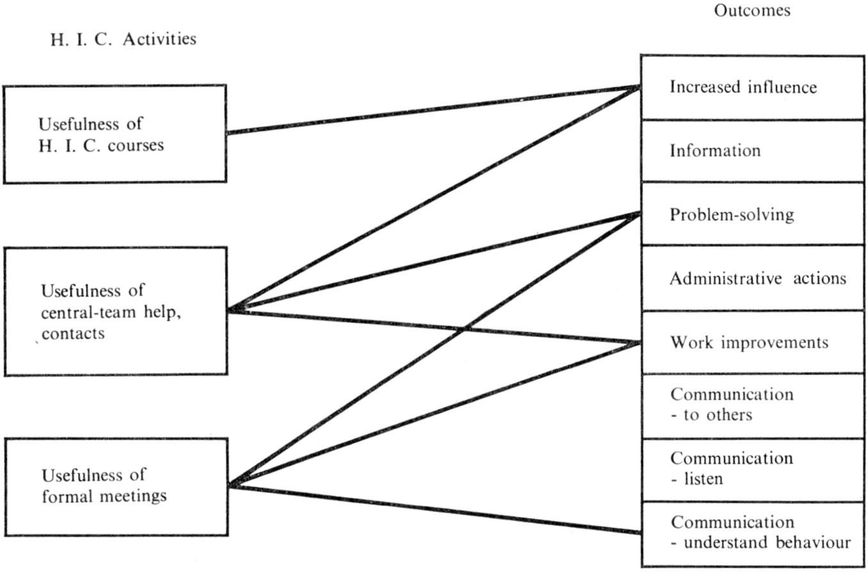


* Direction of causation assumed to be L → R; all relationships positive.

mined in part by the Project programmes, activities, and materials supplied by Revans and the central team. These include the courses given, the reading materials supplied, the meetings set up, and the advice and help given by the central-team members and students (see *Figure 15-2*). So far, we have seen that there are, on the average, some limited outcomes from the H.I.C. Project. However, whatever the degree of outcomes resulting from the overall Project, one may ask participants themselves to evaluate some of the aspects of the programme, so as to get an idea of the value of various activities to them irrespective of their value as judged by the particular criteria we have chosen.

*Figure 15-2* shows the rated value or 'usefulness' of the courses, and aspects of the courses, given during the H.I.C. Project. The ratings for the aspects of the month-long (operational) course seem to conform to the more descriptive, qualitative, views expressed by hospital-team members in discussions and interviews. The study papers are rated lowest (mean of 2·7, or less than 'some' usefulness), the formal lectures are rated considerably higher (mean of 3·6), and the informal discussions and the week spent at another hospital (during the practice project) are rated most highly, showing 'much' usefulness (3·9 and 3·8 respectively). The two items dealing with the three-day (appreciation) course are also rated relatively highly (3·7, 'much' usefulness).[1]

In addition to the relatively high ratings for the practice project and the informal aspects of the appreciation course and operational course items, there are two other items in *Figure 15-2* with relatively high 'usefulness'.[2]

FIGURE 15-2 *The Usefulness of H.I.C. Project Courses and Programmes*

(A diagram of mean responses superimposed on actual questionnaire items)

How useful have *you personally* found each of the following aspects of the H.I.C. project? (Circle one number for each line)

*Usefulness:*

| | | *Very much* | *Much* | *Some* | *Little* | *None* | *Not Done* |
|---|---|---|---|---|---|---|---|
| F90 | The formal lectures and formal activities at the month-long course (3.6)* | 5 | 4 | 3 | 2 | 1 | x |
| F91 | The informal contacts and discussions at the month-long course (3.9) | 5 | 4 | 3 | 2 | 1 | x |
| F92 | The week spent at another hospital (3.8) | 5 | 4 | 3 | 2 | 1 | x |
| F93 | The study papers used at the month's course (2.7) | 5 | 4 | 3 | 2 | 1 | x |
| F94 | The material presented at the 3-day appreciation course (3.7) | 5 | 4 | 3 | 2 | 1 | x |
| F95 | The informal contacts and discussions at the 3-day appreciation course (3.7) | 5 | 4 | 3 | 2 | 1 | x |
| F96 | H.I.C. conferences at which several hospitals have reported on their activities (3.1) | 5 | 4 | 3 | 2 | 1 | x |
| F97 | Informal contacts and discussions with people at *other* H.I.C. hospitals, since the month or appreciation course (2.6) | 5 | 4 | 3 | 2 | 1 | x |
| F98 | Meetings at your hospital with H.I.C. central team members (3.3) | 5 | 4 | 3 | 2 | 1 | x |
| F99 | Help given by Central H.I.C. staff in carrying out studies in your hospital (3.6) | 5 | 4 | 3 | 2 | 1 | x |
| F100 | Help given by Brunel student(s) in carrying out studies at your hospital (3.7) | 5 | 4 | 3 | 2 | 1 | x |
| F101 | Feedback meetings held at the Centre (3.1) | 5 | 4 | 3 | 2 | 1 | x |
| F102 | H.I.C.-initiated contacts with 'experts' from outside the hospital (work study experts, personnel from technical colleges, universities, etc.) (2.7) | 5 | 4 | 3 | 2 | 1 | x |
| R192 | How useful did you find London School of Hygiene meetings? (3.0) | 5 | 4 | 3 | 2 | 1 | x |

* The mean response for all respondents ($N=28$ to 62) is given at the end of each item.

TABLE 15-1 *Relationships between the Usefulness of Some H.I.C. Programmes and Course Aspects*

($N = 13$ to 29 individuals)

| | | *Usefulness of Course Aspects* | | | | |
|---|---|---|---|---|---|---|
| *Usefulness of H.I.C. Programme* | *Month formal F90* | *Month informal F91* | *Week project F92* | *Study papers F93* | *3-day material F94* | *3-day informal F95* |
| F96 Conferences | ·61** | ·44** | ·41** | ·55** | ·60** | ·61** |
| F101 Feedback meetings | ·49** | ·27 | ·09 | ·29 | ·75** | ·73** |
| R192 LSH meetings | ·04 | ·45** | ·46** | ·38* | ·72** | ·55** |
| F97 Contact with others | ·34 | 50** | ·29 | ·51** | ·22 | ·22 |
| F98 Meetings with central team | ·48** | ·53** | ·26 | ·10 | ·37* | ·03 |
| F99 Help of central team | ·28 | ·36* | ·28 | ·07 | ·50** | ·04 |
| F100 Help of students | ·40* | ·69** | ·19 | ·22 | ·79** | ·70** |
| F102 Contacts with 'experts' | ·19 | ·25 | ·06 | ·28 | ·64** | ·44* |

* Significant at a probability less than 10 per cent, two-tailed test.
** Significant at a probability less than 5 per cent, two-tailed test.

These are the 'help given by the Central H.I.C. staff in carrying out studies' at the hospitals, and similar help given by students attached to the hospitals (means of 3·6 and 3·7 respectively).[3]

A number of other aspects of the H.I.C. Project are rated somewhat lower, clustering nearer the middle point on the scale ('some' usefulness, with means from 3·3 to 3·0). These include meetings at the hospitals with central-team members, regional conferences at which several hospitals reported on their activities (the first series of Project meetings), the 'feedback' meetings at The Hospital Centre (the third series of Project meetings) and the London School of Hygiene meetings (fourth series of Project meetings).[4]

The two remaining items – namely informal contacts and discussions with people at other H.I.C. hospitals, and H.I.C.-initiated contacts with 'experts' from outside the hospital – are rated relatively low in usefulness. Both of these activities seem to have occurred relatively infrequently (26 per cent and 32 per cent, respectively, of all team members ringed 'not done'), and when these activities did occur, the ratings are not very high. The relatively low rating for contacts with 'experts' is perhaps due to the mixed reception that hospitals got from some technical colleges in the attempts by the H.I.C. Project to gain their co-operation. On the other hand, the relatively low rating of usefulness for contacts with other H.I.C. hospitals (item F97) is less understandable, and perhaps rather unfortunate, as one of the stated key aims of the H.I.C. Project was to encourage this kind of relationship between hospitals (see the Introduction to this volume). In the event, however, we shall see from our data that increases in the usefulness of this activity apparently would not have increased H.I.C. outcomes.[5]

The usefulness ratings for different aspects of the courses are consistently and positively associated with one another (r=0·33 to 0·68). No doubt this is partly because the items come close together on the questionnaire with a resulting response-set co-variance, and partly because it is difficult to distinguish different aspects of the courses.

Similarly the ratings for the usefulness of meetings, contacts, and sundry help provided by the central team are also all positively associated (r=0·28 to 0·78). *Table 15-1* shows the relationships between these two groups of usefulness ratings. The usefulness of the post-course conferences is consistently related to the usefulness of aspects of the courses, but the usefulness ratings for various activities provided by the central team show less consistent relationships with aspects of courses. In addition, there appears to be no connection between the usefulness of the week-long project or of the study papers, and any of the non-course activities.[6]

The next four tables provide some information on how the usefulness of different H.I.C. programmes might be related to various criteria of H.I.C. success. *Table 15-2* seems to indicate that those seeing the course activities

TABLE 15-2 *Relationships between the Usefulness of Course Aspects and First–Survey Criteria*

($N=23$ to 29 individuals)

| | First survey criteria | | | | | | | | |
|---|---|---|---|---|---|---|---|---|---|
| *Usefulness of courses aspects* | *Team knowl prob F72* | *Solve problems (hosp) F76* | *Help set right F78* | *Solve problems (own) F87* | *Get R's to solve F79* | *Info abt hosp F82* | *Info abt assoc F83* | *Incr infl gen F85* | *Incr infl assoc F86* |
| F90 Month formal | ·41** | ·24 | ·25 | ·11 | ·11 | ·43** | ·35* | ·23 | ·18 |
| F91 Month informal | ·36* | ·13 | ·34* | ·31 | −·09 | ·52** | ·29 | ·22 | ·07 |
| F92 Week project | ·17 | ·39** | ·50** | ·56** | ·22 | ·34* | ·61** | ·36* | ·30 |
| F93 Study papers | ·07 | ·27 | ·28 | ·30 | ·01 | ·26 | ·58** | ·21 | ·17 |
| F94 3-day material | ·17 | ·30 | ·34* | ·52** | ·18 | ·42** | ·57** | ·17 | ·44** |
| F95 3-day informal | ·02 | ·63** | ·41** | ·59** | ·34* | ·11 | ·38* | −·00 | ·10 |

* Significant at a probability less than 10 per cent, two-tailed test.
** Significant at a probability less than 5 per cent, two-tailed test.

TABLE 15-3 *Relationships between the Usefulness of some H.I.C. Programmes and First Survey Criteria*

($N$=34 to 64 individuals)

| *Usefulness of H.I.C. programmes* | | *First survey criteria* | | | | | | | | |
|---|---|---|---|---|---|---|---|---|---|---|
| | | *Team knowl prob F72* | *Solve problems (hosp) F76* | *Help set right F78* | *Solve problems (own) F87* | *Get R's to solve F79* | *Info abt hosp F82* | *Info abt assoc F83* | *Incr infl gen F85* | *Incr infl assoc F86* |
| F96 | Conferences | ·13 | ·33** | ·29** | ·34** | ·11 | −·02 | ·12 | ·18 | ·19 |
| F101 | Feedback meetings | ·28* | ·30** | ·34** | ·40** | ·20 | ·16 | ·08 | ·12 | ·23 |
| R192 | LSH meetings | ·12 | ·22 | ·36** | ·41** | ·13 | ·04 | ·22 | −·06 | ·20 |
| F97 | Contact with others | ·23 | ·01 | ·22 | ·22 | ·00 | ·26* | ·26* | ·11 | ·24 |
| F98 | Meetings with central team | ·34** | ·24* | ·34** | ·47** | ·16 | ·28** | ·19 | ·22* | ·33** |
| F99 | Help of central team | ·31** | ·26** | ·38** | ·56** | ·31** | ·17 | ·20 | ·12 | ·36** |
| F100 | Help of students | ·30* | ·28* | ·44** | ·53** | ·23 | ·34** | ·21 | ·19 | ·30* |
| F102 | Contacts with 'experts' | ·17 | ·05 | ·36** | ·41** | ·18 | ·32* | ·20 | ·34** | ·34** |

* Significant at a probability less than 10 per cent, two-tailed test.
** Significant at a probability less than 5 per cent, two-tailed test.

TABLE 15-4 *Relationships between the Usefulness of Course Aspects and Second Survey Criteria*

($N$=21 to 29 individuals)

| *Usefulness of course aspects* | | *Second survey criteria* | | | | | | |
|---|---|---|---|---|---|---|---|---|
| | | *Admin action R214* | *Worth of actions R215* | *Improved work R239* | *Improved work R304* | *Change-commun RC100* | *Change-listen RC260* | *Change-aware RC420* |
| F90 | Formal aspects – month course | ·21 | ·09 | ·11 | ·28 | ·57** | ·44** | ·48** |
| F91 | Informal aspects – month course | −·17 | ·05 | ·22 | ·62** | ·26 | ·11 | ·21 |
| F92 | Week project | ·27 | ·40** | ·40* | ·47** | ·31 | ·19 | ·39* |
| F93 | Study papers | ·42** | ·11 | ·25 | ·39** | ·55** | ·29 | ·42** |
| F94 | Formal aspects – 3-day course | ·23 | ·14 | ·48** | ·64** | −·16 | ·07 | −·05 |
| F95 | Informal aspects – 3-day course | ·28 | ·41* | ·43** | ·42** | ·05 | ·26 | ·22 |

* Significant at a probability less than 10 per cent, two-tailed test.
** Significant at a probability less than 5 per cent, two-tailed test.

as 'useful' also claim acquisition of more information and (not so consistently) also more solving of problems.

*Table 15-3* presents a more definite pattern of significant correlations, and indicates that the usefulness of meetings and of contacts and help provided by central-team members is quite consistently associated with the solving of problems. Less consistent relationships obtain between ratings of usefulness and ratings of (a) increased influence over associates, or (b) increased knowledge by the hospital team of problems in the hospital.

So far, it appears that something about the courses – their 'usefulness' – may facilitate the acquisition of information about the functioning of associates and others in the hospital. This is not very surprising in a course that is multi-disciplinary and requires hospital associates to spend at least several days together going over material, and attempts to communicate a great deal of information by lectures and discussions.

There is less evidence that certain aspects of the course (especially the week-long practice project) facilitate problem-solving in the hospitals. No doubt more than course attendance is required for much problem-solving to occur. The relationships between problem-solving and the usefulness of activities involving the central team may provide the beginnings of an answer to what 'more' is required. Some aspects of central-team behaviour may enhance the solution of problems within the hospital (for more details see Chapter 17).

The next two tables provide some evidence on the relationship of courses and other H.I.C. programmes to administrative action in the hospitals and to changes in work behaviour and in communication behaviour. There is some evidence in *Table 15-4* that those finding the courses useful (and especially the week-long practice project) are also those making changes in their work behaviour. However, the most surprising set of relationships in the table is between course usefulness and changes in communication behaviour. The significant correlations are found primarily in connection with the formal aspects of the month course. Those finding this activity useful are individuals seen by their colleagues as improving their communication behaviour. Rating the three-day course as 'useful' makes no difference to communication changes, however.

The main implication to be drawn from *Table 15-4* is that a course with the characteristics of the H.I.C. month-long operational course, offers a great potential for changes in the communication behaviour of participants. In fact, it will be seen that the correlations here obtained, with communications change variables, are some of the highest correlations to be found in this examination of the sources of communication change. It is unfortunate that more detailed and objective course measures are not available, so as to explain just what is meant by 'useful'.[7]

*Table 15-5*, the last in this series of tables on the relationship between H.I.C. programmes and H.I.C. outcomes, shows that the usefulness of meetings, contacts, and help provided by the central team is systematically

TABLE 15-5 *Relationships between the Usefulness of some H.I.C. Programmes and Second Survey Criteria*

($N$=30 to 61 individuals)

| *Usefulness of H.I.C. programmes* | | *Second survey criteria* | | | | | | |
|---|---|---|---|---|---|---|---|---|
| | | *Admin action R214* | *Worth of actions R215* | *Improved work R239* | *Improved work R304* | *Change-commun RC100* | *Change-listen RC260* | *Change-aware RC420* |
| F96 | Conferences | ·20 | ·22 | ·35** | ·44** | ·12 | ·14 | ·32** |
| F101 | Feedback meetings | ·28* | ·29* | ·46** | ·53** | ·04 | ·20 | ·31** |
| R192 | LSH meetings | ·09 | ·01 | ·44** | ·55** | ·01 | ·00 | ·09 |
| F97 | Contact with others | ·10 | ·05 | ·44** | ·54** | ·21 | ·15 | ·27* |
| F98 | Meetings with central team | ·23* | ·08 | ·36** | ·50** | −·03 | ·01 | ·15 |
| F99 | Help of central team | ·23* | ·10 | ·33** | ·36** | −·06 | ·06 | ·24* |
| F100 | Help of students | ·18 | ·16 | ·35** | ·62** | ·04 | ·20 | ·26 |
| F102 | Contacts with 'experts' | ·05 | ·14 | ·24 | ·50** | −·11 | ·12 | ·03 |

* Significant at a probability less than 10 per cent, two-tailed test.
* Significant at a probability less than 10 per cent, two-tailed test.

related to changes in the work behaviour of hospital-team members, even more consistently than was the case for the usefulness of the courses. But by and large, hospital-team members' view of these meetings and other help are unrelated to changes in communication behaviour. The only exception is in the case of changes in the knowledge and understanding of others. Those finding the post-course conferences, or the feedback meetings, relatively more useful are seen by their colleagues as changing and becoming more understanding of the behaviour of other people. While the correlations are not high, it should be remembered that the ratings of change in communications are ratings of 'all change', whatever the source – H.I.C. or not. The other correlations in this table involve criteria or outcomes specific to H.I.C. While the proportion of 'all' communication change created by various meetings may be relatively small, such change may be a direct outcome of these meetings, as are the other outcomes discussed above. We shall return (in Chapter 16) to the relationship between meeting usefulness and increases in awareness and understanding of the behaviour of others.

In summary, we find that hospital-team members generally value the H.I.C. courses quite highly; furthermore, those who see some aspects of these courses as especially useful are also (1) Those who claim increased information from H.I.C. and (2) Those who are seen by their colleagues as improving some of their communication behaviour. Contacts with, and help from, the central-team are also seen as relatively valuable by the hospital-team members, and this view is associated with reports of problem-solving outcomes, as well as changes in work behaviour. However, changes in communication behaviour, with the exception of changes in the understanding of others, seem to be unrelated to the usefulness of central-team help.

In contrast, the various formal meetings run by H.I.C. for hospital-team members seem of relatively low value to the members generally. But those finding these valuable are also those who tend to report problem-solving outcomes. Even more important, the meetings seem to offer the potential for changes in one particular kind of communication activity—the understanding and knowledge of the behaviour of other people. Finally, contact with other hospitals or between hospitals—one of the stated key aims of H.I.C. Project—is rated relatively low in usefulness and such usefulness is unrelated to H.I.C. outcomes.

## HOSPITAL PROJECT PARTICIPATION

Many of the above aspects or programmes of the H.I.C. Project are not unique. Meetings are part of the normal functioning of hospitals and courses part of the normal improvement programme for many professionals, although one may argue that the particular kinds of meetings or courses in H.I.C. are rather different from others. However, what is clearly unusual—

at least in the degree of its emphasis within the H.I.C. Project—is the active participation by hospital-team members in surveys or projects within their own hospitals. Furthermore, where H.I.C. courses or meetings were different from the more usual kinds of courses or meetings for hospital people, was in preparing hospital-team members to carry out project work —by teaching statistics, survey methods, etc.

In this section of the chapter we shall see that participation in projects by hospital-team members seems to be associated with some information outcomes, and also increases of team member communication to others (*Figure 15-3*). However, problem-solving seems to flow not from hospital-

FIGURE 15-3 *Hospital project participation and H.I.C. outcomes**

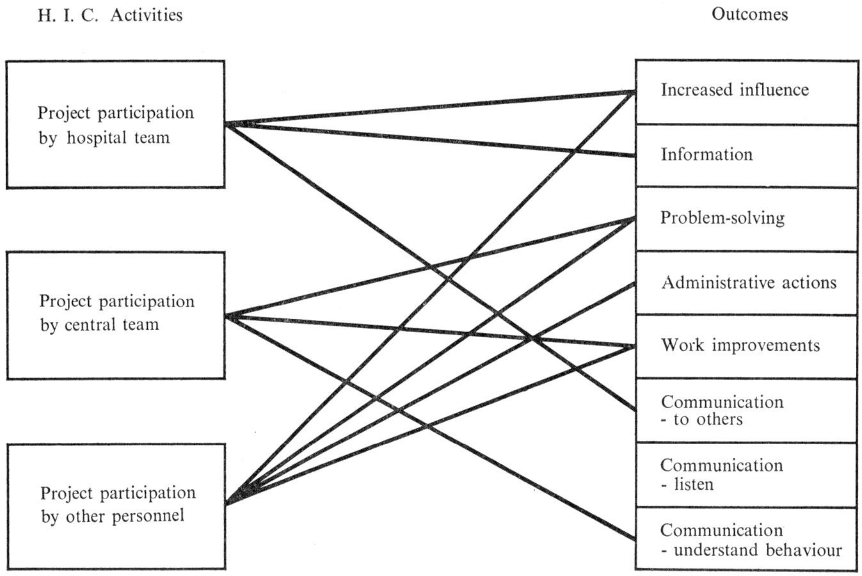


* Direction of causation assumed to be L → R; all relationships positive.

team members' involvement in projects, but from high involvement of the central team, and especially from the involvement of other non-team members in the hospital. On the basis of these relationships, and relationships with other outcomes, it would appear that the project participation by the central team and others in the hospital may be at least as important, if not more important, for H.I.C. success than is hospital-team members' participation.

*Figure 15-4* shows some items included in the first survey to obtain systematic information on the amount of participation by hospital-team members at various different stages of hospital projects. Respondents were asked to indicate 'how much work you, personally, did' on planning, interviewing, report-writing, etc. The relative order of the ratings for these items follows quite closely that given in Chapter 6 on project activities.

FIGURE 15-4 *Amount of Hospital Project Work done by Individuals*

(A diagram of mean responses superimposed on actual questionnaire items)

Now please indicate how much work *you personally did* on each of these activities: (Circle one number on each line)

*I worked on this:*

| | | *A great deal* | *Much* | *Some* | *Little* | *None* |
|---|---|---|---|---|---|---|
| F65 | A. Planning the problem and people to be studied (3.0)* | 5 | 4 | 3 | 2 | 1 |
| F66 | B. Planning the methods used (e.g. the questionnaire or observation methods used) (2.5) | 5 | 4 | 3 | 2 | 1 |
| F67 | C. Carrying out the study (interviewing, observing, etc.) (2.1) | 5 | 4 | 3 | 2 | 1 |
| F68 | D. Analysing the information gathered (2.1) | 5 | 4 | 3 | 2 | 1 |
| F69 | E. Writing the report (1.9) | 5 | 4 | 3 | 2 | 1 |
| F70 | F. Feeding the information back to those studied (2.8) | 5 | 4 | 3 | 2 | 1 |
| F71 | G. Participating in discussion groups with those studied (2.9) | 5 | 4 | 3 | 2 | 1 |

* The mean response for all respondents ($N=59$ to 63) is given at the end of each item.

Hospital-team members tended to participate relatively more during the early, planning stages or the later, feedback stages of projects, than during the intermediate stages.

Another adjacent series of first survey questions (not shown in the diagram) compared the proportions of work done by the hospital team and by the central team. Hospital-team members, in these items, see their team as doing on the average at least 'half' or more of the work at different stages in the hospital projects. 'Most' of the work was done by the hospital team—as opposed to the central team—in the early and late stages of a project, as has been described above. On the other hand, the central team did about 'half' of the work in the middle stages, particularly the work of collecting and analysing the data and writing the report.

A more important point, however, concerns the desire of hospital-team members in this matter. After the above series of questions, respondents were asked, 'Do you think the H.I.C. central staff should have done more work in any of the above activity areas?' Ten per cent of the answers are 'yes', indicating that there was some, but not much, desire for further help.[8] It is our impression from observing and talking to team members informally, that the hospital-team members wanted to do the work themselves, particularly at the earliest planning stages and at the feedback stage. Only in between, in the 'donkey-work' stages as the central team termed them, did hospital-team members want help, if at all. At least during 1967—the time of survey—hospital-team members felt they were doing 'most' of the project work, and for much of it they did not want further help.

In order to gain a more precise idea of the amount of work being done by hospital-team members, the first survey respondents were asked, 'On the average how much time per week have you devoted to H.I.C. matters *since* you went to the H.I.C. (3-day or month) course?' The distribution of responses to this question is given in *Table 15-6*. While there is considerable variation, many team members clearly spent very little time on H.I.C. activity. Over half of all team members spent two hours or less per week on H.I.C. If those saying 'don't know' or not answering the questions are disregarded, over two-thirds spent two hours or less.

TABLE 15-6 *The Average Number of Hours per Week spent on the H.I.C. Project*

| | *Number of hours spent** | | | | | | | | | *DK or NA* | *Total* |
|---|---|---|---|---|---|---|---|---|---|---|---|
| | *0* | *1* | *2* | *3* | *4* | *5* | *6* | *8* | *20* | | |
| Number of respondents | 12 | 12 | 15 | 4 | 6 | 2 | 1 | 2 | 2 | 16 | 72 |
| Percentage of all respondents | 17 | 17 | 21 | 6 | 8 | 3 | 1 | 3 | 3 | 22 | 100 |

* Rounded to the nearest whole number. The mean for the distributions equals 2·7 hours and the median equals 2 hours per week spent in H.I.C.

Clearly, this relatively small amount of time spent on H.I.C. must be considered as one determinant of the relatively low outcomes or low success for H.I.C. which we reported in Chapter 14.

Revans's idea was that participants would spend one-third or more of their time on H.I.C. work, but only two of the seventy-two spent that amount of time, and the great majority of team members fell far below Revans's original expectation. We shall see that time alone is not sufficient to obtain various outcomes from H.I.C., but in our view an adequate amount of time – more probably than was spent here – is a necessary condition for obtaining various outcomes.

The original plan of H.I.C. Project was that hospital-team members should do most of the hospital project work themselves, with only occasional advice by a few central-team members. Above, we reported that hospital-team members, on the average, felt that they generally did 'most' of the project work. However, as the H.I.C. Project developed, it became evident that hospital-team members were not progressing sufficiently quickly on their projects. Some team members seemed reluctant to call in central-team help, but when student help was offered (starting in mid-1966) a number of teams did accept extensive help by students on some of their projects, in addition to the continuing assistance of the permanent central-team staff. A series of questions was asked on the first questionnaire to assess the extent of central-team participation in the work at the hospitals. Although more detailed questions were subsequently asked about the specific kinds of help given by central-team members (see Chapter 17), the items below provide a summary statement of the degree of central-team participation.

Hospital-team members were asked about the influence of various individuals or groups of individuals on the H.I.C. work in their hospital (see *Figure 15-5*), and one of these questions referred to 'the H.I.C. central team—Revans, Smith, Bellaby, Leigh, Barnes and students' (see item F145 in *Figure 15-5*). Another item in the first survey asked, 'How much has the team relied on direction from the central H.I.C. team?' (item F136, *Figure 15-5*). In both cases the average answer is 'some'.

Perhaps the best assessment of the amount of 'influence' by the central team on H.I.C. activities in the hospitals can be made by comparing their influence with that of the hospital-team members *Figure 15-5* shows the central team, on the average, as having less influence than any of the month-course trained operational-team members, and only about the same amount of influence as the supporting-team administrators and nurses, who attended the three-day course. This influence is not negligible, but clearly the central team cannot be said to have 'run' the project work in the hospitals. As was intended, project work was under the primary control of the operational members, and then secondarily of the members of the supporting and central teams.

We shall shortly examine the apparent effects of the central team's influence on H.I.C. outcomes, but first there is one more category of individuals who may have influenced or participated in H.I.C. activities in the hospitals. These are, of course, hospital staff other than team members. Revans (1967) alludes to the question of other hospital staff when he speaks of the 'diffusion' problem—how to get other staff involved in a project (see also the Introduction). It is probably not absolutely necessary to involve other hospital staff in actual project work, particularly in the early stages of projects. Perhaps involvement could be delayed until the feedback stages of projects. However, in light of the frequent protests from hospital teams about lack of time to carry out projects, more involvement of others would have been of practical value as well as relevant to the problem of diffusion.

FIGURE 15-5 *H.I.C. Project Influence of Hospital-team Members and Others*

(A diagram of mean responses superimposed on actual questionnaire items)

For each of the following people, please indicate the *amount of influence* they have had on the *H.I.C. activities* in this hospital. (Do not rate general influence, see next question)

| *The influence of:* | | *Very much* | *Much* | *Some* | *Little* | *Very little* |
|---|---|---|---|---|---|---|
| F139 | Administrative—3-day course member (3.2)* | 5 | 4 | 3 | 2 | 1 |
| F140 | Medical—3-day course member (2.8) | 5 | 4 | 3 | 2 | 1 |
| F141 | Nursing—3-day course member (3.2) | 5 | 4 | 3 | 2 | 1 |
| F142 | Administrative—month course member (4.1) | 5 | 4 | 3 | 2 | 1 |
| F143 | Medical—month course member (3.4) | 5 | 4 | 3 | 2 | 1 |
| F144 | Nursing—month course member (3.7) | 5 | 4 | 3 | 2 | 1 |
| F145 | The H.I.C. central team—Revans, Smith, Bellaby, Leigh, Barnes, and students (3.2) | 5 | 4 | 3 | 2 | 1 |
| F146 | Hospital personnel who have not attended the H.I.C. courses (2.2) | 5 | 4 | 3 | 2 | 1 |
| F136 | How much has the team relied on direction from the central H.I.C. team (2.7) | 5 | 4 | 3 | 2 | 1 |
| F137 | How much has the hospital H.I.C. team involved others in the hospital in planning and carrying out H.I.C. activities? (2.7) | 5 | 4 | 3 | 2 | 1 |

* The mean response for all respondents ($N=50$ to 63) is given at the end of each item. The space at the end of each item was used in the actual questionnaire to give the names of hospital-team members in addition to the tripartite and course identification.

It is our impression that others in the hospital were in most cases only very reluctantly involved in H.I.C. work, if at all. This seemed evident from our earliest observations of the hospital projects.

The data here support these observations. Hospital-team members were asked, 'How much has the hospital H.I.C. team involved others in the hospital in planning and carrying out H.I.C. activities?' – and also asked about the influence of 'hospital personnel who have not attended the H.I.C. courses'. The average response in both cases varies between 'some' and 'little' (see items F137 and F146 in *Figure 15-5*).

In other words, compared to the various hospital-team members, or even the central team, other hospital personnel played a small part in the work of the hospital projects.

*Table 15-7* provides the intercorrelations for the items described above. As one might expect, the extent of participation at one stage of a project is generally related to the extent of participation at other stages, and participation at various stages is consistently related to the estimated weekly number of hours a hospital-team member spent on the H.I.C. Project. Judging from the magnitude of the correlations, participation in hospital projects seems to account for a relatively large proportion of the time devoted to H.I.C. This is probably because participation in one kind of project activity led an individual to participate in other kinds – there was not a great deal of 'specialization' in different stages of projects.

The amount of some kinds of project participation by hospital-team members tends to be negatively associated with central-team participation, as measured by the above central-team items (see *Table 15-7*). Apparently, the more a hospital-team member did in planning methods, collecting data, and writing reports, the less he accepted influence from the central team. Either one team or the other did this work. Presumably, hospital-team members doing this work felt that they had learned their lessons in the courses quite well; in a few cases perhaps, they were already experienced in these matters. They did not need any advice or help from the central team. Still another explanation for these negative correlations is that the nature of certain activities precludes co-operation with the central team or the exertion of its influence. This might be partly true for report writing, but it is likely that the explanation generally lies at least as much in the decision of the hospital-team member himself.[9]

The extent of involvement of other hospital staff, or their influence, appears to be generally unrelated to hospital-team or central-team participation, as measured by the above items. The only exception is participation by hospital-team members in feedback and in discussion groups. The more a team member does in these areas, the more he reports other staff were involved. While it is unfortunate that the participation of hospital-team members in other areas is not correlated with involving other hospital staff, participation in feedback and discussion groups would clearly appear to be desirable if H.I.C. is to involve the whole hospital.

TABLE 15-7 *Relationships among Measures of Hospital Teams and Central Teams' Participation in Project*

(*N*=49 to 65 individuals)

| | F65 | F66 | F67 | F68 | F69 | F70 | F71 | F159 | F136 | F145 | F146 | F137 |
|---|---|---|---|---|---|---|---|---|---|---|---|---|
| F65 Planning the problem | – | | | | | | | | | | | |
| F66 Planning the methods | ·79** | – | | | | | | | | | | |
| F67 Data collection | ·56** | ·72** | – | | | | | | | | | |
| F68 Data analysis | ·57** | ·58** | ·71** | – | | | | | | | | |
| F69 Report-writing | ·50** | ·54** | ·67** | ·73** | – | | | | | | | |
| F70 Feedback | ·53** | ·46** | ·35** | ·59** | ·48** | – | | | | | | |
| F71 Discussion groups | ·28** | ·25** | ·20 | ·34** | ·22* | ·72** | – | | | | | |
| F159 Hours worked at H.I.C. | ·36** | ·47** | ·44** | ·59** | ·56** | ·43** | ·40** | – | | | | |
| F136 H.T. reliance on directions by C.T. | –·09 | –·34** | –·28** | –·09 | –·29** | ·05 | ·13 | –·17 | – | | | |
| F145 Influence of C.T. on H.I.C. activities | –·10 | –·28** | –·30** | ·00 | –·28** | –·02 | ·06 | ·02 | ·68** | – | | |
| F146 Influence of hospital personnel | ·20 | ·10 | ·22 | ·21 | ·03 | ·40** | ·44** | –·09 | ·20 | ·13 | – | |
| F137 Involve hospital personnel | ·05 | –·04 | ·04 | ·14 | ·01 | ·26** | ·21 | –·02 | ·21* | –·01 | ·38** | – |

* Significant at a probability less than 10 per cent, two-tailed test.
** Significant at a probability less than 5 per cent, two-tailed test.

TABLE 15-8 *Relationships between Hospital and Central Teams' Participation in Projects and First Survey Criteria*

($N=52$ to 65 individuals)

| *Participation* | *First survey criteria* Team knowl prob F72 | Solve problems (hosp) F76 | Help set right F78 | Solve problems (own) F87 | Get R's to solve F79 | Info abt hosp F82 | Info abt assoc F83 | Incr infl gen F85 | Incr infl assoc F86 |
|---|---|---|---|---|---|---|---|---|---|
| F65 Planning the problem | ·29** | ·18 | ·17 | ·24** | −·07 | ·24* | ·11 | ·32** | ·18 |
| F66 Planning the methods | ·19 | ·09 | ·14 | ·24* | −·13 | ·31** | ·15 | ·15 | ·04 |
| F67 Data collection | ·13 | ·12 | ·24* | ·27** | −·11 | ·32* | ·31** | ·29** | ·16 |
| F68 Data analysis | ·25** | ·13 | ·17 | ·22* | −·10 | ·35** | ·32** | ·28** | ·18 |
| F69 Report-writing | ·24* | −·05 | ·07 | ·15 | −·14 | ·20 | ·16 | ·28** | ·21* |
| F70 Feedback | ·19 | ·08 | ·17 | ·21* | ·03 | ·22* | ·18 | ·20 | ·16 |
| F71 Discussion groups | ·30** | ·21* | ·16 | ·17 | ·18 | ·27** | ·28** | ·18 | ·08 |
| F159 Hours worked at H.I.C. | ·33** | ·04 | ·11 | ·11 | −·06 | ·46** | ·42** | ·31** | ·26* |
| F136 H.T. reliance on directions by C.T. | ·08 | ·33** | ·27** | ·29** | ·22* | ·08 | ·24* | −·04 | ·16 |
| F145 Influence of C.T. on H.I.C. activities | ·21 | ·22* | ·08 | ·12 | ·08 | ·19 | ·22* | ·01 | ·07 |
| F146 Influence of hospital personnel | −·03 | ·29** | ·25* | ·24* | ·21 | ·20 | ·27** | ·26** | ·24* |
| F137 Involve hospital personnel | ·10 | ·31** | ·25** | ·23* | ·35** | ·11 | ·30** | ·30** | ·28** |

* Significant at a probability less than 10 per cent, two-tailed test.
** Significant at a probability less than 5 per cent, two-tailed test.

Let us turn now to the relationship between project activity and the outcomes of H.I.C. *Table 15-8* shows that participation in various stages of project activity by hospital-team members seems to be associated to some extent with knowledge about problems, and with increases in information, as well as with some increases in influence generally (but not influence over associates). However, by and large, problem-solving outcomes are unrelated to this kind of participation by hospital-team members. The number of hours devoted to H.I.C. per week also shows the same relationships with the various outcomes measured in the first survey.

The relationship of participation to knowledge about problems, information, and increase of influence seems to be strongest for participation in the data analysis stage, and weakest for participation in planning of methods or in feedback stages of projects. In other words, increasing participation of hospital-team members in data analysis might increase their knowledge, information, and influence. However, increasing participation at any stage is not very likely to increase problem-solving outcomes.

Working with central-team members, in contrast, seems to facilitate problem-solving, but not the other outcomes cited above. Central-team influence or involvement seems to make little difference to information outcomes.

Finally, involving other hospital personnel also seems to facilitate problem-solving and also increases the influence of the hospital-team members. These are both very important areas in our view, and if our assumptions about casual directions are correct, the data provide strong reasons for involving other hospital staff in H.I.C. activities – in contrast to what was generally done in H.I.C.

*Table 15-9* shows the relationship between the various measures of project activity and the criteria measured in the second survey. For hospital-team members, only participation in feedback meetings and discussion groups seems to be related to the extent of administrative action resulting from projects. These two project stages are unique in requiring the involvement of others in the hospital, and not surprisingly it is this involvement of others (see items F146 and F137) that is consistently related to the extent of administrative action and the worth of those actions. To implement findings it would appear that involving others, perhaps in discussions and feedback meetings, is necessary.

When it comes to changes or improvements in work, there is some evidence that participation of hospital-team members in various project stages, as well as central-team involvement and the involvement of others in the hospital, are all related or beneficial. However, neither of the measures of improved work shows complete consistent relationships with each of the independent variables. The most consistent set of relationships for work improvement obtains with participation by hospital-team members in those stages involving the participation of others – the feedback and discussion stages. The importance of involving others to obtain practical, concrete

TABLE 15-9 *Relationships between Hospital and Central Teams' participation in Projects and Second Survey Criteria*

($N$=49 to 65 individuals)

| | Second Survey Criteria | | | | | | |
|---|---|---|---|---|---|---|---|
| *Participation* | *Admin action R214* | *Worth of action R215* | *Improved work R239* | *Improved work R304* | *Change-commun RC100* | *Change-listen RC260* | *Change-aware RC420* |
| F65 Planning the problem | ·16 | ·03 | ·12 | ·34** | ·21* | ·21* | ·10 |
| F66 Planning the methods | ·11 | ·05 | ·11 | ·29** | ·23* | ·18 | ·03 |
| F67 Data collection | ·10 | ·05 | ·17 | ·36** | ·23* | ·11 | −·01 |
| F68 Data analysis | ·20 | −·07 | ·26* | ·37** | ·28** | ·10 | ·15 |
| F69 Report-writing | −·01 | −·17 | ·09 | ·30** | ·26** | ·06 | ·03 |
| F70 Feedback | ·40** | ·14 | ·29** | ·25* | ·28** | ·16 | ·21 |
| F71 Discussion groups | ·39** | ·12 | ·36** | ·24* | ·26** | ·06 | ·20 |
| F159 Hours worked at H.I.C. | ·07 | −·10 | ·27* | ·42** | ·30** | ·12 | ·24* |
| F136 H.T. reliance on directions by C.T. | ·24* | ·02 | ·29** | ·08 | −·24* | −·05 | ·14 |
| F145 Influence of C.T. on H.I.C. activities | ·06 | −·15 | ·27** | ·15 | −·09 | ·06 | ·29** |
| F146 Influence of hospital personnel | ·26* | ·36** | ·36** | ·24* | ·01 | ·13 | ·19 |
| F137 Involve hospital personnel | ·28** | ·28** | ·28** | ·05 | −·09 | −·07 | ·05 |

* Significant at a probability less than 10 per cent, two-tailed test.
** Significant at a probability less than 5 per cent, two-tailed test.

outcomes—'work improvements'—is once more demonstrated by the correlations between items F146 and F137 and the relevant outcomes.

The participation by hospital-team members in various project stages also seems to encourage changes in communicating to others. Involving other hospital personnel does not seem to make a difference to these overall changes in communicating, while involving central-team members shows a similar lack of relationship. There is only one exception to the latter. The influence of central-team members on H.I.C. activities is positively associated with increases in understanding, as rated by hospital-team colleagues. We shall see that this relationship is supported by other data in Chapter 17.

Clearly, participation in hospital projects by central-team members and, especially, others in the hospital is more important for problem-solving, action, and work-improvement outcomes than is participation by hospital-team members. For hospital-team members to do project work in the hospital would seem to be valuable when the projects entail the involvement of others in the hospital – especially the feedback or discussion stages.

In summary, ratings of the degree of participation by hospital-team members in projects are relatively high for initial and terminal stages of project activity-planning and feeding-back. At intermediate stages hospital-team members played a less important role, on the average apparently comparable with the central team. The average hospital-team member devoted relatively little time to H.I.C.—two hours per week—but he seemingly did not want much additional help from the central team.

Compared to the operational hospital-team members the central-team on the average had less influence, perhaps about the same as the supporting-team members. Others in the hospital seem to have had considerably less influence than any of the hospital-team members, or the central team. Involving others or diffusing the H.I.C. Project in this way was apparently done to a very small extent.

The correlational evidence indicates that hospital-team members' participation in projects may facilitate increases in the influence of the participants, increases in information about the functioning of others, and knowledge about problems in the hospital, but apparently not the solving of problems. There is also a little evidence that participation in hospital projects may facilitate changes in the work behaviour of hospital-team members, and stronger evidence that it may facilitate changes in the extent hospital-team members communicate with others, though not by listening to them or understanding their behaviour.

In contrast, participation in project work with central-team members does not appear to be similarly related to acquiring information, knowledge, etc. Most importantly, working with and allowing some direction by the central-team, seems to facilitate the solution of problems. The effects of central-team involvement in project work also seem to include changes in hospital-team members' understanding and knowledge about the behaviour of others.

Finally, involving other hospital staff in projects would appear to facilitate problem-solving, administrative actions, work changes, and to increase the influence of hospital-team members—a very formidable array of outcomes.

## FURTHER DETERMINANTS OF H.I.C. SUCCESS

In this section we shall report on a number of further apparent determinants of H.I.C. success. These include various characteristics and behaviour of the hospital-team members themselves, as well as their views of some other aspects of the H.I.C. Project. One of the most important points is the relatively small extent to which hospital-team members made their own work part of the H.I.C. Project, and the great apparent potential of this factor in creating information, problem-solving, and communication outcomes (*Figure 15-6*). We shall also find that several other factors, including central-team support for the hospital-team and H.I.C.-derived improvements in relationships among hospital-team members are good predictors of problem-solving outcomes.

*Figure 15-7* shows the questions and the mean responses for the items in this section, while *Table 15-10* presents the intercorrelations, including

FIGURE 15-6 *Further determinants and H.I.C. outcomes**

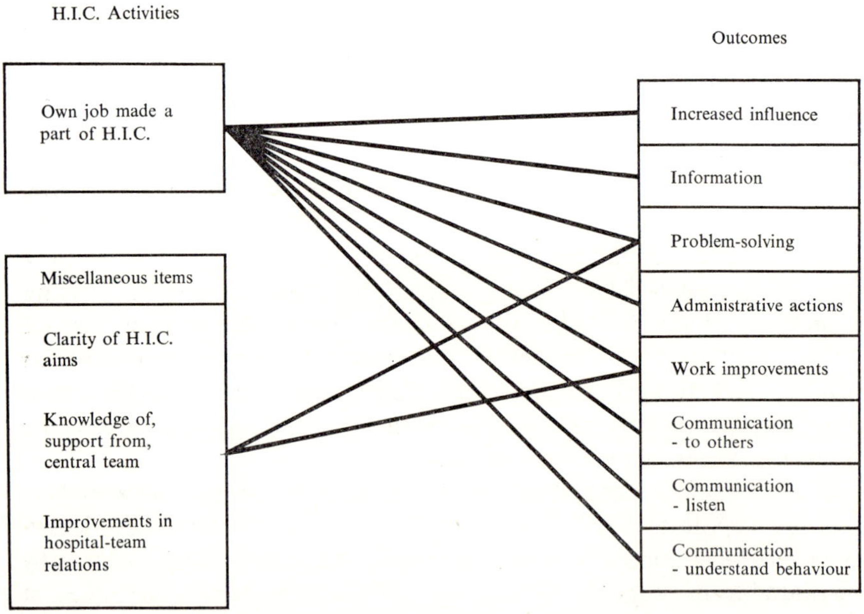


* Direction of causation assumed to be L → R; all relationships positive.

FIGURE 15-7 *Various H.I.C. Characteristics from the Second Survey*

(A diagram of mean responses superimposed on a selection of second survey questionnaire items)

| | | *Very much* | *Much* | *Some* | *Little* | *None* |
|---|---|---|---|---|---|---|
| R26 | How *desirous of changes* in your hospital are you? (4.1)* | 5 | 4 | 3 | 2 | 1 |
| R218 | To what extent did your H.M.C., and other policy-making people, have a favourable attitude towards H.I.C.? (3.6) | 5 | 4 | 3 | 2 | 1 |
| R219 | How *clear* were the aims of H.I.C. during the course? (3.0) | 5 | 4 | 3 | 2 | 1 |
| R220 | How clear later on? (3.5) | 5 | 4 | 3 | 2 | 1 |
| R221 | Were you able to work on your own particular job concerns as part of H.I.C. activities? (2.6) | 5 | 4 | 3 | 2 | 1 |
| R226 | Before, and during, these concrete changes, how much personal *contact* and support did you get from central-team members? (3.2) | 5 | 4 | 3 | 2 | 1 |
| R227 | How much did you generally feel you *knew* what central-team members (including students) wanted? (3.1) | 5 | 4 | 3 | 2 | 1 |
| | How much did each of the following *improve your relations* with the other hospital-team members: | | | | | |
| R229 | The H.I.C. course? (3.5) | 5 | 4 | 3 | 2 | 1 |
| R230 | Feedback meetings at the Hospital Centre? (2.6) | 5 | 4 | 3 | 2 | 1 |
| R231 | Doing projects in your hospital? (3.2) | 5 | 4 | 3 | 2 | 1 |
| R238 | How much interest do you generally display, in joining schemes like H.I.C., or of a similar nature? (3.6) | 5 | 4 | 3 | 2 | 1 |

* The mean response for all respondents (*N*=59 to 83) is given at the end of each item.

TABLE 15-10 *Relationships among Various H.I.C. Characteristics*

($N$=41 to 73 individuals)

| | *R26* | *R218* | *R219* | *R220* | *R221* | *R226* | *R227* | *R229* | *R230* | *R231* | *R238* |
|---|---|---|---|---|---|---|---|---|---|---|---|
| R26 Desire changes | – | | | | | | | | | | |
| R218 HMC favourable | ·06 | – | | | | | | | | | |
| R219 Clear aims (course) | ·42** | ·11 | – | | | | | | | | |
| R220 Clear aims (later) | ·39** | ·11 | ·43** | – | | | | | | | |
| R221 Job part of H.I.C. | ·38** | ·11 | ·16 | ·35** | – | | | | | | |
| R226 Central team support for concrete | ·22** | ·19 | ·22 | ·17 | ·38** | – | | | | | |
| R227 Knew central team desires | ·25** | ·28** | ·30** | ·24* | ·10 | ·52** | – | | | | |
| R229 Improve hospital team – course | –·08 | ·10 | ·19 | ·13 | ·01 | ·13 | ·14 | – | | | |
| R230 Improve hospital team – feedback | ·24** | ·15 | ·15 | ·24* | ·15 | ·52** | ·38** | ·46** | – | | |
| R231 Improve hospital team – projects | ·07 | ·27** | –·12 | ·03 | ·10 | ·36** | ·20* | ·56** | ·49** | – | |
| R238 Interest in schemes | ·35** | –·02 | ·12 | ·21* | ·44** | ·33** | ·28** | –·16 | ·01 | –·02 | – |

* Significant at a probability less than 10 per cent, two-tailed test.
** Significant at a probability less than 5 per cent, two-tailed test.

evidence for a number of interesting relationships. Hospital-team members desiring changes in their hospital (item R26) also report that they are generally interested in joining schemes like H.I.C. (R238), and those reporting either or both of these factors also indicate integration of their own work with H.I.C. activities (R221). This is quite important, for as we shall see, the degree to which one's job is made part of H.I.C. is a good predictor of improvements in communication behaviour. In general, there seems to have been considerable room for greater integration of job and H.I.C., since the average rating for this item is quite low ('some' to 'little', see *Figure 15-7*). Selecting H.I.C. hospital-team members from among those who desire changes, or those who generally display interest in joining similar schemes, might better assure that participants will make their jobs a part of H.I.C. and in so doing, ultimately improve their communication behaviour (see also Chapter 4).

Making one's job a part of H.I.C. is consistently associated with some of the most important criteria of H.I.C. success: solving problems, making changes and improvements in one's job, increasing one's influence over the functioning of others, and most importantly, improving communications behaviour (see *Tables 15-11* and *15-12*). Those who report making their job a part of H.I.C. are seen by their colleagues as communicating more to others, listening more to others, and being more aware of what others are doing. While desiring changes and being interested in improvement schemes are also related to some of these same criteria, and are therefore factors to be enhanced or included in any subsequent H.I.C. Project, they are generally not related to improvements in communication. The only exception is that those who generally join similar projects are also seen by colleagues as increasing their understanding of the behaviour of others.

Two questions on clarity (R219 and R220) were asked in order to obtain objective information on a topic frequent in conversations of hospital-team members. A number of team members claimed to be quite 'in the dark' about the aims of H.I.C., particularly during the course, and this relative lack of clarity during the early stages of H.I.C., compared with later, is confirmed by the average scores for the two items (see *Figure 15-7*). Lack of clarity during the course, however, does not seem to be detrimental to the various outcomes measured here (*Tables 15-11* and *15-12*). It is apparently clarity about H.I.C. aims later on, while projects are being carried out, that is important in solving problems and making work changes (for a further discussion of clarity, see Chapter 19).

Two important questions were asked about hospital-team members and their relations with central-team members—whether they got support from the central team when making 'concrete changes' in their work, and whether they knew what central-team members wanted (R226 and R227). As one might expect, the degree to which a hospital-team member makes his job part of H.I.C. is associated with getting support from the central-team in making work changes (*Table 15-10*). Furthermore, both getting such support and knowing what the central-team wanted are related to problem-solving and making work changes (*Tables 15-11* and *15-12*). This conforms to other analyses in this report (see Chapters 17 and 18), showing that central-team influence is generally beneficial, in terms of problem-solving and work improvement. Also consistent with any other analyses is some evidence that central-team activity is beneficial in changing hospital-team members' reported influence over the functioning of work associates, and, even more importantly, in improving hospital-team members' communication to others and knowledge and understanding of others' behaviour (see *Tables 15-11* and *15-12*).

By and large, the H.I.C. Project restricted its activity to hospitals; it went no higher in the structure of the hospital service. It is therefore of interest to examine briefly the relationship of the hospital management committees to the Project (item R218). These committees can be the most immediate barrier to any major improvement schemes in hospitals, since they hold the purse strings. Hospital-team members were asked for their perception of the degree of HMC favourability towards H.I.C., and not surprisingly, such favourability is positively associated with solving problems in the hospitals, although not with changes in the behaviour of hospital-team members.

One of the aims of the H.I.C. Project was to improve relations among team members—in part to get hospital-team members to act as a 'team'. By working together on the hospital projects they would be more successful in solving various problems in their hospitals, but in the process they would also improve their communications or relations with each other. Later, in Chapter 18, we shall examine some data on the extent to which 'teams' did exist, but here we shall look at some factors that might facilitate better relations among team members.

*Figure 15-7* shows questions on three different sources of improvement in relations among team members: the courses, feedback meetings, and hospital project work (items R229, R230, R231). The feedback meetings seem to have had little effect (for a more detailed evaluation of these meetings, see Chapter 16), while project work and, particularly, the courses seem, on the average, to have improved relations among hospital-team members. The residential nature of the courses probably facilitated improvements in relations. However, it should be remembered that the courses were the first H.I.C. activities producing intensive contacts between team members, and the relatively high rating for courses may be due in part to their being the first H.I.C. activities requiring teamwork. The correlations between the central team's support for concrete changes and improvements in team relations derived from feedback meetings or project activities (*Table 15-10*) suggest that the support received from the central team in those two settings may have enhanced relations. Alternatively, of course, it is possible that causation runs the other way. The creation of good relations may have facilitated the giving of support in these situations.

TABLE 15-11 *Relationships between Various H.I.C. Characteristics and First Survey Criteria*

($N$=42 to 63 individuals)

| | *First survey criteria* | | | | | | | | |
|---|---|---|---|---|---|---|---|---|---|
| *H.I.C. characteristics* | *Team knowl prob F72* | *Solve problems (hosp) F76* | *Help set right F78* | *Solve probs (own) F87* | *Get R's to solve F79* | *Info about hosp F82* | *Info about assoc F83* | *Incr infl gen F85* | *Incr infl assoc F86* |
| R26 Desire changes | ·33** | ·10 | ·31** | ·37** | ·10 | ·25** | ·28** | ·21* | ·30** |
| R218 HMC favourable | ·24* | ·42** | ·48** | ·13 | ·35** | ·26** | ·16 | ·10 | ·14 |
| R219 Clear aims (course) | ·12 | −·04 | ·08 | ·21 | −·10 | −·13 | −·13 | −·09 | ·18 |
| R220 Clear aims (later) | ·04 | ·22* | ·27** | ·30** | ·10 | ·03 | ·16 | −·02 | ·20 |
| R221 Job part of H.I.C. | ·20 | ·29** | ·40** | ·30** | ·10 | ·14 | ·32** | ·30** | ·18 |
| R226 Central-team support for concrete | ·10 | ·25 | ·56** | ·39** | ·16 | ·03 | ·25 | ·29** | ·39** |
| R227 Knew central-team desires | ·17 | ·40** | ·53** | ·41** | ·38** | −·05 | ·07 | ·13 | ·38** |
| R229 Improve hospital-team course | −·07 | ·05 | ·06 | ·14 | ·03 | ·31** | ·16 | ·24* | ·12 |
| R230 Improve hospital-team feedback | ·09 | ·22 | ·34** | ·33** | ·22 | ·29** | ·35** | ·21 | ·32** |
| R231 Improve hospital-team projects | ·02 | ·25* | ·29** | ·23* | ·13 | ·41** | ·36** | ·26* | ·27** |
| R238 Interest in schemes | ·15 | ·20 | ·20 | ·16 | ·20 | −·21 | ·05 | ·21 | ·25** |

* Significant at a probability less than 10 per cent, two-tailed test.
** Significant at a probability less than 5 per cent, two-tailed test.

TABLE 15-12 *Relationships between various H.I.C. Characteristics and Second Survey Criteria*

($N$=53 to 82 individuals)

| *H.I.C. characteristics* | | *Second Survey Criteria* | | | | | | |
|---|---|---|---|---|---|---|---|---|
| | | *Admin action R214* | *Worth of actions R215* | *Improved work R239* | *Improved work R304* | *Change-commun RC100* | *Change-listen RC260* | *Change-aware RC420* |
| R26 | Desire changes | ·32** | ·14 | ·28** | ·31** | ·07 | ·02 | ·14 |
| R218 | H.M.C. favourable | ·10 | ·28** | ·14 | ·15 | −·03 | ·02 | ·02 |
| R219 | Clear aims (course) | ·30** | ·15 | ·22* | ·15 | −·11 | ·01 | ·10 |
| R220 | Clear aims (later) | ·31** | ·31** | ·41** | ·35** | ·07 | ·15 | ·20* |
| R221 | Job part of H.I.C. | ·56** | ·24** | ·46** | ·39** | ·24** | ·25** | ·38** |
| R226 | Central-team support for concrete | ·48** | ·19 | ·23* | ·28** | ·14 | ·21 | ·35** |
| R227 | Knew central-team desires | ·30** | ·12 | ·21** | ·27** | −·01 | ·15 | ·10 |
| R229 | Improve hospital-team – course | −·15 | ·07 | ·29** | ·39** | −·00 | −·00 | ·05 |
| R230 | Improve hospital-team – feedback | ·12 | ·01 | ·46** | ·55** | ·05 | ·05 | ·20* |
| R231 | Improve hospital-team – projects | −·00 | ·05 | ·37** | ·52** | ·35** | ·19 | ·18 |
| R238 | Interest in schemes | ·29** | ·14 | ·34** | ·22* | ·10 | ·12 | ·25** |

* Significant at a probability less than 10 per cent, two-tailed test.
** Significant at a probability less than 5 per cent, two-tailed test.

In any event, improvement in relations with other team members is associated with reports of a number of outcomes. For feedback- and project-derived improvement in relations, there are correlations with problem-solving, increases in information about work associates, and increases in influence over work associates (*Table 15-11*). The correlations with work improvements are also quite high (see *Table 15-12*), providing some possible confirmation of the importance that the H.I.C. Project placed on improving relations among team members.

While there is only one significant correlation between improvement in team relations and changes in communication behaviour, the correlation—between project-determined improvements in team relations and improvements in communicating to others—supports and amplifies similar correlations found above (*Table 15-9*) between the extent of participation in projects and improvement in communicating to others. Presumably, in discussing findings, as well as planning projects, and so on, team members are able to develop and improve relations between one another and are able to communicate more freely to others.

In summary, potentially the most important factor, because of its general absence in the H.I.C. Project, and because of its high and systematic relationships with criteria of H.I.C. success, is the extent to which hospital-team members made their work a part of the H.I.C. Project. The extent to which this was done is positively associated with problem-solving, administrative action, and changes in work practices. Most importantly, involving one's work in H.I.C. is relatively highly associated with ratings by colleagues of improvements in several different kinds of communications behaviour.

Other variables associated with problem-solving or making changes in one's work are: (1) the favourability of the HMC to the H.I.C. Project (at least as seen by hospital-team members), (2) the clarity of H.I.C. aims, (3) knowing what the central team wanted, as well as (4) getting support from the central team, and (5) the building of good relations among members of the hospital team. All of these could be prospective points for improvement in any subsequent H.I.C. Project, particularly if problem-solving and work improvements are desired ends.

## NOTES

[1] Because the ratings of the month (operational) and three-day (appreciation) courses were made by different groups of respondents, it is not altogether proper to compare the relative levels of ratings. There is always the possibility that different kinds of individuals have different standards when rating something as vague as 'usefulness'. Examination of ratings by attenders of each course for identical items in the questionnaire – especially where the criterion to be rated is vague – shows that appreciation-course attenders tend to be rather more 'optimistic' or positive than operational-course attenders. Thus,

if one were to take this bias into account, the near equality of ratings for operational and appreciation courses would have to be modified. The operational course is somewhat more 'useful' than the appreciation course, according to this line of reasoning.

[2] Two-day course ratings are available for items comparable to numbers F94 and F95. Because only 10 or 11 ratings were obtained, and because of the possible difference in rating standards used by attenders of the two-day course (possibly more 'pessimistic' than attenders of either of the other courses), the findings are very tentative. The 'material presented' at the two-day course was of 'some usefulness' (mean of 3·2) and the 'informal contacts and discussions' between 'some' and 'much' (mean of 3·5). While these are lower ratings than for the other courses, the ratings are probably not greatly different when one takes into account the possible bias in rating standards. If one can place any confidence in ratings by only ten individuals, one might also conclude that the informal aspects were of more usefulness than the formally presented material.

[3] The responses for the item on students came from only some of the hospitals, since only the first group of students had completed their work at the time for the collection of this data. Some 31 per cent of all hospital team members ringed 'not done' for this item.

[4] Some 26 per cent of all hospital-team members ringed 'not done' for the item on feedback meetings. The second survey item on LSH meetings did not include a 'not done' alternative, but the non-response rate was 35 per cent.

[5] Following the questionnaire items listed in *Figure 15-2*, a question was asked to establish whether any of the activities had had any harmful effects on the hospital. Two individuals answered 'yes', both from the same hospital. 'Meetings at the hospital with H.I.C. central-team members' and 'help given by H.I.C. staff in carrying out studies in your hospital' were cited.

[6] Some of these relationships may be interpreted in the following terms: The post-course conferences were meant to continue the work of the courses, and the content consequently overlapped. Central-team activities were not such a direct carry-over of course activity, in part because most central-team members were not present at the courses.

[7] When hospital-team members were asked during the first survey what they personally got out of the course, only three people said they got nothing or mentioned only negative aspects of the course. The remainder mentioned a great variety of different positive aspects of the course they attended, for example:

'I now view certain problems in much different light, and much more often think of using, for example, statistical material to try to get answers or to find out if problems actually exist.'

'Knowledge of techniques used in getting people's real opinions.'

'Learned about other hospitals' problems from chatting with other people.'

'Some knowledge of what social science is all about.'

'Better understanding of my own hospital because I was living with [other team members] and so we chatted.'

'It made you see yourself in a role ... from the other person's angle.'

'Contact with other administrative, medical, and nursing people and the exchange of ideas.'

'Got to know each other as people out of uniform – as human beings – not over an office desk.'

'Gave us a taste to know more.'

'The course taught me very clearly the techniques we were taught to do.'

'A much more scientific approach to the analysing of problems.'

'We jump to conclusions so often – we know the reason, even the solution. [I've learned that] ... it turns out the real cause is often something different.'

[8] The seven individuals came from only three hospitals. The activities on which more help was wanted were particularly 'carrying out the study' and 'analysing'. There was most satisfaction on the two planning items, and on the feedback item. No one, or only one person, wanted more help from the central team during these project stages.

[9] See Chapter 18 for further data showing that when operational doctors were highly involved, central-team participation in projects tended to be excluded.

# 16 *The Project meetings*

Evaluation of the Project meetings is limited primarily to the third, or 'feedback', series of meetings, as they came to be known. This series attracted more time and effort than any of the others. In addition, the greatest amount of data for analysis and evaluation is available for this series. Some data on the London School of Hygiene meetings will also be presented in the tables and some mention made of the second series of Project meetings, primarily because they both serve as a contrast to the 'feedback' meetings and thus as an additional source of understanding of them.

We shall assume two possible major goals for the feedback meetings: (1) learning information about hospital projects and about hospital matters, and then acting on the information in order to solve problems, and (2) learning about oneself and other hospital participants, and thereby becoming better and more sensitive communicators. The observational data and correlational analyses suggest that effects in the area of information and problem-solving are not much in evidence, but that the meetings did have

FIGURE 16-1 *Meeting activity and H.I.C. outcomes**

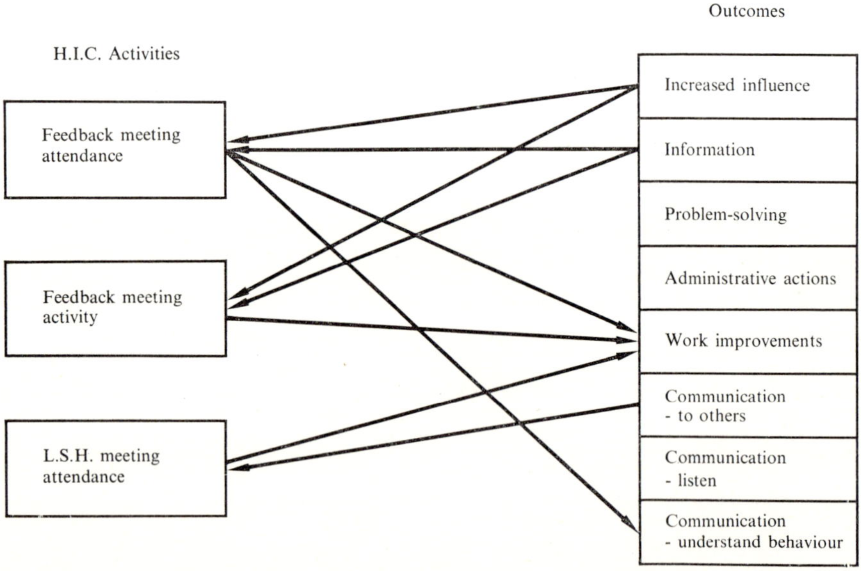


* Assumed direction of causation shown by arrows; all relationships positive.

effects in improving the communications behaviour of attending hospital-team members.

Our data suggest that information and increased influence outcomes obtained from project participation may determine attendance at feedback meetings rather than the reverse (see *Figure 16-1*). Problem-solving is not associated with attendance or activity at the feedback meetings, but reports of work improvements are in part apparent consequences, as are increases in understanding of the behaviour of others in the hospital.

## THE DATA

Our assessment of the meetings is based, first, on general non-systematic observations at meetings. A member of the evaluation team was present at most of the meetings held after May 1966.[1] Furthermore, typescripts made from tape-recordings of the presentations and discussions during the meetings were used to study and review the interactions that occurred (for an exploratory content-analysis using these data, see Appendix 16A).

In addition, the first survey of hospital-team members included a question on the usefulness of 'feedback' meetings and the second survey included a question on the usefulness of the London School of Hygiene meetings (see items F101 and R192 in Chapter 15). The questionnaire items were supplemented by discussions with several hospital-team members, and by a series of formal, directed interviews of six hospital-team members and of three central-team members much involved in the feedback meetings.

Finally, the convener of the feedback meetings has provided attendance data for the feedback and LSH meetings. These measures of attendance, together with a measure of 'contributions' obtained from the transcripts of feedback meetings, are the basic 'objective' indicators of meeting activity presented in the tables of this chapter.[2]

The first of the measures of meeting activity (item FF16) consists simply of the number of attendances at feedback meetings by each hospital-team member. The range is 0 to 7 attendances; one-third of team members attended no meetings at all. The median number of meetings attended is 1, and the mean 1·8.[3]

Item FF19 is also a measure of attendance at feedback meetings, but is based on only those attendances with a hospital team colleague of the same professional group. For example, a nurse's score would be based on the number of times she attended feedback meetings with another nurse from her hospital team. The range for this variable is 0 to 5. Some 68 per cent attended no meetings with a colleague of their own professional group, and the median number of such attendances was 0 (mean=0·6).

The number of contributions at feedback meetings (item (FF24) is obtained from transcripts, with a score of one assigned for each uninterrupted statement or question made. Those not attending any meetings are eliminated from the analysis. The range is 0 to 304 contributions (8 per cent of hospital-team members attending feedback meetings made no contribution), and the median number of contributions is 62 (mean=44).

Item FF37 is the number of attendances at LSH meetings. The range is 0 to 6 attendances, with 29 per cent of team members attending none, and the median is 1 attendance (mean=1·5).

*Table 16-1* provides the intercorrelations among the meeting activity measures and the usefulness measures (the latter are described in more detail above in Chapter 15). Attendances and contributions at feedback meetings and attendances at LSH meetings are generally highly intercorrelated, but for the most part unrelated to either of the usefulness measures. The latter point is quite interesting – perhaps what is 'useful' from these meetings does not accumulate over a number of meetings. One attendance leads to a rating of usefulness as high as the rating based on more than one attendance.

## AIMS AND OUTCOMES

We are told above (Chapter 7) that the aims and intentions of the Project meetings were 'to provide an opportunity for hospital teams to learn from and support each other by sharing information'. But one may ask a further question: to learn (or to share information about *what*?)

A number of H.I.C. Project participants felt that a major purpose of the third series of meetings was to learn about 'feedback', or how one reports back to respondents what was said in a survey. However, while this was the explicit aim, the time devoted to the problem of feedback was quite small. It is true that this content increased over time, but it is our impression that it was never at a very high level in the feedback meetings.[4]

Another somewhat related aim is indicated in the convener's suggestion (in an interview) that one criterion of success for these meetings would be the convening of meetings in the hospitals not only for project feedback but for 'sharing information'. Again, it appears that relatively little time and effort during the meetings was devoted to this. This is important, for amounts of time and effort expended are very significant indicators of the *real* goals of meetings (Warriner, 1965).[5]

The time and effort expended during meetings suggest that learning about hospital projects and the information derived from projects is of some importance, because at least the first hour and a half of each meeting were devoted to a formal, extended presentation of data and data-gathering methods. Subsequently, much of the discussion would amplify the data report and cover previous project activities and plans for the future.

Another possible goal of the feedback meetings was learning about hospital problems that were not specifically studied by H.I.C. For example, a very interesting and, apparently, useful discussion for a number of hospital

TABLE 16-1 *Relationships among Meetings Measures*

($N$=38 to 72 individuals)

| | | *FF16* | *FF19* | *FF24* | *F101* | *FF37* | *R192* |
|---|---|---|---|---|---|---|---|
| FF16 | Number of feedback meetings attended | – | | | | | |
| FF19 | Number of feedback meetings attended with team member of same tripartite division | ·45** | – | | | | |
| FF24 | Number of contributions at feedback meetings | ·59** | ·35** | – | | | |
| F101 | Rated usefulness of feedback meetings | ·14 | ·26* | ·13 | – | | |
| FF37 | Number of LSH meetings attended | ·61** | ·22* | ·26* | ·17 | – | |
| R192 | Rated usefulness of LSH meetings | ·11 | ·03 | ·09 | ·37** | ·11 | – |

* Significant at a probability less than 10 per cent, two-tailed test.
** Significant at a probability less than 5 per cent, two-tailed test.

participants centred upon the use of Addressograph materials for the medical records department. Other aspects of hospital technology came up during the feedback meetings from time to time. One way of viewing this area of concern in the feedback meetings might be to term it 'how other hospitals are doing things'. It is the broadening of the work horizons of hospital members by exposing them to other hospital members.

Some objective evidence about the effort expended during feedback meetings on hospital project discussion and on general non-H.I.C. hospital problems is provided by a content analysis of tapes from some of the feedback meetings (see Appendix 16A). Projects and hospital matters took up the bulk of the discussion at these meetings. However, the evidence suggests that while hospital team members seemed more interested in hospital matters (and increasingly so, over the course of the meetings), the central team (excluding the convener) seemed much more interested in the hospital projects. Perhaps hospital-team members wanted to learn about one thing – hospital matters generally – but central-team members intended that they should learn about something else – hospital projects.

A separate analysis of meeting 'process' (also in Appendix 16A) shows that exchanging information and opinions was the most common activity in meetings, and that decision-making or discussions about action were relatively infrequent. So whatever the main topic, instead of moving from diagnosis of problems to discussions and decisions about solutions (Bales and Strodtbeck, 1951; Kelley and Thibaut, 1970), the meetings seemed to go 'round and round', as one hospital-team member put it. From these kinds of meetings one might perhaps expect increases in information about doing hospital projects or about general hospital matters. However, action on hospital project matters and action on general hospital problems are not highly likely outcomes from the feedback meetings, judging from the absence of any overt emphasis on these matters.

*Tables 16-2* and *16-3* provide further evidence about the role of the feedback meetings in producing various outcomes. *Table 16-2* shows that feedback meeting activity is correlated with obtaining knowledge about hospital problems and acquiring information about hospital functioning (variables F72, F82, and F83). However, the 'usefulness' of feedback meetings is not correlated with the information outcomes. The fact that this is not so, while other 'usefulness' variables may be correlated with these kinds of outcomes (see Chapter 15), lends some support to the inference that acquiring information causes feedback meeting activity, but not necessarily the reverse. Those attending relatively more feedback meetings do report more learning, but those saying the meetings are more 'useful' do not learn any more or less. Perhaps learning (i.e. project 'success') leads to attending feedback meetings, but not necessarily to perceptions of meeting 'usefulness' or further learning within the meetings.

Whatever the causal direction for the relationships between information outcomes and feedback meeting activity, *Tables 16-2* and *16-3* provide

TABLE 16-2 *Relationships between Meetings Measures and First Survey Criteria*

($N$=42 to 69 individuals)

| | *First survey criteria* | | | | | | | | |
|---|---|---|---|---|---|---|---|---|---|
| *Meetings measures* | *Team knowl prob F72* | *Solve problems (hosp) F76* | *Help set right F78* | *Solve problems (own) F87* | *Get R's to solve F79* | *Info abt hosp F82* | *Info abt assoc F83* | *Incr infl gen F85* | *Incr infl assoc F86* |
| FF16 Number of feedback meetings attended | ·11 | −·07 | ·08 | ·12 | −·04 | ·33** | ·25** | ·28** | ·24** |
| FF19 Number of feedback meetings attended with team member of same tripartite division | ·33** | ·15 | ·11 | ·28** | ·30** | ·26** | ·29** | ·25** | ·42** |
| FF24 Number of contributions at feedback meetings | ·43** | ·05 | ·01 | ·22 | −·02 | ·32** | ·24 | ·31** | ·20 |
| F101 Rated usefulness of feedback meetings | ·28* | ·30** | ·34** | ·40** | ·20 | ·16 | ·08 | ·12 | ·23 |
| FF37 Number of LSH meetings attended | ·17 | −·22* | −·02 | −·05 | −·14 | ·09 | −·02 | ·02 | ·01 |
| R192 Rated usefulness of LSH meetings | ·12 | ·22 | ·36** | ·41** | ·13 | ·04 | ·22 | −·06 | ·20 |

* Significant at a probability less than 10 per cent, two-tailed test.

** Significant at a probability less than 5 per cent, two-tailed test.

TABLE 16-3 *Relationships between Meetings Measures and Second Survey Criteria*

(*N*=40 to 71 individuals)

| | | *Second survey criteria* | | | | | | |
|---|---|---|---|---|---|---|---|---|
| *Meetings measures* | | *Admin action R214* | *Worth of actions R215* | *Improved work R239* | *Improved work R304* | *Change-commun RC100* | *Change-listen RC260* | *Change-aware RC420* |
| FF16 | Number of feedback meetings attended | ·09 | −·02 | ·24* | ·45** | ·27** | ·15 | ·37** |
| FF19 | Number of feedback meetings attended with team member of same tripartite division | ·11 | ·03 | ·50** | ·35** | ·11 | −·04 | ·30** |
| FF24 | Number of contributions at feedback meetings | ·01 | −·16 | ·12 | ·32** | ·16 | ·01 | ·13 |
| F101 | Rated usefulness of feedback meetings | ·28** | ·29* | ·46** | ·53** | ·04 | ·20 | ·31** |
| FF37 | Number of LSH meetings attended | ·11 | −·07 | ·24* | ·46** | ·34** | ·45** | ·42** |
| R192 | Rated usefulness of LSH meetings | ·09 | ·01 | ·44** | ·55** | ·01 | ·00 | ·09 |

* Significant at a probability less than 10 per cent, two-tailed test.
** Significant at a probability less than 5 per cent, two-tailed test.

little evidence for a relationship between problem-solving, or administrative action outcomes, and feedback meeting activity. Attending more feedback meetings did not seem to help team members in solving problems, nor did solving problems in their hospitals lead them to attend more feedback meetings.

So far we have seen that the feedback meetings do not seem to facilitate problem solving or other kinds of action in the hospitals. Furthermore, meeting activity, as measured by attending and participating in discussions, is related to acquiring information, but it is quite possible that the latter leads to, or causes, the former.

There is still another important kind of outcome from the feedback meetings. In all of these contacts and discussions with others during the feedback meetings, it is possible for the meeting participants to learn something about themselves, including how other individuals react to them. There are a number of terms for groups with aims of this sort, some of which are 'T (for training)-groups', or 'sensitivity training groups' in which one becomes more 'sensitive' to others as well as to one's own behaviour (see Schein and Bennis, 1965), and 'Tavy', for Tavistock groups (see Chapter 7, and also Rice, 1965). While most of the consciously stated aims of feedback meetings pertained to projects or problems, and much of the content of the meetings leads us to infer the sharing of project or hospital information as their primary aim, there are strong reasons for identifying the sharing of 'behavioural' information – and changing the people involved in the meetings (see Chapter 3) – as another, possibly conflicting, primary aim.

Firstly, the overall goals specified by H.I.C. for the Project meetings (see Chapter 7) are compatible with those one may expect of a T-group. Furthermore, the second series of meetings was in fact set up as what the convener has called a 'Tavy-type' group (see Chapter 7). In structure (small size, one and a half hour's duration, weekly meetings, 'safe' meeting-place away from hospitals, etc.) and leader behaviour (lack of direction initially, subsequent directiveness in pointing out feelings, frustrations, avoidance of here-and-how, etc.), the second series of meetings was similar to the small 'study groups' run by the Tavistock Institute. The interpersonal dynamics within the second series of meetings were also similar to those found in 'Tavy-groups': unease, silence, avoidance of the 'here-and-now', and hostility to the convener.

When the earlier, second series of meetings proved to be 'not satisfactory', (see Chapter 7), they were modified by the convener along the lines suggested by hospital-team members.[6] According to the background notes circulated to participants in the first meeting of the third series, 'the day should be structured, with time for presentation by one or more hospital teams followed by time for general and group discussion'. However, while the hospital-team members structured the meetings with the presentations of projects, the convener also continued the work of examining behaviour begun in the course of the earlier series of meetings – the 'Tavy-type group'.

The convener's role during the third, feedback, series of meetings was, as the term 'convener' suggests, primarily that of arranging or preparing for the meeting by sending out invitations and so on, and seeing that the meeting came to a close sometime at the end of the day. In between, the convener commented on process. Requests for information or help were turned back to the hospital participants, and attention focused on emotional aspects of the group. In addition, the convener conformed to the 'Tavistock' model by refraining from discussing the group with other central-team members outside the meetings.[7]

The analysis of feedback meeting tapes (Appendix 16A) provides some support for these general observations. The convener, more than other central-team members asked for opinions and made points on various matters concerning the emotions or feelings of individuals. In contrast to the other central-team members, she also refrained from making suggestions about decisions or actions.

While there was this leadership by the convener, the amount of discussion about 'emotional' matters did not apparently increase over the course of the entire series of meetings, at least as evidenced by the four transcripts sampled (Appendix 16A). Our general impression is that the relatively large size of the feedback meetings – much larger than the limit of 12 usually placed on T-groups – and the continuing throughput of 'new' individuals prevented much disclosure of 'sensitive' matters in the meetings, and hindered members from opening up and exposing their work problems to others.[8] Whatever the causes, by the criterion of discussion of 'emotional' issues the feedback meetings do not appear to have been very successful. However, while the level of achievement may not have been very great, there is some correlational evidence that the feedback meetings, or something similar, may be of potential benefit in this area.

*Tables 16-2* and *16-3* provide some data bearing on the matter of behavioural changes possibly resulting from feedback meetings in their function as a 'Tavy-type' group. *Table 16-2* shows increases in influence are associated with feedback meeting activity, while *Table 16-3* shows changes in work behaviour or work improvements and also increases in understanding and knowledge of the behaviour of others are associated with feedback meeting activity, and with rated usefulness of feedback meetings.

Again, it is not possible to specify the causal priorities here, but the differential correlations between activity and usefulness in relation to the outcomes suggest that, of the correlates of feedback meeting activity, work improvements and increases in understanding may be outcomes of, or are at least caused in part, by participation in feedback meetings. Those who attended relatively more meetings and saw them as relatively more useful also report more improvements in their work and are seen by colleagues as having increased their understanding and knowledge of the behaviour of others.

Perhaps not very much change in such understanding was created by feedback meeting activity (if in fact our causal inferences are correct), since the level of these outcomes is typically not very high (see Chapter 14), and the correlation between attendance and change in understanding is not very high either. However, the relationship is one of the relatively few in this evaluation study involving a change in communications behaviour, and so, however slight in magnitude, it is important in providing a lead for further efforts in improving hospitals.

To summarize, we have seen that one of the purposes of the feedback meetings was to change people, in a sense to make 'better communicators' out of them. Correlations provide some evidence that changes in work behaviour and changes in understanding about the behaviour of others may be due to feedback meeting activity.

Somewhat related to the T-group emphasis of the feedback meetings – and its aim of changing people, are a number of aims for the feedback meetings which may be termed 'changing or creating relationships'. First of all, some members of the central and hospital teams mentioned the feedback meetings as an opportunity to introduce new co-opted team members to the H.I.C. Project and to provide a substitute source of stimulation, since they had missed the course and Revans's introduction to the Project. This purpose may have been achieved; at least attendance did not create a sufficiently negative effect to prevent the subsequent re-attendance of these new team members at later feedback meetings. However, a number of hospital people, not team members, were brought along at subsequent stages of the H.I.C. Project and to some of the later feedback meetings. Sometimes these individuals did not attend subsequent meetings, and several of our hospital-team interviewees or informants indicated that the apparent aimlessness of the feedback meetings had confused these later visitors and that they left the meetings with no further incentive to attend.

Another explicitly stated goal in the creation of the third series of meetings was to obtain the support of the senior hospital-team members (the supporting team). However, only a very small percentage of all attendances were by supporting-team members and, on the average, at any one meeting, only one or two of the ten hospital teams had members of both operational and supporting teams in attendance. It is therefore likely that little improvement in relations between supporting and operational teams was obtained in this way (also, see the rating for item R230 in *Figure 15-7*).

However, when supporting-team members were somehow induced to attend, it may have been quite useful. Some related evidence is provided by the correlation, in *Table 16-1*, between attending feedback meetings with a member of one's own tripartite division and the rated usefulness of the feedback meetings ($r=0{\cdot}26$). Furthermore, such attendance is correlated with problem-solving variables (*Table 16-2*) as well as with the other outcomes related to simple numbers of meetings attended. Finally, attending with a member of one's own tripartite division is associated with reducing tension with one's immediate colleagues and involving other hospital staff in projects (items F34 and F137, r=0·23 and 0·22, respectively, both significant at less than 10 per cent).

In short, scattered evidence suggests that the feedback meetings apparently did not achieve much in the way of improving relationships among team members because supporting-team members could not be induced to attend. However, when such attendance occurred, relationships were improved (tension, for example, was reduced).[9]

## THE LONDON SCHOOL OF HYGIENE MEETINGS

We have not had much to say about the London School of Hygiene meetings. At this point we shall summarize the relevant correlational data presented in *Tables 16-1, 16-2,* and *16-3,* and we shall provide a brief assessment of the effects of the LSH meetings on the H.I.C. outcomes studied by the evaluation.

Attendance at the LSH meetings is highly associated with attendance at the feedback meetings (*Table 16-1*). Those who attended one kind of meeting attended the other. Those who found one kind of meeting useful also found the other kind useful, but LSH attendance is not correlated with the rated usefulness of LSH meetings. The latter correlation, or lack of correlation, may indicate that additional attendances at LSH meetings were not motivated by increments in the usefulness of the meetings for hospital or Project functioning, but, rather, continued attendance was due to some other factor or expectation – such as expecting to learn from others or to make contacts with others.

Attendance at LSH meetings is not correlated with informational outcomes or problem-solving, but it is correlated with work changes and, quite highly, with ratings by colleagues of the attenders' improvement in communications behaviour (see *Tables 16-2* and *16-3*). However, since usefulness ratings are not correlated with communication changes, we suspect that communication changes lead to attendance, but attendance has no 'use', at least not for communication change. On the other hand, it is quite possible that LSH attendance in some way facilitates improvements in one's work. Most likely the causal sequence works both ways. Perhaps – and this is speculation – hearing 'success stories' of others at the LSH meetings somehow served as an inspiration for work changes. Attendance at LSH meetings is positively associated with seeing contacts with other hospitals in H.I.C. as relatively useful (item F97, r=0·33).

However, one wonders how enduring these work improvements (reported in items R239 and R304) are, or how they are seen by others in the hospital, since those attending LSH meetings tended not to involve others in their hospital in H.I.C. activities (item F137, $r=-0{\cdot}31$). One would guess that some of the reported work improvements presumably resulting from LSH attendance were made unilaterally, rather than together with co-workers in the hospital. In conclusion, then, this is perhaps a relatively pessimistic assessment of the LSH meetings, but no worse than what the hospital-team members themselves give (see item R192 in *Figure 15-2*), as well as other observers (see Chapter 7).

In conclusion then, we see that the aims of the feedback meetings may be several: learning how to 'feedback', how to hold meetings, or how to share information; exchanging information and learning about specific project activities in the hospitals and hospital problems generally; and learning about, and becoming more sensitive to, members of other professional groups. Aside from the sheer content to be learned, the feedback meetings could have had the general aim of changing the people involved in the meetings (changing attitudes and behaviour in one or more of the above areas) and improving relations among the H.I.C. Project participants in the hospitals.

The existence of these aims may be ascertained from various statements of purpose, but even more important and probably more valid, is the inference of aims from what really happened. From the content of the meetings and the things most often discussed, it would appear that learning about hospital functioning and about the hospital projects was important to hospital-team members and some central-team members. But the purposes expressed by, and the behaviour of, the key central-team member in this situation – the convener – suggest that learning about, and changing, people were equally important.

The correlational evidence indicates that the exchanging of project and hospital information apparently did not facilitate any problem-solving and (less certainly) did not increase the knowledge or information of team members. Rather, team members seem to have come to meetings because they had acquired knowledge (by means of projects) that they wished to impart to others. The prospect of presenting a report at a meeting may well have served as an incentive to do project work, but actual attendance does not seem to have resulted in more knowledge relevant to team members' hospitals. Perhaps this is why team members see feedback meetings as not very useful (see Chapter 15).

However the relationship between feedback meeting activity and increases in understanding of other people suggests that the meetings (and probably the T-group aspects of the meetings) did have value in this area, and seem to offer considerable further potential.

Not much in the way of improving relations among team members – or, apparently, improving relations with other people in the hospitals – was achieved by feedback meeting activity. This appears to be due at least in part to the difficulty of getting supporting-team members to attend. But there is evidence that attendance at these meetings with colleagues from one's own tripartite division (i.e. usually with a supporting-team member) may facilitate the improvement of some relationships.

In addition to the relatively low rating of usefulness given to the London School of Hygiene meetings by hospital-team members (Chapter 15), we find in this chapter that the correlational evidence does not give rise to any optimism regarding outcomes from further extension of meetings of this nature.

## NOTES

[1] In order to mitigate the threatening aspects of the evaluator's presence, the observation included occasional participation (see Weick, 1968, p. 371). But apart from one small exception – at the end of the meetings in the third series – this participation was of a very minor kind. Most of the interventions were of the nature of requests for the repetition of a comment ('I couldn't hear that') or, less frequently, for simple non-evaluative and unthreatening information about project activities in the hospital ('when did you start your data collection?').

[2] It is perhaps of interest to recount the development of evaluation efforts in connection with the feedback meetings. These started out as just another series of meetings and seemed to be neither more nor less successful than the other kinds of meetings in the H.I.C. Project. Care was taken to observe the meetings and to obtain typescripts of the proceedings, but no special analysis was planned.

However, as it became clear that considerable effort would be devoted by H.I.C. to these meetings, plans were made for a content analysis of transcripts and for correlations of attendance data. Unintentionally, but fortunately at least in one respect, the relatively 'objective' attendance and transcript analyses did not become available until after an extensive report of the informal observations had been made. This is fortunate in that the rather limited and crude correlational analyses and the exploratory transcript analyses do, for the most part, independently corroborate impressions obtained from observations of meetings and other informal sources of data.

[3] This measure and the other measures of meeting activity are based on a maximum of 72 team members. Other, new, team members are not included here, but at most they attended only one or two of the later meetings in any of the series. The frequency distribution for this measure and others derived from meeting records (all such measures are prefixed "FF") are given in Appendix 14A.

[4] One difficulty which may have hindered the discussion of feedback was the limited view held by many Project members of what feedback entailed. Researchers often make the mistake of viewing feedback as action after data has been collected – i.e. feedback is reporting results back to the respondents. However, feedback may be viewed more comprehensively as a process that begins very early in any survey or project to achieve change. If the investigator is to do this he must learn what respondents or organizational participants think of him and the change effort, and he must be able to modify his behaviour accordingly (see, e.g., Sofer, 1961, Argyris, 1960). That is, the investigator must himself get feedback from respondents on how they view him and the project, and he must then give feedback *to* them on what he

sees. A comprehensive view of feedback encompasses a continual interplay between social units in close contact. Feedback refers to the functioning of parts of a 'system'.

More precisely, according to this view the investigator should go to his contacts (and potential respondents) and begin the process of getting and giving feedback quite early. Rather than presenting the aims of his study to contacts in the organization at his first meeting with them, the investigator would do well to ask what they think of the study: 'Perhaps you've heard about the study and I'd like to tell you about it in some detail, but first I'd like to know what you've heard and what you think about it.' The investigator would then follow this up with exploration of the individual's feelings about the project, and he would go into the perceptions of the participant regarding his own needs and their articulation with the project. The investigator can then correct misperceptions (i.e. give the respondent 'feedback'), and he can also reassess his own procedures. It would seem that the earlier feedback, or the evaluation of perceptions and responses, is given, the sooner individuals can begin to change their perceptions and responses. Of course, feedback can be too hasty or it can elicit resistance (see Chestler and Flanders, 1967), and feedback is not always desirable.

[5] Further evidence on the matter of feedback and discussion groups as topics for discussion and action is provided by the correlations between the measures of activity in H.I.C. feedback meetings and the measures of participation in discussion groups and feedback meetings in the hospital (item F70, see Chapter 15). Participation in hospital feedback meetings is correlated with attendance at H.I.C. feedback and LSH meetings ($r=0{\cdot}22$ to $0{\cdot}32$) but not their rated usefulness. The fact that usefulness is not correlated with participation in feedback meetings in the hospital, may indicate that attendance at the H.I.C. feedback meetings followed upon participation in feedback meetings in the hospital, rather than 'useful' attendance at H.I.C. feedback meetings preceding and determining participation in hospital feedback meetings.

Our interpretation is that team members successful in their hospital projects – in the sense of doing feedback of project data – would attend feedback meetings at the Hospital Centre to report on their success but these individuals would not necessarily report the latter meetings as 'useful' – which they would have done if they were facilitative of project success.

However, whatever the causal priorities there, hospital discussion activity is not significantly correlated with any of the meeting activity variables. The latter finding suggests that feedback meeting participation may not facilitate the setting up of, or participation in, new discussion groups in hospitals, as hoped by the convener. However, this cannot be more than a tentative inference, since the question on hospital discussion groups referred to groups set up in the special context of hospital projects.

[6] The major reason for the ending of the second series of meetings apparently was the entrance into the group of central-team members who did not have any T-group experience. Just when frustrations and anxieties were building up because of the need to deal with the 'here-and-now', several members of the central team began to attend the meetings. These individuals had not attended T-groups before nor were they given a detailed briefing by the convener on the purposes and procedures of the group beforehand. As a result, these central-team members supported the hospital-team members in the evasion of the 'here-and-now', and encouraged their turning towards the discussion of hospital projects, and the study of the literature on feedback, as reasons for ending the current course of meetings.

[7] Others in the central team had no experience of T-groups and consequently

assumed that the meetings (both second and third series) would be devoted to the H.I.C. Project in general and the hospital projects specifically. It is difficult to judge just how much effect this conflict of expectations had on the hospital participants. In time, the conflict did become apparent, at least to central-team members, and they initiated a meeting in which the convener presented her views and others theirs. Up to this time there had been no general discussion within the central team about the goals of these meetings and what particular means towards those goals should be adopted. While no concrete changes came out of this meeting, the opportunity to express views and discuss their ramifications seems to have reduced the conflict.

Only towards the end of the feedback series of meetings did the conflict reappear. One of the other central-team members played a more active role, as measured in numbers of contributions, and attempted to develop a process of problem-solving to deal with the difficulties of feedback, and especially getting action, that were then developing in the hospitals. In the last few meetings, this activity focused on the possibility of a more structured examination of problems. Study questions resulted (see Chapter 7), but further attempts at implementation of this more structured approach were followed by the termination of the meetings.

[8] Of the total attendances, 40 per cent were by individuals who attended only 3 or fewer of the 7 meetings, and 71 per cent by individuals who attended 4 or fewer of the 7 meetings.

[9] There are a number of further ways in which the feedback meetings could, and probably in part did, facilitate H.I.C. aims. Rather than the learning or informational purposes mentioned above, the feedback meetings may be seen as having a motivational purpose (e.g. the meetings 'provided continuity and rejuvenated us a bit', according to one hospital-team member). As well as having a motivational basis on the individual level, the meetings may have served symbolic and integrative functions for the group as a whole. 'Keeping the body alive,' said one hospital-team member. According to a central-team member, the meetings created a sense of identification with the Project that served the function of keeping it alive. Unfortunately, aside from the comments by hospital-team members, we have no evidence, and certainly no systematic evidence, about achievements in this area. However, it is possible that these motivational and integrative functions may have facilitated some of the apparent outcomes of meetings described above.

Also, for some central-team members, and for the members of the evaluation team, the meetings provided a very useful opportunity to acquire information about the progress of hospital projects, as well as about hospital functioning generally. Finally, the feedback meetings provided an opportunity to make contacts with Project members during the course of the day.

# 17 *The central team*

In this chapter we take a closer look at the different kinds of activities carried out by the central team. Not originally expected to play a major role in the Project, the central team, including students, came to be an important component of H.I.C. The questions we ask here are: 'What did the central team do?' and 'What should the central team do in order to maximize various outcomes?'

We shall divide the helping activities of the central team into three different kinds: (1) providing information for a diagnosis, (2) providing advice or assistance in making changes, and (3) actually making changes, especially in people. The central team emphasized the first kind of activity, as the hospital teams desired, but correlational data suggest that the latter kinds of help are more effective in creating a wide range of outcomes – especially problem-solving and action outcomes (for some relationships, see *Figure 17-1*).

All twenty-one central-team members working on the H.I.C. Project for two months or more were interviewed for the evaluation. Open-ended

FIGURE 17-1 *Central-team activity and H.I.C. outcomes**

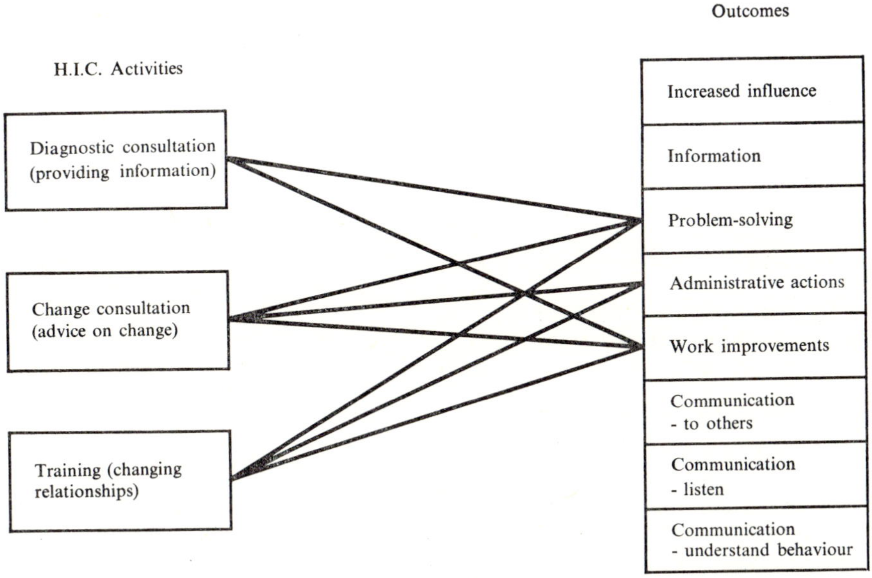


* Direction of causation assumed to be L → R; all relationships positive.

FIGURE 17-2 *Central-team Activity—Rated by all Central-team Members*
(A diagram of mean responses superimposed on questionnaire items)

How *important* do you see the following as aspects of your role in the hospitals? ('Important' here means time spent or priority and emphasis put on the task.) For each aspect of your role please *circle* the proper number according to how you *actually* have performed your role. Then go back and put an 'X' through the proper number according to how you personally feel you *ought* to perform your role.

| | | *Extremely important* | *Very important* | *Somewhat important* | *Only a little important* | *Not important at all* |
|---|---|---|---|---|---|---|
| C1 | Provide information by digging it up (3.9, 3.9)* | 5 | 4 | 3 | 2 | 1 |
| C5 | Help to manage changes coming out of findings (2.1, 3.3) | 5 | 4 | 3 | 2 | 1 |
| C6 | Provide technical advice or assistance to team in their search for information (3.1, 3.8) | 5 | 4 | 3 | 2 | 1 |
| C8 | Teach team members how to gather data (2.2, 3.1) | 5 | 4 | 3 | 2 | 1 |
| C9 | Evaluate the accuracy, importance, and usefulness of data gathered (3.0, 3.7) | 5 | 4 | 3 | 2 | 1 |
| C10 | Provide psychological support to team members (3.1, 3.9) | 5 | 4 | 3 | 2 | 1 |
| C14 | Provide assistance in using data to implement changes (2.7, 4.2) | 5 | 4 | 3 | 2 | 1 |
| C15 | Evaluate the efficacy of changes made as a result of projects (1.7, 3.4) | 5 | 4 | 3 | 2 | 1 |
| C16 | Encourage the hospital team to work as a team (2.4, 3.9) | 5 | 4 | 3 | 2 | 1 |
| C17 | Improve relations between team and others (2.6, 3.8) | 5 | 4 | 3 | 2 | 1 |

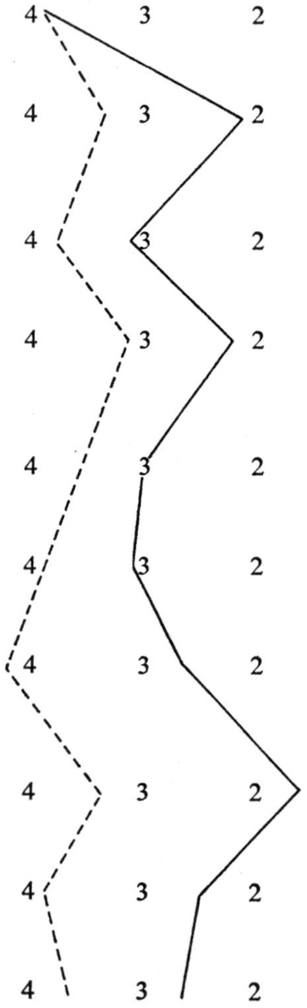

*The mean response for all respondents ($N$=19 for 'actual', $N$=18 for 'ought') is given at the end of each line. The first score is the mean for 'actual', the second score, for 'ought'. The former is diagrammed by a solid line, the latter by a broken line.

interview questions were distributed beforehand, and responses were tape-recorded by evaluation interviewers. Respondents were also given some paper-and-pencil rating scales to be returned subsequently. The present analysis utilizes data from the nineteen respondents interviewed during the last four months of 1967, while the two students joined in the Project in 1968 are excluded.

*Figure 17-2* shows some ratings of different kinds of activities performed as part of the role of the central-team members. By means of the averages shown in the diagram, we shall obtain an overall picture of the activity of the central team, as seen by its members.

The actual performance of central-team members emphasized a number of activities that may be termed 'diagnostic consultation'. That is to say, some of the most important activities of the central team were to 'provide information by digging it up', to 'provide technical advice ... in the search for information', and to 'evaluate the accuracy ... of data collected'. All of these activities are by way of making a diagnosis. Another important activity, but not part of 'diagnostic consultation', was providing psychological support.

Relatively little emphasis was given by central-team members to (a) 'change consultation' or (b) 'training people'. By 'change consultation', we mean advice or indirect help in the implementation of changes, such as 'providing assistance in using data to implement changes', 'evaluating the efficacy of changes made', and more ambiguously, 'helping to manage changes'.

By 'training people' we mean changing behaviour or relations between people, and, this too, received relatively little attention from central-team members. Examples of training people are teaching team members how to gather data, encouraging work as a team, and improving relations between the team and others.[1]

Another way of describing this emphasis by the central team on diagnostic consultation, instead of change consultation or training people, is to say that relatively 'low-risk' activities were favoured (Harrison, 1970). There is relatively low risk to the hospitals in getting diagnostic advice. Such advice can be accepted or rejected and, in any event, the effects of the advice on any management action are liable to be indirect and subject to considerable modification by the managers. Advice about changes and changing behaviour or relationships are more directly linked to action, or imply actions themselves. In these activities, hospital staff open themselves to a greater risk of adverse effects. Some changes or actions are irrevocable; the harm cannot be undone.

From the point of view of the change-agent, or the central-team member, change consultation and training people are risky also. The typical central-team member was a university student or one who had recently graduated from university, and his relevant work experience, if any, was in research. Understanding, or diagnosis, could be given relatively more easily than prescriptions or advice for action, and rather more easily than training or changing activity.

Central-team members' views of their ideal role, or how important each of the various activities should be, are also shown in *Figure 17-2*. Most activities are rated as ideally having consistently high importance. This may be interpreted in several ways. Those activities most performed in actuality (diagnostic consultation) are seen by central-team members as requiring only a little greater emphasis, while those least performed required considerably increased emphasis. That is to say, central-team members may have felt there should be a greater balance among activities. Alternatively this pattern of ideal role preferences may be interpreted as a desire to move (within the limitations of their capabilities) to the more 'risky' and seemingly more effective change consultation and training activities.

It is also of some interest to examine the roles of the two somewhat different kinds of central-team members – students and senior (or 'permanent') members. *Figure 17-3* shows that the relative emphasis on diagnostic activities in actual role behaviour holds good separately for both groups of central-team members. In both cases, three of the four most important activities are gathering information, evaluating data, and providing technical advice. That is, both students and permanent central-team members concentrated on diagnosis and avoided change consultation or training activities.

The ideal role activity of both groups is given in *Figure 17-4*. In distinction from the different emphasis actually placed on diagnosis compared with change consultation and training, the students and permanent central-team members saw their desired role activities in the three areas as equally important. One possible explanation for this pattern is that both groups saw the need to include training and change consultation activities, if hospital-team members were to benefit from H.I.C. At least one of the more senior central-team members felt this quite strongly, but it is our impression that some of the ideal levels of activity were rated without either full awareness of the precise needs for change in the hospitals or the relevant competencies and skills needed within central-team members. In our view, the ratings of the ideal levels of activity are high, and consistently high across different activities, because most central-team members, including students, were dissatisfied about the results of what they were doing and they wanted to do 'more' in all areas. Only the 'ceiling' on the scale prevented even higher ratings.

Hospital-team members also rated the same ten items, using a slightly modified scale (see *Figure 17-5*). Instead of rating the importance of an activity in terms of time spent and emphasis, hospital-team members rated how much was done – 'very much', 'much', etc. There is agreement with the central team in seeing diagnostic consultation as the activity most performed by the central team. The most highly rated three items, in order,

**FIGURE 17-3** *Central-team Actual Activity—Rated by Senior and Student Central-team Members*

(A diagram of mean responses superimposed on questionnaire items)

How *important* do you see the following as aspects of your role in the hospitals? ('Important' here means time spent or priority and emphasis put on the task.) For each aspect of your role please *circle* the proper number according to how you *actually* have performed your role. Then go back and put an 'X' through the proper number according to how you personally feel you *ought* to perform your role.

| | | *Extremely important* | *Very important* | *Somewhat important* | *Only a little important* | *Not important at all* |
|---|---|---|---|---|---|---|
| C1 | Provide information by digging it up (3.3, 4.3)* | 5 | 4 | 3 | 2 | 1 |
| C5 | Help to manage changes coming out of findings (2.4, 1.9) | 5 | 4 | 3 | 2 | 1 |
| C6 | Provide technical advice or assistance to team in their search for information (3.4, 2.9) | 5 | 4 | 3 | 2 | 1 |
| C8 | Teach team members how to gather data (2.7, 1.8) | 5 | 4 | 3 | 2 | 1 |
| C9 | Evaluate the accuracy, importance, and usefulness of data gathered (3.0, 3.0) | 5 | 4 | 3 | 2 | 1 |
| C10 | Provide psychological support to team members (3.3, 3.0) | 5 | 4 | 3 | 2 | 1 |
| C14 | Provide assistance in using data to implement changes (2.9, 2.6) | 5 | 4 | 3 | 2 | 1 |
| C15 | Evaluate the efficacy of changes made as a result of projects (2.3, 1.3) | 5 | 4 | 3 | 2 | 1 |
| C16 | Encourage the hospital team to work as a team (3.1, 1.9) | 5 | 4 | 3 | 2 | 1 |
| C17 | Improve relations between team and others 2.4, 2.7) | 5 | 4 | 3 | 2 | 1 |

* The mean response for respondents ($N=7$ senior staff, 12 students) is given at the end of each line. The first score is the mean for senior members, the second score, for students. The former is diagrammed by a solid line, the latter by a broken line.

FIGURE 17-4 *Central-team Ideal Activity—Rated by Senior and Student Central-team Members*

(A diagram of mean responses superimposed on questionnaire items)

How *important* do you see the following as aspects of your role in the hospitals? ('Important' here means the time spent or priority and emphasis put on the task.) For each aspect of your role please *circle* the proper number according to how you *actually* have performed your role. Then go back and put an 'X' through the proper number according to how you personally feel you *ought* to perform your role.

| | | *Extremely important* | *Very important* | *Somewhat important* | *Only a little important* | *Not important at all* |
|---|---|---|---|---|---|---|
| C1 | Provide information by digging it up (3.6, 4.2)* | 5 | 4 | 3 | 2 | 1 |
| C5 | Help to manage changes coming out of findings (3.3, 3.3) | 5 | 4 | 3 | 2 | 1 |
| C6 | Provide technical advice or assistance to team in their search for information (3.9, 3.7) | 5 | 4 | 3 | 2 | 1 |
| C8 | Teach team members how to gather data (3.1, 3.0) | 5 | 4 | 3 | 2 | 1 |
| C9 | Evaluate the accuracy, importance, and usefulness of data gathered (4.3, 3.4) | 5 | 4 | 3 | 2 | 1 |
| C10 | Provide psychological support to team members (4.0, 3.8) | 5 | 4 | 3 | 2 | 1 |
| C14 | Provide assistance in using data to implement changes (4.3, 4.1) | 5 | 4 | 3 | 2 | 1 |
| C15 | Evaluate the efficacy of changes made as a result of projects (3.6, 2.9) | 5 | 4 | 3 | 2 | 1 |
| C16 | Encourage the hospital team to work as a team (4.1, 3.7) | 5 | 4 | 3 | 2 | 1 |
| C17 | Improve relations between team and others (3.3, 4.1) | 5 | 4 | 3 | 2 | 1 |

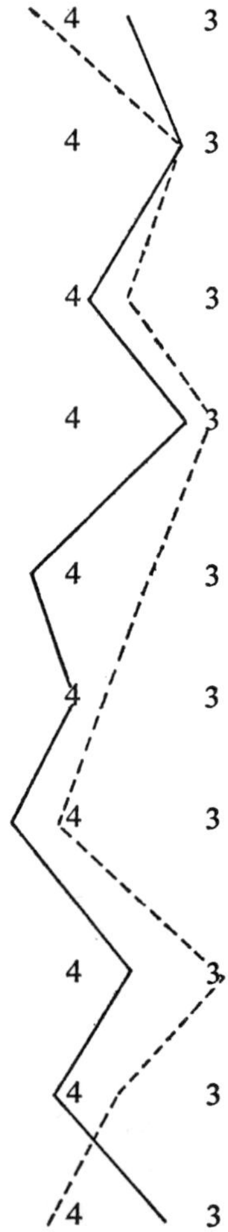

* The mean response for respondents ($N$=7 senior staff, 12 students) is given at the end of each line. The first score is the mean for senior members, the second score, for students. The former is diagrammed by a solid line, the latter by a broken line.

FIGURE 17-5 *Central-team Activity—Rated by Hospital-team Members*

(A diagram of mean responses superimposed on second questionnaire items)

For each of the following items, please indicate how much the *central team* (*including students*) *did for you*. Then, indicate how much you *would like* a team of helpers to do if another similar project were to be done. (Please ring one answer for each line)

| | *How much did the central team (including students):* | *Very much* | *Much* | *Some* | *Little* | *None* |
|---|---|---|---|---|---|---|
| R260 | Provide information by digging it up? (3.5, 3.8)* | 5 | 4 | 3 | 2 | 1 |
| R263 | Help to manage changes coming out of findings? (2.5, 2.9) | 5 | 4 | 3 | 2 | 1 |
| R266 | Provide technical advice or assistance to you in the search for information? (3.6, 3.7) | 5 | 4 | 3 | 2 | 1 |
| R269 | Teach you how to gather data? (3.4, 3.5) | 5 | 4 | 3 | 2 | 1 |
| R272 | Evaluate the accuracy, importance, and usefulness of data collected? (3.6, 3.8) | 5 | 4 | 3 | 2 | 1 |
| R275 | Provide psychological support? (3.2, 3.3) | 5 | 4 | 3 | 2 | 1 |
| R278 | Provide assistance in using data to implement changes? (2.8, 3.3) | 5 | 4 | 3 | 2 | 1 |
| R281 | Evaluate the efficacy of changes made as a result of projects? (2.4, 3.5) | 5 | 4 | 3 | 2 | 1 |
| R284 | Encourage the hospital team to work as a team? (3.1, 3.3) | 5 | 4 | 3 | 2 | 1 |
| R287 | Improve relations between team and others? (2.8, 3.3) | 5 | 4 | 3 | 2 | 1 |

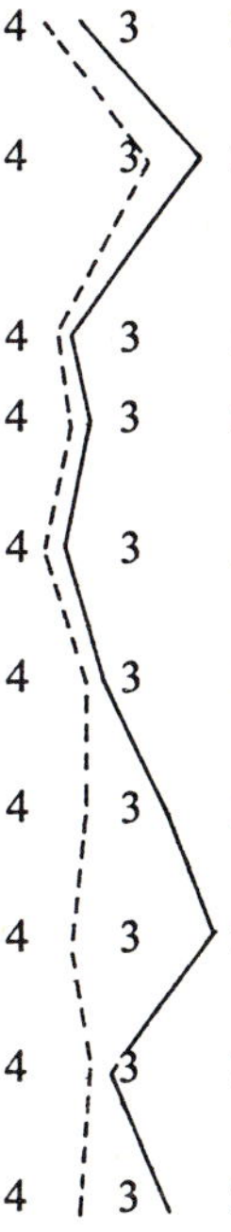

* In the original question format given to respondents, each item was followed on a separate line by 'How much would you like?' The first score in parenthesis after an item is the mean rating for the item, and the second score is the mean rating for the amount hospital-team members 'would like'. These are diagrammed, respectively, by a solid line and a broken line. The respondents for each item vary from 68 to 73 individuals.

are: providing technical advice in the search for information, evaluating data, and providing information.

However, the extent and pattern of central-team activity desired by the hospital team seems somewhat different from that desired by the central team itself. While central-team members would give more or less equal emphasis to all activities, the hospital-team members would still emphasize diagnosis consultation above the other two areas.

Another way of viewing hospital-team desires is that they are quite close – in level as well as in differential emphasis – to their views of what was actually provided. Help in diagnosis was provided and should continue to be provided, but change consultation less so. There are only two major exceptions to the general congruence between what was provided and what was desired. Two activities among those we have termed change consultation are rated quite low for actual provision, but rather higher in terms of what hospital-team members would ideally like (also see the recommendations in Chapter 4). Increasing both of these change consultation activities – providing assistance in using data to implement changes and evaluating the efficacy of changes – would presumably entail relatively low risk for hospital-team members. 'Evaluating' would still be providing hospital-team members with information – evaluative information in this case. While the 'assistance' in the other activity is not specified, presumably it could also entail handling 'data'. Neither of these activities would seem, on the face of it, to be as 'dangerous' or risky as managing changes, or changing relationships involving team members.

*Table 17-1* shows that the relationships among central-team activity variables are all quite high. The more hospital-team members reported receiving one kind of help from central-team members, the more they reported receiving other kinds of help. These rather high intercorrelations could be because hospital-team members had difficulty in distinguishing or rating separately the various kinds of help provided. That is to say, the high interrelationships may reflect response set. Consequently, differential degrees of correlation with other variables must be interpreted cautiously.

*Table 17-2* shows the relationships between central-team activity variables and the criteria from the first survey. The most general and consistent finding in the table is that problem-solving outcomes seem to be related to all of the different kinds of central-team activity variables, and especially to what we have termed change consultation and training people. There is also some evidence that acquiring information about close work associates (item F83) is also related to these latter kinds of central-team activity. However, with minor exceptions it would appear that the other variables in the table – such as knowledge about problems, increased information about the hospital, and also increased influence – are unrelated to the central-team activities measured here.

A general conclusion from the table is that central-team activity seems primarily to facilitate action outcomes (items F76, F78, F87, and F79 in *Table 17-2*), not cognitive outcomes such as knowledge about problems. The hospital teams, as they often told us, did not learn very much new information from the surveys done by the central team. Instead, the data here show that the informational or diagnostic aspects of surveys done by central-team members may have facilitated problem-solving by hospital-

TABLE 17-1 *Relationships among Central-team Activity Variables*

($N=65$ to 73 hospital-team members)

| | | *R260* | *R263* | *R266* | *R269* | *R272* | *R275* | *R278* | *R281* | *R284* | *R287* |
|---|---|---|---|---|---|---|---|---|---|---|---|
| R260 | Dig up information | – | | | | | | | | | |
| R263 | Manage changes | ·40** | – | | | | | | | | |
| R266 | Technical advice in search | ·62** | ·59** | – | | | | | | | |
| R269 | Teach team to gather data | ·24** | ·40** | ·34** | – | | | | | | |
| R272 | Evaluate data | ·45** | ·50** | ·73** | ·48** | – | | | | | |
| R275 | Provide psychological support | ·44** | ·45** | ·56** | ·59** | ·60** | – | | | | |
| R278 | Assist use of data for change | ·52** | ·55** | ·56** | ·31** | ·50** | ·50** | – | | | |
| R281 | Evaluate changes | ·45** | ·62** | ·56** | ·39** | ·64** | ·59** | ·60** | – | | |
| R284 | Encourage work as a team | ·44** | ·45** | ·47** | ·26** | ·42** | ·53** | ·60** | ·60** | – | |
| R287 | Improve team – other relations | ·41** | ·53** | ·60** | ·34** | ·52** | ·52** | ·60** | ·64** | ·70** | – |

* Significant at a probability less than 10 per cent, two-tailed test.
** Significant at a probability less than 5 per cent, two-tailed test.

TABLE 17-2 *Relationships between Central-team Activity and First Survey Criteria*

($N=49$ to 54 individuals)

| | *First survey criteria* | | | | | | | | |
|---|---|---|---|---|---|---|---|---|---|
| *Central-team activity* | *Team knowl prob F72* | *Solve problems (hosp) F76* | *Help set right F78* | *Solve probs (own) F87* | *Get R's to solve F79* | *Info about hosp F82* | *Info about assoc F83* | *Incr infl gen F85* | *Incr infl assoc F86* |
| R260 Dig up information | ·04 | ·36** | ·44** | ·26* | ·31** | ·02 | ·10 | ·20 | ·21 |
| R263 Manage changes | ·14 | ·28** | ·38** | ·36** | ·29** | ·18 | ·27** | ·04 | ·15 |
| R266 Technical advice in search | ·17 | ·25* | ·22 | ·20 | ·36** | ·09 | ·08 | ·05 | ·21 |
| R269 Teach team to gather data | ·42** | ·27* | ·50** | ·44** | ·27* | ·17 | ·18 | ·24* | ·08 |
| R272 Evaluate data | ·26* | ·22 | ·24* | ·27** | ·37** | ·16 | ·18 | ·11 | ·32** |
| R275 Provide psychological support | ·33** | ·20 | ·34** | ·31** | ·23 | –·02 | –·03 | ·13 | ·19 |
| R278 Assist use of data for change | ·10 | ·54** | ·44** | ·52** | ·27* | ·02 | ·36** | ·09 | ·35** |
| R281 Evaluate changes | ·19 | ·44** | ·45** | ·29** | ·27* | ·15 | ·23* | ·09 | ·20 |
| R284 Encourage work as a team | ·10 | ·39** | ·39** | ·35** | ·34** | ·06 | ·29** | –·06 | ·08 |
| R287 Improve team – other relations | ·08 | ·36** | ·33** | ·24* | ·30** | ·21 | ·31** | ·03 | ·15 |

* Significant at a probability less than 10 per cent, two-tailed test.
** Significant at a probability less than 5 per cent, two-tailed test.

team members, rather than improved their fund of information.

Alternatively, while providing information or advice about information does not seem to have helped the hospital-team members in any cognitive way (see item F83 in *Table 17-2*), there is some evidence that helping them to act, or changing their ability to act, would seem to have provided these outcomes. This is important, for if one views the primary aim of H.I.C. as giving hospital people increased information on their situation in the hospital, the best way to do it is not by directly giving them information, but rather by helping them make changes in their situation, or even increasing their ability to make these changes. In other words, the best way to learn how something works is not to study it, but to try to change it.

The same point would seem to hold for action outcomes. The data show that information facilitates problem-solving, but even better than information is help in changing – whether it is advice and assistance for problem-solving or whether it is training – actually changing people and their relationships. These data make clear the great importance of the central-team activities that we have termed change consultation and training people.

The next table (*Table 17-3*) shows the relationships between central-team activities and second survey criteria. On the left-hand side of the table, we see that the central-team activities associated with administrative actions, as in the case of problem-solving (*Table 17-2*), seem to be either change-consultation or training activities. If one desires administrative actions, then advice about making changes or about action, and the actual changing of people or the relations between people, would appear to be helpful.

Regarding work changes, almost all of the ten central-team activities seem to be beneficial. Only evaluating data and teaching the team how to gather data show inconsistent relationships with work improvements. In our view these findings are quite reasonable. Work improvements, at least of the minor sort that are the frequent outcomes of the hospital projects, may be facilitated by many different kinds of central-team help – whether diagnostic or change consultation or, most naturally, training people. Merely providing information may be sufficient for a hospital-team member who is ready and able to change. However, it is our view that major changes in work behaviour that are more than minor administrative rearrangements and involve central or pervasive aspects of individuals' behaviour, require change consultation and, especially, training at an intensive level not frequently found in the H.I.C. Project. The next set of data provide some evidence bearing on the requirements for basic changes in hospital members.

The right-hand side of *Table 17-3* shows an almost complete absence of relationships between central-team activity and changes in the communication behaviour of hospital-team members. The only exception is a correlation 'suggestive' at the 10 per cent level. It is difficult to explain the absence of relationships in the light of the earlier demonstration of the effects of certain central-team variables – at least on the knowledge and

TABLE 17-3 *Relationships between Central-team Activity and Second Survey Criteria*

($N$=54 to 73 individuals)

| | | Second survey criteria | | | | | | |
|---|---|---|---|---|---|---|---|---|
| *Central-team activity* | | *Admin action R214* | *Worth of action R215* | *Improved work R239* | *Improved work R304* | *Change-commun RC100* | *Change-listen RC260* | ***Change-aware RC420*** |
| R260 | Dig up information | ·14 | −·01 | ·37** | ·35** | −·01 | ·10 | ·09 |
| R263 | Manage changes | ·20* | ·10 | ·35** | ·39** | −·08 | ·00 | ·09 |
| R266 | Technical advice in search | ·16 | ·00 | ·34** | ·23* | −·12 | ·10 | ·11 |
| R269 | Teach team to gather data | ·15 | ·02 | ·10 | ·28** | ·13 | ·09 | ·20* |
| R272 | Evaluate data | ·14 | ·04 | ·20* | ·27** | ·02 | ·12 | ·15 |
| R275 | Provide psychological support | ·23* | −·02 | ·20* | ·29** | −·03 | ·05 | ·13 |
| R278 | Assist use of data for change | ·49** | ·32** | ·46** | ·32** | −·05 | ·07 | ·15 |
| R281 | Evaluate changes | ·25** | ·13 | ·40** | ·42** | −·05 | ·03 | ·08 |
| R284 | Encourage work as a team | ·33** | ·22* | ·36** | ·33** | −·07 | −·09 | −·03 |
| R287 | Improve team – other relations | ·33** | ·23** | ·42** | ·33** | ·05 | ·14 | ·20 |

* Significant at a probability less than 10 per cent, two-tailed test.
** Significant at a probability less than 5 per cent, two-tailed test.

understanding by hospital-team members of others (see item RC420 in *Tables 15-9* and *15-12*). The only explanation would seem to be that the effects of central-team activity on communications are so minimal that indices of separate kinds of activities (as in *Table 17-4*) fail to show the barely significant relationships found when a summary measure of central team activity is used (e.g., F145 in *Table 15-9*). The general point is clear, however: differing provision of the particular kinds of central-team activities measured here seem to make no discernible difference in communication behaviour.

In summary, the hospital-team members feel, as do the central-team members, that much of the helping activity carried out in H.I.C. was by way of providing information or advice on getting information – what we have termed diagnostic consultation. Less was done in the way of providing advice on making changes or in the way of 'training people', or actually making changes. The data indicate that the central team want to emphasize these activities just as much as the diagnostic consultation activities. Hospital-team members, also, want to get more help from the latter two kinds of activities. But the order of emphasis would still be diagnostic consultation first, change consultation second, and training people last. Our interpretation is that the kinds of help relatively preferred by the hospital team are less risky or dangerous – more within the competence of the helpers, and less demanding or threatening to those being helped.

The extent of central-team activity, of whatever kind, measured here, is positively associated with problem-solving and the making of work changes by hospital-team members. In addition, several change consultation and training activities seem particularly highly related to problem-solving and work changes, to administrative action, and to acquisition of information about the functioning of work associates. In other words, change consultation and training people would appear to be more beneficial for a wide range of outcomes, compared to diagnostic consultation. This is despite the fact that hospital-team members seem to prefer diagnostic consultation to the other activities. Finally, it would appear that central-team activity, as we have measured it here, is not associated with changes in communication behaviour.

## NOTES

[1] Two McQuitty (1964) cluster analyses of the intercorrelations of the ten items provide some empirical support for our differentiation of central-team helping activities. In the ratings of the ten items by hospital-team members, there is good support for the distinctions. The three items we have labelled diagnostic consultation, the three items labelled change consultation, and two of the three items labelled training activities, are in fact more closely related

to each other than to other kinds of activities, although the differences in magnitude of the correlations are very slight. In the central-team ratings, there is also some correspondence between clusters and the terms used here – for two of the three clusters. Perhaps the terms are a better description of the way help received by hospital-team members was organized, than a description of the way central-team individuals organized their helping activities.

# 18 *Hospital projects*

The last four chapters have provided an analysis of the functioning of individuals in the H.I.C. Project. In this chapter, we shall supplement this with an analysis by hospital projects. Some of the data from Chapter 15 will be utilized, but in a different fashion, and some new data will be introduced. In this way, we shall be able to supplement and buttress some of the foregoing conclusions, as well as attempt to provide some conclusions concerning the hospital projects on which H.I.C. participants spent so much time.

In this chapter we shall see that hospital project outcomes were apparently most evident in terms of administrative actions, less so in terms of the morale of project respondents, and least of all in terms of improvements in the work of those hospital-team members carrying out the project. Project actions (see *Figure 18-1*) seem to be facilitated by 'clear' data and by the central team, rather than the hospital team, doing data collection, analysis, and report writing. The extent to which the hospital-team members

FIGURE 18-1 *Hospital project determinants of hospital project actions**

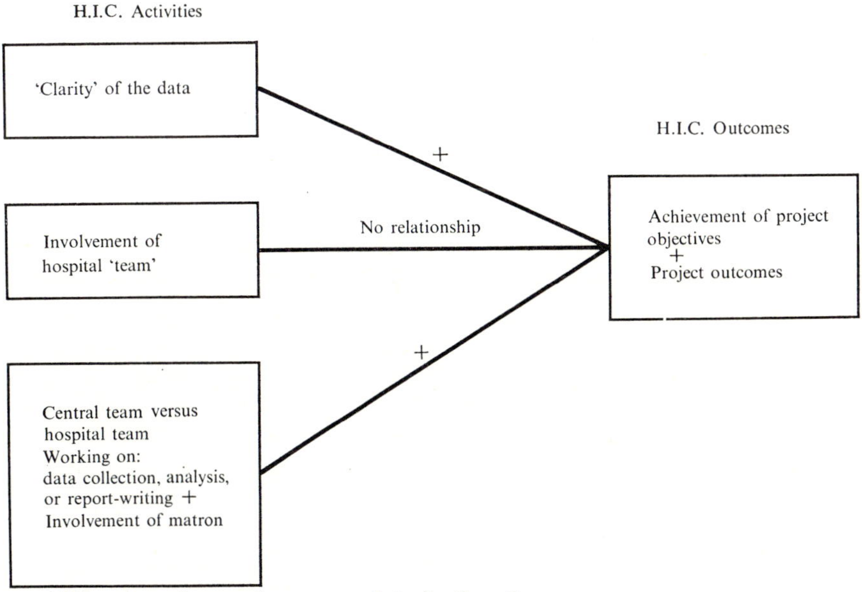


* Direction of causation assumed to be L → R.

were involved as a team does not seem to make a difference, although matron's involvement does. We shall see that improvements in the work of hospital-team members (see *Figure 18-2*) are apparently facilitated by projects with 'unclear' data and by discussing data with hospital staff and others – and especially by using the data to make comparisons among different respondents.

FIGURE 18-2 *Hospital project determinants of hospital-team members' work improvements**

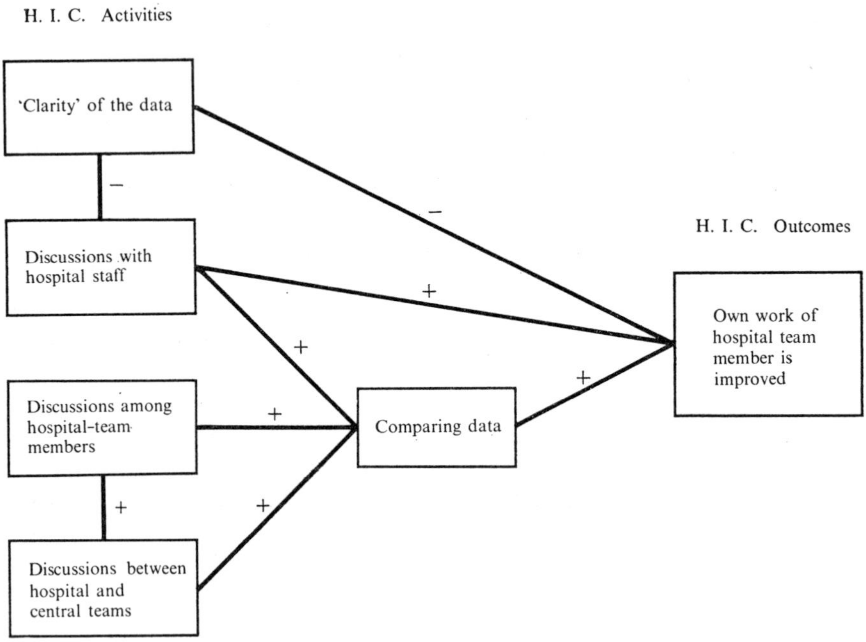


* Direction of causation assumed to be L → R.

## THE PROJECT DATA

Some of the project data to be discussed here were obtained from the second survey of hospital-team members, towards the close of the H.I.C. Project (for full details on this survey, see Chapter 14). Each interviewee was asked how much he was involved in each of the projects carried out in his hospital (see *Figure 18-3*). Those involved in a project to 'some' extent, or more, were then asked to answer three further questions about the outcomes or results of that particular project. In this way, ratings of involvement and outcomes were obtained for each of the thirty-eight projects (these items and indices based on the items are identified by variable numbers prefixed 'PR').

In the middle of the written questionnaire for the second survey, respondents were asked to indicate the project with which they had the greatest

FIGURE 18-3 *Hospital Project Outcomes as Rated by Hospital-team Members*

(A diagram of mean responses superimposed on reinterview questionnaire items)

| Project: (*1 of 38 project titles supplied here*) | | *Very much* | *Much* | *Some* | *Little* | *None* |
|---|---|---|---|---|---|---|
| PR425 | How much were you involved with this project? (2.8)* | 5 | 4 | 3 | 2 | 1 |
| *How much did this project:* | | | | | | |
| PR500 | Achieve its *objectives*? (3.4) | 5 | 4 | 3 | 2 | 1 |
| PR538 | Improve the *work or morale of the respondents* (i.e. those being studied) or of their department? (2.9) | 5 | 4 | 3 | 2 | 1 |
| PR596 | Improve *your own work* in some way? (2.5) | 5 | 4 | 3 | 2 | 1 |

* The mean response for all projects ($N$=36 to 38) is given at the end of each item. Project scores for item PR425 are based on 5 to 11 respondents per project, with a median of 8. Project scores for items PR500, PR538, and PR596 are based on 1 to 8 respondents per project, with a median of 3.

familiarity, and the greatest contact with the data and information produced. Respondents supplied the name of this project and then answered a series of questions on the project. Twenty-seven different projects, out of the total of thirty-eight projects, were selected by respondents, and this is the maximum number of cases used in analyses involving these variables (identified by the prefix 'PU', for 'project data utilization'). These twenty-seven projects, and the respondents providing data on them, are of course a biased sample – being relatively more successful projects and relatively more involved respondents. Nevertheless, the projects selected do cover more than three-quarters of all projects, and in this sense they provide some evidence about the hospital projects as a whole.

Finally, some additional data on 'project procedures' – on who did various kinds of project work, how long it took, what was done in terms of numbers of meetings – were obtained from H.I.C. files and from 'key' informants, in both hospital and central teams, for each project (these variables are identified by the prefix 'PP').

## PROJECT OUTCOMES

In general, hospital-team members viewed hospital projects as (a) achieving objectives on the average, 'much' to 'some', (b) morale effects, 'some', and (c) effects on their own work, 'some' or 'little' (see *Figure 18-3*). The rather small effects on hospital team members' 'own work' are paralleled by similar findings in the second survey questionnaire showing that the effects of the H.I.C. Project on the work of hospital-team members were generally moderate ('some') (e.g. see results for item R304, Chapter 14). The ratings for project effects on respondents' morale or on respondents' work are better, but still not very promising. It is only for the achievement of unspecified project 'objectives' that the ratings are relatively high – high in terms of the face-value content of the response alternative ('much' to 'some') and high relative to other ratings in the evaluation surveys. However, we shall have to wait until intercorrelations and other data are examined to learn the meaning of the achievement of project objectives.

Another measure is obtained from the items dealing with project data utilization. At the end of this series of questions in the second survey questionnaire, respondents were asked 'how much administrative action on your part resulted?' (item PU48). The response for the average project was 'some', (mean of 2·9, based on the usual scale from 5='very much' to 1='none').

The extent objectives were achieved is quite highly related to the extent project respondents were affected (r=0·72) and to the extent of 'administrative actions' (r=0·61), suggesting that the hospital-team members saw the objectives of projects in these terms. Probably administrative actions are the most likely way in which the 'work or morale of the respondents' would be affected (r=0·50). During informal talks with hospital-team members, we occasionally encountered denials that projects were intended to change anything, but we were impressed that most of the projects seemed to be aimed at improving the functioning of others. These data seem to lend support to this view.[1]

While achieving objectives seems to be related to actions and effects on project respondents, it is not related to effects on their own work (r=0·09). Neither is the extent of administrative actions or the extent of effects on respondents related to effects on their own work (r=−0·03 and 0·16, respectively). In other words, these other outcomes apparently have nothing to do with personal outcomes for the hospital-team members – their work is generally not related to the achievements of the hospital projects. We have, in fact, encountered some team members whose work has been improved, and they feel that the objectives of their project have been, to some degree, attained. But a considerable number of others apparently find little connection between project outcomes and their own work.

If some of these relationships are examined for project outcomes rated separately by administrators, doctors, and nurses, a clearer picture emerges. For each of the three groups, the correlations between the achievement of project objectives and respondent effects are high and significant (r=0·60, 0·84, and 0·73, respectively). In other words, one could say that the objectives of project activity are seen by each of these groups as including respondent effects. But the correlations between objectives and 'own work' effects, and between respondent effects and 'own work' effects, are inconsistent across the three groups.

For nurses there is a strong relationship between all three ratings, and for administrators less so (correlations significant at less than 10 per cent). For doctors, while projects that achieve objectives are often projects in which respondents are positively affected (the two ratings are correlated), neither kind of project is necessarily one in which their own work (that of medical-team members) is improved. In other words, it would appear that project objectives and effects on respondents overlap, or are related, for all three groups of team members. However, when it comes to the projects improving their own work, nurses to some degree, administrators to a lesser degree, and the doctors still less, see this as somehow related to project objectives and project effects on respondents.[2]

In conclusion, the responses by hospital-team members to various project criterion measures present a rather equivocal picture of success. In terms of the achievement of objectives, the average project is rated 'some' to 'much'. The effects of projects on respondents are at a rather similar level – there are 'some' effects. It is in the realm of effects on their own work that hospital-team members are rather pessimistic. While they are willing to attribute some success to projects in terms of 'objectives' being achieved, and to a lesser degree, staff morale improved, hospital-team members tend to see relatively little effect on their own work.

The next sections of this chapter will examine some of the factors associated with varying degrees of project success, so that they may be emphasized and outcomes improved in any further H.I.C. Projects.

## USING DATA FROM HOSPITAL PROJECTS

Perhaps the simplest view of what determines project success is the information obtained. Do hospital team members get 'good' information, and do they talk it over with their colleagues and then act?

If the aim of the H.I.C. Project was for hospital-team members to obtain some clear information about their hospitals, the ratings by hospital-team members seem to provide some evidence of success. When asked 'how much was the data clear and understandable?', they answered 'much' to 'some'. Using a base of 27 projects, and a rating scale from 'very much' (scored 5) to 'none' (scored 1), the average is 3·8. 'Was the data invalid (misinformed gripes, untrue, etc.)?' is answered 'little' (mean of 2·2). The existence of 'valid criticisms in the data' was rated 'some' to 'much' (mean of 3·5).

However, respondents gave a relatively low rating to the question 'how much were you able to compare your data with data from other hospitals or other parts of your hospital?' – the average response was 'little' (2·1). This is one of the lowest ratings in our evaluation study for an item that, on *a priori* grounds, would appear to reflect a very useful and desirable activity.

Finally, there was 'much' to 'some' discussion of 'findings' between hospital-team members and various others (discussion with hospital-team members, a mean score of 3·7; with others in the hospital, 3·4; and with central-team members, including students, 3·3).

*Table 18-1* shows the intercorrelations among these variables. While many of the variables are not related to each other, there are a number of interesting relationships. The extent the data are 'clear' is negatively correlated to (and, in our view, probably in part determines) the amount of discussion between hospital-team members and others in the hospital. Discussion among hospital-team members flows from or, more likely, determines 'valid criticisms in the data', while hospital-team members may turn to central-team members for discussion when the data are 'invalid, misinformed gripes, untrue, etc.'

Discussion with any of the three categories of people listed perhaps helps hospital-team members to compare their data with data from other hospitals or other parts of their own hospitals. Finally, discussion with other hospital-team members and discussion with central-team members are related, but the extent of either kind of discussion is unrelated to the extent of discussion with others in the hospital.

*Table 18-2* shows several relationships suggestive of ways in which certain outcomes may be facilitated. First of all, improving 'own work' seems to occur to the extent that the available data are not clear! Comparing data and discussing the results with others in the hospital also seem to facilitate improvements in 'own work', according to the answers by hospital-team members to these questions (see, e.g., Lorsch and Lawrence, 1969). Finally, the achievement of objectives is associated with 'clear data' and 'valid criticisms'. Several of these determinants of various outcomes are uncorrelated with each other (or negatively associated, in one case), even though they are correlated with the outcomes, so there is some scope for those who might wish to improve project outcomes by changing the ways in which hospital projects are carried out and the ways in which the project information is handled.

If we assume that making changes in one's 'own work' is perhaps rather more desirable than 'achieving objectives' in the sense of administrative action, then 'unclear' data would seem to be preferable to clear, particularly if the lack of clarity leads to discussions between team members and others in the hospital. The extent of these discussions and discussions with central-team members, as well as with discussions among the hospital team, are related to making comparisons with data. These would seem to be the key activities that one would emphasize in order to achieve 'own work' effects for hospital-team members, given our causal assumptions are correct. In corroboration, we have seen above (Chapter 15, *Table 15-9*)

TABLE 18-1 *Relationships among Project Data Variables*
($N$=27 projects)

| | *PU26* | *PU30* | *PU34* | *PU40* | *PU42* | *PU44* | *PU46* |
|---|---|---|---|---|---|---|---|
| PU26 Clear data | – | | | | | | |
| PU30 Invalid data | ·11 | – | | | | | |
| PU34 Valid criticisms | –·16 | ·04 | – | | | | |
| PU40 Comparing data | –·18 | ·04 | ·22 | – | | | |
| PU42 Discuss – hospital team | –·04 | ·28 | ·49** | ·32* | – | | |
| PU44 Discuss – hospital staff | –·46** | –·16 | ·04 | ·54** | ·24 | – | |
| PU46 Discuss – central team | –·24 | ·38** | ·29 | ·46** | ·49** | ·28 | – |

* Significant at a probability less than 10 per cent, two-tailed test.
** Significant at a probability less than 5 per cent, two-tailed test.

TABLE 18-2 *Relationships between Project Data Variables and Project Criteria*

($N$=26 to 27 projects)

| | | *Project criteria* | | | |
|---|---|---|---|---|---|
| *Project data variables* | | *Own work improved PR596* | *Respondents affected PR538* | *Administrative actions PU50* | *Objectives achieved PR500* |
| PU26 | Clear data | −·51** | ·12 | ·31 | ·45** |
| PU30 | Invalid data | −·00 | −·04 | ·08 | ·06 |
| PU34 | Valid criticisms | ·35* | ·56** | ·24 | ·41** |
| PU40 | Comparing data | ·53** | ·04 | ·12 | ·22 |
| PU42 | Discuss – hospital team | ·13 | ·02 | ·35* | ·18 |
| PU44 | Discuss – hospital staff | ·49** | −·08 | ·15 | −·04 |
| PU46 | Discuss – central team | ·32* | −·17 | ·00 | −·07 |

* Significant at a probability less than 10 per cent, two-tailed test.
** Significant at a probability less than 5 per cent, two-tailed test.

that involving other hospital staff in projects, and participating in discussion groups and feedback meetings with them, is associated with reports by hospital-team members that they have made changes or improvements in their work behaviour. The key points added here would seem to be the usefulness of having 'unclear' data, so that discussion comes before (bilateral action), and also the usefulness of making comparisons with one's data – in a sense, making evaluations and, hopefully, in the process becoming aware of the various priorities and considerations involved in one's work and that of others.

## TEAM-MEMBER INVOLVEMENT IN PROJECTS – THE HOSPITAL TEAM

The hospital team, a group of co-operating top hospital staff who would carry out projects and participate in H.I.C. activities together, was to be one of the key elements in the H.I.C. Project. By looking at hospital-team members' ratings of their involvement in projects (item PR425), we can establish whether there were 'teams' – in the sense that all of those selected for a hospital team were in fact highly involved and participated in the projects within their hospital. The next step is then to examine what difference generally high involvement, or working as a 'team', makes for the outcomes of projects. Above we examined the effects of the project data and discussions of data on project outcomes – here we examine the effects of hospital-team members' involvement on project outcomes.

First of all, let us look at the average involvement of hospital-team members in projects. Asking each member of a hospital team about the degree of his involvement in each hospital project produces an average of 'some' (see *Figure 18-3*). While the idea of H.I.C. may have been to involve several hospital-team members in a project, it appears that it was not always possible for every member to become highly involved in a project.

In terms of numbers, between one and two (an average of 1·6) hospital-team members were involved 'very much' in the average project, and another one or two members were involved at least 'much' in the average project. Thus the rating of 'some', obtained by averaging the involvement of all the team members in a hospital does not reflect general apathy, but rather that some hospital-team members involved themselves in some projects but not others.

A breakdown by different kinds of team members is also instructive. In the average project, only about one supporting-team member was involved 'some' or more (a mean of 1·1 individuals) and nearly three others (1·8 original operational-team plus 1·0 co-opted-team members) were involved 'some' or more.

It would appear that supporting-team members were generally not really

TABLE 18-3 *Relationships between Project Involvement and Project Criteria*

($N$=19 to 38 projects)

| | | *Project criteria* | | | |
|---|---|---|---|---|---|
| *Involvement of* | | *Own work improved PR596* | *Respondents affected PR538* | *Administrative actions PU50* | *Objectives achieved PR500* |
| PR425 | Total hospital team | −·07 | −·12 | −·02 | ·13 |
| PR432 | 3-day course team | ·19 | ·02 | ·05 | ·05 |
| PR439 | Month-course team | ·18 | −·24 | −·32 | −·09 |
| PR466 | 3-day administrator | ·18 | −·14 | ·12 | ·06 |
| PR467 | 3-day doctor | ·08 | ·08 | −·12 | −·11 |
| PR468 | 3-day nurse | ·19 | ·31 | ·36 | ·53** |
| PR469 | Month-course administrator | −·14 | −·54** | ·01 | −·43** |
| PR470 | Month-course doctor | ·26 | −·09 | −·40** | ·08 |
| PR471 | Month-course nurse | ·23 | ·06 | −·44** | ·12 |

* Significant at a probability less than 10 per cent, two-tailed test.
** Significant at a probability less than 5 per cent, two-tailed test.

part of an overall hospital 'team' in the sense of being at least somewhat involved in projects. Similarly, not all operational-team members were involved in all of the projects in their hospitals. Instead, perhaps two out of the three operational-team members were involved to a meaningful degree in any particular project. If the notion of a 'team' is important, then the data suggest this apparent lack of involvement as one of the problems facing any future H.I.C. Project.[3]

What then, are the relationships between the involvement of various team members and the various project outcomes (*Table 18-3*)? First of all, somewhat surprisingly, there seem to be no general relationships between the involvement of groups of team members, and the attainment of various different project outcomes. Secondly, there are no relationships between the involvement of groups of team members (or the involvement of individuals) and ratings of effects on the work of the team members themselves – at least in terms of ratings summed over all individuals.[4]

Thirdly, however, there are a number of relationships between involvement and some specific criteria. The degree of involvement by the matron (i.e. supporting-team nurse) in a project is positively associated with the ratings of the achievement of objectives, while the degree of involvement of operational-team members, or at least, of some specific members at this operational level, seems to be negatively associated with some outcomes. Namely, the involvement of the operational-team doctor and the operational-team nurse is negatively associated with administrative action outcomes, and involvement of the operational-team administrator also negatively with the achievement of objectives.[5]

The next section will consider why the involvement of certain hospital staff should have these various effects. At this point, it should be sufficient to say that the involvement of hospital-team members was not uniformly high for most projects. Several team members might be highly involved in a project but usually not all were. In other words, there was not really a hospital 'team'. Furthermore, there are no relationships between the involvement of all team members and various project outcomes. The extent to which hospital teams were a 'team', in the sense of all being involved in a project, seems to make no difference to project outcomes. Only the involvement of a few specific hospital team members seems to make a difference.

## SELF-HELP, CENTRAL-TEAM HELP, AND PROJECT OUTCOMES

A basic dilemma of the H.I.C. Project concerned *who* was to do the actual work in hospital projects. The earliest views were that H.I.C. was to be a 'self-help' project and that benefit would only accrue to hospital staff if they themselves were to study their problems. Hospital staff were to devote perhaps one-third of their working hours to this study. They were to learn research methods and then proceed to do studies. This was not, in fact, feasible, or at least representations on this point by the hospital-team members impelled the central team to make available student help, as well as their own help, in carrying out projects. In this section we shall explore some evidence bearing on the actual distribution of efforts in projects, and we shall then relate these differences to project success. For what kinds of outcomes is it better that central-team members collect and analyse data and write reports, and for what kinds of outcomes is it better that hospital team members do the work?

In order to answer these questions, a measure to discriminate between hospital-team and central-team activity was constructed. The relevant information was obtained from H.I.C. files and 'key' informants for each of the thirty-eight projects. Four separate measures were constructed: who collected the data, who kept the data, who analysed the data, and who wrote the report.

Numbers were assigned to six separate degrees of self-help. At one extreme, hospital-team members might be involved in the project activities, and they would get other non-team members in the hospital involved as well. This would be a project at the further remove from 'central-team help'. Alternatively, the hospital team as a whole, but not others in the hospital, might carry out certain project activities. Both of these extremes, however, were quite rare.

The bulk of the project activities were carried out by a part of the hospital team, or (showing less hospital involvement), by students assigned to the hospitals, or (showing even less hospital-team involvement) non-student central-team members. Finally, a very few activities were carried out by some outside 'experts'. Some ninety per cent of the projects were done by (a) one or more hospital-team members, (b) students, or (c) other central-team members.

Roughly equal numbers of projects were done by each of these three categories of staff; and if one considers students as central-team members, then one would conclude that data collection, data analysis, and report writing were most often done by people other than hospital staff. Thus, H.I.C. was not, (at least in terms of the 'donkey work' of surveys) a 'self-help' project.[6]

In *Table 18-4*, we see that the extent to which the hospital team did the work at various project stages is inversely, and consistently, associated with the extent of administrative action and the achievement of objectives. In other words, if you want 'actions', and 'objectives' achieved, the central team should do the project work (see also *Figure 15-1*, Chapter 15).

Above, we saw that involvement of the supporting-team nurse (matron) in project work seemed to facilitate the achievement of objectives, and the involvement of the operational-team doctor seemed to be detrimental to administrative action. The degree of involvement of these specific hospital-

TABLE 18-4 *Relationships between Hospital/Central-Team Project Activity and Project Criteria*

($N$=23 to 35 projects)

| *Hospital/Central-team project activity* | *Project criteria* Own work improved PR596 | Respondents affected PR538 | Administrative actions PU50 | Objectives achieved PR500 |
|---|---|---|---|---|
| PP36 Hospital collected data | ·33* | −·05 | −·36* | −·14 |
| PP45 Hospital analysed data | −·02 | −·13 | −·49** | −·32* |
| PP46 Hospital kept data | −·09 | −·34* | −·46** | −·36** |
| PP48 Hospital wrote report | −·12 | −·15 | −·39* | −·36** |

* Significant at a probability less than 10 per cent, two-tailed test.
** Significant at a probability less than 5 per cent, two-tailed test.

team members is in fact related to the extent of hospital-team or central-team activity. Matron's involvement is inversely related to hospital activity ($r=-0{\cdot}43$ to $-0{\cdot}59$ according to the different stages of work), and the operational-team doctor's involvement is positively related to overall hospital activity ($r=0{\cdot}35$ to $0{\cdot}48$). This suggests that the involvement of specific hospital staff members and the balance of hospital-team or central-team activity at different stages of a project are operating jointly in affecting project outcomes. The relevant correlations are all of similar magnitude, so there appears to be no causal priority for one set of determinants or the other.

Apparently some projects have relatively high hospital-team activity, and the involvement of the operational-team doctors is associated with this relatively high activity by the hospital team as opposed to the central team. To put it alternatively, when the operational-team doctors are highly involved in a project, hospital staff (probably the doctor) do the project work and the central team plays a smaller role in the work of the project. For other projects the central team takes on a greater share of the work, and in these the matron tends to be relatively highly involved.

Most importantly, it is these latter projects, and not the former, that are relatively more successful in terms of action outcomes and achievement of objectives. We shall find the general relationship found in this section repeated a number of times in the evaluation study, using different kinds of measures. Central team help seems to be essential if hospital-team members are to solve problems by means of the H.I.C. Project (see Chapters 15 and 17).

In summary, a set of data with projects as the referents was collected to provide additional evidence for some of the conclusions obtained from individual-level analyses, and also to provide more information focused squarely on the hospital project, its effects, and the determinants of these effects.

We conclude that the primary objective of projects appears to be not improving the work of team members themselves, but rather affecting the work of others – the respondents studied in the projects. As one might expect with this emphasis, ratings show that the average hospital projects achieved relatively little in the way of effects on the work of team members. While the average project achieved more in the way of administrative actions and effects on respondents in projects, it was still only 'some'.

The data obtained from hospital projects or surveys were generally quite 'clear', but this is not unquestionably desirable. 'Unclear' information apparently discourages direct administrative action by hospital-team members, and instead encourages discussions with other non-team staff in the hospital, thereby possibly facilitating subsequent changes and improvements in the work practices of hospital-team members. Very little in the way of comparative assessments was made with project data, and if this can be improved in subsequent projects (presumably by means of discussions among hospital-team members, others in the hospital, and central-team staff), then the work practices of hospital-team members may also be improved.

There was really no 'hospital *team*' in the sense of all six or eight members being highly involved in each project. There was not even an operational *team* in which the three trained hospital staff worked together on the hospital projects. On the average, one or two operational-team members were moderately or highly involved in a project, with perhaps one supporting-team member. However, the absence of a team does not seem to have affected the direct outcomes from projects one way or the other, at least in terms of the four criterion measures used here.

Rather more important is whether it was hospital-team or central-team members who did the work at various stages of a project. The extent to which the central-team members, rather than hospital-team members, analysed data, wrote the report, and so on, is positively associated with the extent of administrative action and the degree to which hospital-team members themselves see 'objectives achieved'. That the central team did the work is not the whole story, however, since matrons tended to be highly involved in projects when central-team members did project work, and this involvement, also, is associated with achieving objectives. Similarly, the involvement of the operational doctor is highly associated with hospital-team staff doing a project rather than the central team, and this involvement of the operational doctor is also associated with the relative 'failure' of projects to achieve objectives.

These relationships by no means present the full story about the optimal arrangements of central-team co-operation with hospital-team staff, but they do emphasize that if 'actions' and problem-solving activities are desired from H.I.C., then an important factor is the central team carrying out a portion of the survey or project work in the hospitals.

## NOTES

[1] Those denying action as an end seemed to have in mind diagnosis as the project aim, but since they did not have any responsibility for the functioning of those studied, nor were working to a brief given by those responsible, they found it hard to hold an aim other than that of obtaining information as a simple matter of curiosity. While the majority of projects did have some action in view, this is not to say that the alternative actions had been thoroughly considered beforehand. Our impression is that many of the hospital-team members doing projects with action aims simply assumed that, once information was obtained, the correct and proper actions would be known and, barring financial and other constraints from above, the actions would be within their capabilities. That is to say, actions were the objective of most hospital projects – actions that would for the most part flow directly from the information obtained, so that in a sense obtaining information would almost be equivalent to attaining the objectives.

[2] Another way of viewing the intercorrelations between the various ratings is in terms of agreement about the same object of the rating. Only in the case of achieving objectives is there some evidence of agreement. Project respondent, and (understandably) 'own work' effects are not rated similarly across projects by the three tripartite divisions. For this reason, we shall report any relationships for specific ratings that deviate from the relationships obtained with composite indices.

[3] Furthermore, intercorrelations show that the average involvement of the supporting team taken as a whole (the three original members listed in *Table 18-3* plus any later co-opted supporting staff) and the average involvement of the operational team (three original members plus any later joiners) are not correlated. Neither is the involvement of particular team members, or subgroups of team members, highly associated. The only exceptions are a correlation between the average involvement of the supporting-team administrator and the supporting-team nurse, and a correlation between the average involvement of the operational-team nurse and the operational-team doctor.

[4] Own work effects, separately rated by the three different professional groups, do show some interesting relationships with involvement variables. First of all, the involvement of the operational-team doctor is positively associated with ratings of effects on their own work by doctors. Similar correlations do not obtain for administrators' or nurses' involvement and their ratings of own work effects. Perhaps the involvement of doctors is associated with their taking a major role in studies and creating studies of their own work, while the administrators and nurses, when highly involved in a project, tend to study others – often the work of others on the ward – and not their own work.

The involvement of the supporting-team administrator seems to be associated with effects on the 'own work' of all supporting team members. Furthermore, the involvement of operational-team members is positively associated with effects on the work of administrators, and there is a suggestion that the involvement of supporting-team members is also positively associated with the effects on the work of the administrators. Finally, nurses' involvement, or the involvement of others, is not related to 'own work' effects for nurses.

The best interpretation for these various relationships would seem to be that when a senior administrator becomes involved in a project, the effects touch the work of other team members at senior levels, since administrators are often in a central position to affect these others. Senior administrators, through virtue of their central administrative and co-ordinating function, also have their own work affected when a number of team members from different tripartite divisions are jointly involved in a project (i.e. when *all* supporting-team members, or *all* operational-team members are involved).

Doctors, by virtue of their relative autonomy (that is, the absence of control by other individuals), have their own work affected only if they themselves are highly involved in a study. One can only speculate that perhaps nursing involvement shows no relationships with 'own work' effects because they have neither a central administrative function nor sufficient autonomy to study their own work.

[5] An examination of the involvement of the supporting-team administrator in relation to ratings of respondent effects, and objectives, *separately* rated by administrators, doctors, and nurses, shows that only the ratings by doctors are significant and negative. That is, the more the operational-team administrator is involved in a project, the lower the doctor ratings of respondent effects and achievement of objectives. The same holds for the involvement of the supporting-team administrator and the doctor ratings of respondent effects and achievement of objectives. The more these administrators were

involved, the less these outcomes were obtained, at least in the eyes of doctors.

[6] These items concerning who did the project work at various stages are generally highly positively related, as one might expect. If the hospital team, rather than the central team, gathered the project data, they also analysed the data, and so on. Also, it would appear that earlier in the life of the H.I.C. Project there was a tendency for hospitals, rather than the central team, to do studies, as shown by significant positive correlations with a measure of the time at which projects were started (i.e. '1' was assigned to the first project to be done in H.I.C., '2' to the second, and so on). This early emphasis on work by hospitals conformed to the original philosophy of the H.I.C. Project. Later, it became evident to Project staff, including the central team, that the philosophy was impracticable, and that central-team members would have to provide significant help for hospital teams and do much of the survey work themselves. This was a Project-wide decision, not something that happened hospital by hospital. That this interpretation is appropriate is suggested by the absence of significant correlations for 'time projects started *by hospital*'. In other words, not all 'first' projects for a hospital were done by the hospital team – some 'first' projects were not carried out until students joined the H.I.C. Project. But most of the early projects done in the first half-year of the H.I.C. Project were done by the hospital teams.

# 19 *Evaluation conclusions*

We shall start this chapter by briefly reviewing the highlights of the analyses in the last seven chapters. We shall examine what proved to be relatively effective in the H.I.C. Project and what proved to be relatively ineffective, and we shall try to draw up a model of relationships between various activities and various outcomes.

However, after making suggestions for minor revisions in H.I.C. – i.e. suggestions based on these analyses – we move to a consideration of the place of the H.I.C. Project in the wider context of other kinds of change efforts. We shall attempt to make some judgements about the value of the H.I.C. Project in relation to these alternative efforts or programmes, and to this end, we shall utilize the dimensions from Chapter 3. In addition we shall examine the organizational strategy of the H.I.C. Project – the strategy for covering some of the essentially organizational characteristics of the H.I.C. hospitals – and we shall examine the sequential operation of the H.I.C. Project – how the process of change was handled in the Project.

## A SUMMARY OF OBJECTIVE EVALUATION FINDINGS

A comparison (Chapter 12) between length of patients' stay in the individual hospitals and the regional averages showed no significant changes. However, this comparison was very crude, being based on yearly averages and very broad categories of patients, and it may not have been sensitive enough to discern some changes that did in fact occur. An examination (Chapter 13) of staff turnover and absenteeism also seemed to show no discernible H.I.C. effects. Looking at those staff involved in the H.I.C. Project, there seemed to be no clear-cut long-term effects on morale, either over the years of high H.I.C. activity or as a result of the more limited hospital project activity.

However, there is evidence from questionnaire data (Chapter 14) that some aspects of communication behaviour in the broadest sense changed and improved among some project participants. The average participant claimed to have made 'some' improvements in his work and have solved 'some' of his problems at work, although these effects are not readily quantifiable in a comparative fashion. Increases in communicating to others, listening to others, and being aware of the dynamics of behaviour of others, were also seen in some of the hospital-team members by their colleagues. However, these changes were not very great and, furthermore, the measurement is based on a sum of 'all' changes occurring during the period of the H.I.C. Project, including, apparently, changes created by other contemporaneous improvement programmes or 'normal' improvements.

Taking all hospital-team participants into account, and looking at all members of staff groups involved with H.I.C., the effects of the Project seem modest, at least in the light of the original expectations regarding hospital improvement.

Despite the relatively modest overall level of outcomes, however, there was considerable variation in reported H.I.C. achievements. Using questionnaire data we have examined some of the factors determining the outcomes obtained. If the input level of certain determinants were to be increased, a repetition of the H.I.C. Project might be more fruitful in terms of outcomes. Instead of the average team member reporting 'some' problem-solving, for example, he might report 'much', with 'some' the exception.

This kind of tinkering with the Project does, of course, assume that all other things are equal, an assumption that is often not tenable. For example, an increased emphasis on central-team help to hospitals (such as increased 'change consultation' or 'training') might entail hiring a larger central team, and this in turn might adversely (or beneficially) affect the integration and morale of the team, and, ultimately, the learning situation provided for hospital-team members. In other words, the suggestions for improving H.I.C. are made with the reservation that unintended or concomitant effects of changes are not included in the present analysis. The list of inputs to be modified is a list of specific, limited changes only.

Later in this chapter we shall examine the H.I.C. Project as one of a number of different kinds of organizational change projects, and we shall consider modification of the Project in a more general sense. The main thrust of this Project was technological and 'rationalistic'; what if a project with a non-rational, normative base were attempted? This is the basic kind of question to which we shall turn later.

Assuming that the H.I.C. Project is more or less unchanged in broad structure and emphasis, what specific factors might be changed to improve outcomes? The correlational analyses in Chapters 15 to 18 have provided a number of suggestions. *Table 19-1* presents some of the main factors found to be related to the outcomes under study.

First of all, which of the various inputs seem to be of value in improving the H.I.C. Project generally? We see from the table that one of the most generally useful factors or inputs is the extent to which hospital-team members make their job a part of the H.I.C. Project. Increasing this factor in a new H.I.C. Project would be expected to yield increased information, problem-solving, work improvements, increased influence, and improved communication. No other input listed in *Table 19-1* seems to be of such general potential value, although increasing the influence of 'other hospital staff'

TABLE 19-1 *Summary of Relationships between H.I.C. Inputs and Outcomes**

| | *H.I.C. outcomes* | | | | | | |
|---|---|---|---|---|---|---|---|
| *H.I.C. inputs* | *Information; knowledge* | *Problem-solving; action* | *Work improvements* | *Increased influence* | *Improved communication To* | *Improved communication From* | *Understand* |
| Usefulness of: | | | | | | | |
| Courses | + | | + | | | | |
| Central team | | ++ | ++ | + | | | |
| Meetings | | ++ | ++ | | | | + |
| Hospital project participation by hospital-team members | + | | + | + | ++ | | + |
| Central-team influence on hospital projects | | + | + | | | | |
| Influence of other hospital staff on hospital projects | | ++ | + | ++ | | | + |
| Hospital-team members make their job part of H.I.C. | + | ++ | ++ | + | + | + | + |
| Central-team activity: | | | | | + | + | + |
| Diagnostic consultation | | + | ++ | | | | |
| Change consultation | | ++ | ++ | | | | |
| Training | | ++ | ++ | | | | |
| Feedback meeting activity, attendance | | | ++ | | | | + |
| LSH meeting attendance | | | ++ | | | | |

++=Consistent positive relationships. +=Inconsistent positive relationships.

* The table provides entries only for those relationships with inferred causal directions from 'input' to 'output'. Relationships with the reverse causal direction (e.g. some relationships between 'outcomes' and meeting activity 'inputs') are deleted. See Chapter 16 for details.

on hospital projects seems to be related to a number of different useful outcomes.

Alternatively, one might examine a certain outcome, such as problem-solving, to see what inputs would be particularly useful in this direction. Thus one would want to emphasize participation in projects by other hospital staff, and by the central team, instead of participation in projects by the hospital-team members, to obtain problem-solving outcomes.[1] 'Change consultation' and 'training' by central-team members would be particularly useful in this respect.

To obtain greater communications outcomes, such as listening to others and being aware of, and understanding, the dynamics of their behaviour, one would also emphasize central-team influence on projects, and hospital-team members being active in feedback meetings. *Table 19-1* is, of course, an oversimplified picture of the findings and the reader searching for suggestions for factors to emphasize in a 'new' H.I.C. Project would best reread Chapters 15 to 18.

The findings in *Table 19-1* suggest that the new and unusual aspects of the H.I.C. Project were perhaps not so successful as its more conventional aspects. The hospital teams were to 'learn by doing' under their own direction as well as under the direction of the central team. A more typical organizational development project would have had the central team (the 'change-agents') in possession of rather more influence than in the H.I.C. Project, and we have seen in the evaluation that this influence is associated with a number of positive outcomes for the hospital teams and their hospitals.

Similarly, the usual organizational development project would have change-agents spending much of their time on what we have termed 'training' activities (Chapter 18). This was not envisaged as a major role for the central team – one need only consider their lack of experience in this area – but we have found that training activities, more than the prescribed diagnostic consultation activities, are associated with positive H.I.C. outcomes.

The emphasis in H.I.C. was the collection of data by surveys, and somewhat less time and effort were devoted to various kinds of meetings and discussion groups. Again, the evaluation data indicate the positive value of discussion – at least the discussion in the feedback meetings – compared to collecting and analysing survey data.

The emphasis in H.I.C. was on surveys by top staff of others in their hospitals – they were to become survey technicians or survey researchers. Yet the evaluation data indicate that very unscientific studies – contaminated by the influence of other hospital staff, including perhaps even respondents, and contaminated by hospital-team members studying their own work – facilitated various positive outcomes. In other words, the less like survey researchers, and the more like action-researchers or change-agents, the hospital-team members were, the better the results in terms of individual and organizational improvements.

The explanation of all this would appear to be relatively simple. The H.I.C. Project was attempting to create changes in people – changes in the attitudes towards communication, changes in morale, and so on. Instead of taking an indirect approach to such changes by starting with the use of survey technology, the H.I.C. Project would have been more efficient by acting as an organizational development project with a major component directly attempting such changes in people.

In other words, the H.I.C. Project should, perhaps, have been modified by bringing in a relatively influential central team (influential in terms of knowledge, experience, seniority, possession of sanctions), a central team that would work on the emotional and normative aspects of hospital-team members and hospitals, that would dispense with surveys for the most part and would utilize discussion groups to make hospital-team members look at their own work activities and to involve others in the hospital in the developing change programme. A more traditional organizational development project might result, but so might some of the successful outcomes at times achieved by such projects (Greiner, 1965).

However, a hint at the more likely outcome of such a modification of the H.I.C. Project is provided by the reaction of hospital-team members to the second series of Project meetings. These meetings were rather similar in structure and procedure to the sensitivity training groups often used as part of organizational development. It may be recalled that the reaction to these groups was rejection and a desire for more structured, less emotionally oriented groups for the discussion of survey data.

In fact, hospital-team members (a) did not appear, from our observations, to welcome more central-team help or influence (Chapter 15); (b) did not desire relatively more 'training' in contrast to 'diagnostic consultation' from the central team (Chapter 17); (c) did not find the feedback meetings, or any meetings, very useful (Chapter 15); and (d) did not seem to want to involve other hospital staff in survey activity or to wish to look closely at the shortcomings of their own work (Chapter 15). In other words, a modification of the H.I.C. Project along the lines of an organizational development project would not be feasible without consideration of hospital-team members' desires – which seemed generally opposed. For some tentative answers to this dilemma we must take a more intensive look at the H.I.C. Project as a whole – relying on descriptions by central-team members and others, as well as the evaluation survey, for data – and we must look at the H.I.C. Project in relation to other kinds of change projects.

There are several ways of looking at the relative lack of achievement or outcomes of the H.I.C. Project. The validity of the model, the appropriateness of the situation, and the skill in implementation are, of course, almost inextricably interwoven, making any definitive analysis of such a 'natural' experiment extremely difficult (Seashore, 1964). Was the project invalid in its conception or were there shortcomings in its implementation? To put it very simply, perhaps the inputs were inappropriate or insufficient. Were, for example, the situations selected so difficult to change and improve that any reasonable amount of input would be inadequate?

There is also a temporal dimension to all this, and perhaps the inputs may have been appropriate at one time, but not later. Or is it a more complex problem of the 'mix' of the inputs at any one time? Alternatively, the links between preliminary efforts, intermediate outcomes, and subsequent outcomes may have been inappropriately specified or implemented.

## TECHNOLOGY, STRUCTURE, PEOPLE, AND TASK

Let us try to gain some perspective on these questions by returning now to the distinctions made in Chapter 3. In the view of the evaluator, the H.I.C. Project was an attempt to change the technology in hospital organizations, particularly the communication technology, and thereby change the people in the organizations and their structural arrangements, and finally to improve task outcomes. The H.I.C. Project is atypical of projects directed at 'people' because it starts with technology as a change target, and it is also atypical of technological change efforts because it aims eventually and explicitly at changes in people. Thus, the Project broke new ground in attempting to articulate technology with other focuses of change.

We shall now examine each of these focuses of change in the H.I.C. Project, so as to discern whether alternative approaches to change might be more or less desirable. First of all, what were the gross outcomes of the interventions in technology, people, and structure, as these systems were described in Chapter 3? The technology for gathering information did change in most hospitals, at least during the period the Project was active. Survey teams, composed to varying degrees of hospital staff and central-team members, gathered information on a great variety of matters; and we saw in Chapter 15 that hospital-team members' participation in survey activities was correlated with increased knowledge about the functioning of others and about problems in the hospital. But the relationship of this information to patient-care was something less than clear. The Project staff did not specify any model for the effects of particular information on care, nor did hospital-team members themselves have any model to guide their desire for information. The most specific model seemed (see Chapter 12) to be that information about or affecting 'staff morale' would in some way improve patient-care. However, in Chapter 13 we have described the absence of research evidence for a causal link between morale and organizational effectiveness.

Perhaps most importantly, the changes in the technology for gathering information, and the changes in information available, were only temporary. The technology of the hospital seems to have changed relatively little in most of the hospitals, in the long run. While in one hospital there seems to be a more or less permanent skilled survey team that is made use of by others, in other hospitals the survey apparatus seems to be in disuse. In addition to the implementation of the survey technique, there have been a number of other minor technological change efforts in the hospitals; however, these are generally quite minor in relation to the organization as a whole (changes such as the installation of a bell to summon patients to the casualty officer, the provision of a new kind of porter's trolley, and so on).[2] Some of these minor technological changes may have affected patient-care, but probably only in a very limited and most indirect fashion. Improvements in the information system may have been of greater benefit to the hospital, but not beyond the duration of the Project, since the teams and the survey technology were generally not used subsequently.

But perhaps technological improvements in the communication system had desirable ramifications within the hospital structure. There have, in fact, been a moderate number of structural modifications such as the holding of more frequent meetings between matron and students, or the institution of regular meetings between the hospital department heads. One hospital has started a messenger service. Hospital-team members claim more contact with one another, also. However, no hospital made any changes of the magnitude, for example, achieved by Pantall and Elliot (1968) in the reorganization of the top staff structure at East Birmingham Hospital.

Finally, there are changes in people to consider. The evidence for changes in the morale of hospital project participants is relatively limited, but even if there were major changes, one would still have to find a way in which morale affects patient-care in any direct fashion. There were also changes in communication behaviour, but they were apparently limited primarily to certain hospital-team members, especially operational-team nursing and administrative members.

In summary, with neither technology, nor people, nor structure showing major pervasive changes in the organizations, it is not over surprising that our crude measures of task performance, or patient-care, do not show any signs of improvement, whichever general model for the sequence of effects one uses.

It would seem to make sense if the H.I.C. Project, or its successors, were to give more attention to changes in people if, in fact, this is one of the goals of the Project. That is to say, rather than attempt to change them indirectly, by means of technology, or in addition to such attempts, direct change should be encouraged. However, without a clear model of relations between changes in people and improvement in task outcomes, the usefulness of such work on changing people must still be questioned. In addition, there is a major difficulty in making a direct approach to changing people, because client resistance is liable to be fairly high. That is to say, it may not be legitimate in hospitals for change-agents to undertake any of the various kinds of activities commonly used to change people, such as T-groups, encounter groups, and so on.[3]

We shall return to this matter after reviewing the H.I.C. Project in terms of the dimensions described in Chapter 3 – cognitive/emotional and objective/subjective orientations, balance of influence between change-agent and client, clarity of Project means and ends, and the extent of organizational strategy. To anticipate several sections that follow, we see the H.I.C. Project as more or less typical of many technological change efforts. The Project primarily emphasized 'cognitive' inputs and consequences as well as an 'objective' focus of change. Technological change efforts are also typically characterized by unilateral influence relationships between change-agents and clients. This was true of the H.I.C. Project, but the degree of imbalance in the influence relationship was surely unusual. The influence of the change-agents in their field of expertise, the area of technology, was very highly circumscribed in this Project. The H.I.C. Project was generally characterized by clients with a high degree of self-direction in Project activities and with a high degree of direction by these clients over many change-agent activities as well. Finally, the H.I.C. Project was characterized by a great deal of obscurity with regard to the ends (especially organizational ends) of the improvement activity as well as the links between ends and means. In contrast, the means – the various items of survey technology – were closely specified, in fact, perhaps more so than in some other technological change programmes.

## COGNITIONS AND EMOTIONS

The reader will have seen from previous chapters that the H.I.C. Project, in keeping with the 'technological' characterization we have given it, and in keeping with other change programmes of a technological nature such as operational research, was eminently cognitive in orientation. Cognitive means of change were used, and the cognitive aspects of people were emphasized as focuses of change. Information was provided in the hope that the resulting understanding ('intelligibility' according to Revans) would ultimately affect actions.

Emotions were recognized, but in a limited fashion. The absence of knowledge, according to Revans, leads to anxiety. Emotional resistance to change was also mentioned, but, by using self-direction, such resistance to outside attempts at change was to be avoided. But probably the most potent emotion in the hospital situation – anxiety regarding authority – was handled in the H.I.C. Project in a prescriptive fashion. Hospital-team members were to 'cast off' their authority in their H.I.C. Project relationships. In summary, the H.I.C. Project, as conceived, was to emphasize the cognitive aspects of people as means and targets of change.

In practice, the Project accepted the need for change in emotional behaviour. Although hospital project activity with its emphasis on collecting information was pre-eminent, the central team gradually became aware of the need to 'change attitudes', and the younger central-team members especially came to discuss frequently among themselves the need for more 'democratic attitudes' at the top of the H.I.C. hospitals. Similarly, one of the senior central-team members emphasized, in speaking of the change process, that one has to 'hurt' in order to change – that one cannot change without 'feeling' it. These are some of the points within the Project that displayed a concern for emotional changes, but to the extent that the central team lacked influence over the hospital-team members or others in the hospital – and we saw that this was generally the case – the attempts at looking at emotions in addition to the cognitive emphasis on surveys by Revans, could not be implemented.

If we agree that many organizational problems are located at the emotional level of individual functioning, (and there are a large number of practising change-agents who feel that this is so),[4] we can readily accept that the H.I.C. Project had relatively little effect in improving matters in the client organizations. Furthermore, it is felt by some analysts that the crucial problem in hospitals, and also the crucial deterrent to any amelioration of these problems, rests respectively in anxieties and the defences induced by anxieties (Menzies, 1960; Revans, 1964b).

These points may explain why the average hospital-team member typically reported that he learned nothing 'new' from the surveys. Team members were already aware of the problems, they claimed, and they wanted to know how to change people – other people, not themselves. Analysis of the ratings of feedback meetings – with their limited but consistent emphasis on the examination of emotional matters (see Chapter 16 and Appendix 16A) indicates some support for the hypothesis of the efficacy of emotional orientations in change efforts. Meetings were not consciously seen as 'useful', but there was continued reattendance by some hospital-team members (despite explicitly denied 'usefulness', given in an informal interview setting), and correlations show that attendance was associated with problem-solving.

Similarly, the apparent efficacy of the influence of central-team members, in facilitating various problem-solving outcomes, may be interpreted in part as due to their concern with the feelings of hospital-team members (and with providing 'psychological support') as well as their concern with changing the 'authoritarian' values of hospital-team members (suggested by objective ratings not reported here, as well as interview comments). There was not much influence available to or utilized by central-team members, but the relationship of such influence with desirable outcomes may be interpreted in terms of emotional orientation. Although this view is not firmly based on objective survey evidence, it does suggest one direction any subsequent project might wish to take to increase various outcomes – a more 'emotional' orientation.

## OBJECTIVE AND SUBJECTIVE ORIENTATIONS

The H.I.C. Project was also eminently 'objective' in orientation. People in the project were often viewed as objects. We have seen how hospital projects were usually studies of other people; hospital-team members tended not to study their own work as part of the H.I.C. Project (Chapter 15). From the beginning, in the assembling of hospital-team members, and in the recruitment of central-team members for that matter, there seemed to be relatively little consideration of attitudes, of how individuals felt about one another or related to each other. The main considerations for selection were the jobs, the roles they would fill, or the position they held in the hospital.

The central team, however, put effort into the examination of its work and its developing relationship with the hospitals and hospital teams. But this attention to 'process' seemed to arise primarily because of problems and difficulties, including resignations of staff and ineffectual change efforts. In fact, the central-team members were criticized by a number of hospital people for being so introspective and concerned with themselves that their view of their work was rather distorted by the apparent over-emphasis on shortcomings and inadequacies.

This perhaps only illustrates the difficulty of such an examination of process (Schein, 1969). Skills in this area are acquired by rather lengthy training and experience (see also Lippitt *et al.*, 1958). The student members of the central team, however, remained with the project only some six months, while the average senior central-team member stayed only about a year. There was not much time for learning, particularly in the light of the immense task – ten hospitals – faced by the central team. As has been indicated in Chapter 5, the previous training and experience of the central team did not provide any background in process observation.

Even given skills in this kind of work, the use of an outside consultant or observer to provide validation of process observations by the change-agent is indispensable (Schein, 1969). Consideration was given to the use of the evaluation team in this role, but in the view of the advisory committee, it would have been undesirable to 'contaminate' the working of the Project, or the evaluation either, by providing such feedback on Project functioning, whether process or outcomes. Consequently, for the various reasons given above, the change-agents (central team) were at some disadvantage in trying to take a process, or even an adequate subjective, approach to their Project activities. Undoubtedly, a valid subjective orientation by the change-agents would have been most helpful to their work.

Those being changed in the hospitals, the hospital-team members who were themselves to change others in the hospital, generally shunned the subjective approach. The hospital teams attempted to be most 'objective' in their studies (for examples, see Chapter 6). We have seen that they tended infrequently to study their own work or to make 'their job' a part of the

H.I.C. Project (Chapter 15). Neither did the hospital team, as a team, study the work of any one of its members. In point of fact, there usually was not enough of a 'team' (Chapter 18) to permit firm comment on whether there was a focus internal or external to the team, in terms of the projects undertaken.

Probably it is most accurate to say that the individual members of the hospital team tended in many cases to select projects rather distant from their personal interests – rather distant from the 'top'. There were no studies of the nursing office as such, for example. Often, when wards were studied, linking individuals in the nursing office would be overlooked. There were even cases where departments were studied, and the department heads, or those individuals closest to the hospital-team members, were omitted.

Of course, in taking an objective approach, the hospital-team members were only following the example of their training courses. The questionnaires provided there were for the study of ward staff, not top people like themselves. The collection of data by means of 'objective' survey instruments – rather than the use of subjective rating scales or the use of participant observation – was emphasized. Finally, the hospital teams spent the practice week using their survey skills in another hospital, not their own. It was not surprising that the central team subsequently had difficulty in getting hospital teams to move away from the study of individuals who were distant from the top staff in the hospital. We have seen that to the extent that the central team was successful in this, and hospital-team members followed any predilections to study 'their job', the outcomes of project work were enhanced (Chapter 15).

## INFLUENCE RELATIONSHIPS

One might have expected that the central team, being required to use some of their survey knowledge in helping run surveys, would have influenced the composition of the hospital teams as well as the portions of the hospital the team was to study with the survey technology. That is to say, the central team might suggest where and how the survey technology of H.I.C. might be implanted in the information system of the hospital. However, the central team usually had little influence over the diagnostic process, since only after a project – including the team composition, those to be studied, the topics to be investigated, and so on – was decided upon, did the hospital team come to the central team for advice on methodology. It was assumed that the hospital-team members knew where the problems lay, knew the nature of the problem and its sources, and also where its solution might be found (see Schein, 1969). The central team had to accept the influence of the hospital team in structuring projects in this manner, despite the fact that the decisions were often made against the better judgement of the central team. The philosophy of the Project, as the central team saw it, was that the central team should not be 'directive' towards the hospital team.

Those carrying out a typical technological change project do not, in fact, have very much influence, since their final recommendations can always be rejected by management – no matter how good the diagnosis, analysis, or report. The technologist only has influence in being able to present an analysis with some cogent recommendations, it being assumed that they will be accepted by a rational manager to the extent that they fit in with his goals and other organizational needs. However, the influence of the central team was even more circumscribed than in the usual technological change project. It was assumed in the H.I.C. Project that recommendations for action would come from hospital-team members themselves, and only in the area of survey methodology might they wish to take advice and to be influenced by the central team. For this reason, the central-team members, in analysing the survey data from hospital projects, often left hospitals with a report consisting of raw data or data summaries, not interpretations and recommendations. Only in the later stages of the H.I.C. Project did the central team consistently try to influence hospital teams over the use of the survey results.

What influence the central team did have, at least during the early and middle stages of the H.I.C. Project, was in deciding which particular data collection and analysis procedures were to be utilized. Later on, the central team had more influence, since they often undertook these tasks, as well as providing advice on which were the best to use. However, this influence was often of little value, for at the feedback stage of projects the central team once more abstained from 'directiveness' towards the hospital-team members. The central team usually waited to see if the hospital team would invite them to a feedback meeting, which, if held, had usually been decided upon by the hospital teams themselves. Thus the application of methodology by the central team could come to nothing if the hospital did not want to do feedback or to act on findings. Even if there was feedback and action, however, one had to assume that the hospital team had chosen wisely in deciding on doing the project, that they had performed an appropriate diagnosis, etc., before approaching the central team.

One might view this patterning of influence relationships – in which hospital-team members decided on a project, central-team members provided the methods and often carried them out, and hospital-team members decided on, and carried out, feedback in the hospitals – as being very rational. The hospital-team members had complete control over hospital matters about which they knew best – over what problems should be studied, and over what help they should be given in order to solve the problems. On the other hand, central-team members had control over those things which they had studied and knew well, namely project methods.

In point of fact however, central-team members did know a little about hospitals, and at the very least they could provide an outsider's more objective view of matters, even if their only data were those provided by hospital-team members. At best, as has been indicated above, the central team could have played a vital role in selecting projects to be done (in terms of the location in the information system, and in terms of content to be studied) and could have played an important role in the utilization of data by feedback or even in action. The evaluation survey evidence (Chapters 15, 17) indicates that the central team's influence on project activity – in a number of ways, including not only what we have termed diagnostic consultation or change consultation, but also training – seems beneficial for various outcomes. It would appear, in short, that any further H.I.C. Projects might best be structured so that central-team members are enabled and encouraged to influence hospital-team members much more actively.

What are some of the possible problems involved in encouraging this new set-up in terms of influence? In addition to losing some volunteers and to losing some hospital-team motivation, as we have described in Chapter 3, there is the danger that the central team may influence the 'wrong' things. That is to say, if central-team members are to have influence, they must be experts in some sense; they must know what they are talking about when they try to influence things in a particular direction. Most importantly, they must be 'experts' in the sense of knowing when they are ignorant about something.

These possible problems and shortcomings must be balanced against the beneficial effects such a change will have on the central team. Giving central-team members some influence will improve their morale, and it is likely to improve their learning and performance as well. By having some control over the situation, they are likely to think through the situation and make choices for which they will feel responsible and involved, and, on the basis of feedback, they will learn whether these choices have been appropriate or not.

What then of the influence of the hospital-team members? The data show that there were variations in the influence of the various members of a team over H.I.C. matters (Chapter 15). When these survey data are combined with informal observations of hospital-team meetings at the hospitals, an interesting picture emerges. Revans had advocated that the hospital-team members should cast off their authority, but their behaviour in meetings indicated that this was not so easily done. Those hospital-team members in a subordinate relationship to others on the team, namely the administrative and nursing members of the operational team (especially the nurses), generally refrained from active behaviour in such situations. Deference was often almost complete. Apparently both parties to a relationship found it difficult to cast off authority. Those with superior status could not afford to lose face by making mistakes in the presence of their juniors, while the juniors themselves were in a very threatening situation which immobilized any innovative behaviour. In a sense, it was as Revans had described from his earlier research. Hospital-team members were immobilized and could not communicate, and so anxiety was maintained and the immobilization reinforced.

How does one break into this self-reinforcing cycle of immobilization, anxiety, and lack of communication? The survey information about the hospitals was of no help here. Rather, a secure situation had to be provided (and this was in fact recommended by Revans). Instead of, say, holding Project meetings in the office of a superior, the subordinate's office or a neutral site should be used. In a secure situation, the influence of central-team members could have made an impact, both by providing an example (since they too were in a low authority position) and by direct attempts at supporting low-status members. These actions, of course, require central-team influence and even 'directiveness'. The usual way in which this system was broken down, in fact, was by central-team influence outside the direct interaction situation, often by students operating in the hospital over a lengthy period of time. They would coach the more junior hospital-team members or other junior staff in the hospital and they would also make direct appeals to the senior hospital-team member on behalf of the more junior. This was often done by students who had time and access to these contacts by virtue of their residence in the hospitals; the students, moreover, were not so clearly impressed by the Project policy regarding 'directiveness' set up by Revans and supported by the advisory committee (and probably their anti-authoritarian values also made a difference). We are suggesting here that greater influence on the part of the central team, and also greater influence by some more junior hospital-team members (and other hospital personnel) may have been more productive of H.I.C. outcomes.

All this is not to say that the hospital team should have little influence, or that the senior members of the hospital team should abdicate their influence. It is unrealistic to expect hospital-team members to cast off all the influence derived from their normal position of authority in the hospital, particularly in any meetings taking place in the hospital situation. Differences in influence will continue to exist and must exist, especially where there are differences in values and in views of organizational goals and approaches to those goals, such as the differences among the different professions in the hospital. Ideally, there should be high, more or less equal influence from both the central team and the hospital teams. We have cited research evidence (Chapter 3) indicating that gains in influence by one group need not be at the expense of another. We shall say more below about the efficacy of such a situation where there is mutual influence and mutual collaboration.

## CLARITY OF PROGRAMME

The lack of clarity in the Project is perhaps the most universally agreed assessment by observers, whether from central team, hospital team, or outside. The central team felt unsure of themselves throughout the Project, because of their inability to fathom what Revans had in mind when he spoke of 'communication' and their subsequent inability to agree among themselves when they began individually to develop various approaches towards what and how to change in the hospitals.

In contrast, the Project tended to become clearer to hospital-team members after the training courses were given (although a few explicitly volunteered the information in evaluation interviews that they were not clear about it even after the courses ended). The concrete activities of carrying out the surveys in the hospitals gave clarity and structure to the Project. However, there was little questioning of how surveys would improve matters until after the data had been gathered, at which point doubts about where and how the Project would proceed arose again.

Perhaps a better model of the links between the survey efforts and the desired end of improved communication might have demonstrated to H.I.C. participants the shortcomings of many surveys.[5] Improvement in communication could not be expected to flow from the mere demonstration of the existence of a problem. As Likert (1967) has indicated, many surveys focus on 'end-result' or sometimes 'intervening' data – on, for example, feelings of dissatisfaction with the food in the canteen, or tensions and poor co-ordination between medical records and the wards. But using surveys for measuring these phenomena is nothing more than charting a fever. 'Causal' variables must be examined also, if therapeutic efforts are to be launched.

Measurement of causal factors, however, may not be sufficient to produce improvements. Some causal or contributing factors cannot be easily altered, at least in the short run. Thus dissatisfaction with food that stems from physical segregation of staff into separate status categories can only be wholly improved by renovation of physical facilities.

What is needed, then, is data on the forces that facilitate or hinder change in intervening or causal variables. While we have no adequate theory of how to produce change, there are models suggesting some of the important parameters. In our example, complaints about food could have many sources, but it is likely that an assessment of status and authority relations inside the dining situation as well as measurement of communication patterns and work interdependence relations would be of use. One should also consider that resistance to change in one staff group may arise from the high functional value of separation from other staff and the value of expressing solidarity and exchanging information during meal-times. But if another way of meeting these needs can be found, resistance can be reduced. Finally, all this needs to be viewed in the context of who will propose what changes to whom. Forces for change are, of course, very dependent on relationships between change-agents and the system to be changed.

We have touched on only some of the variables possibly relevant to this problem, but the main point should be clear. Without a careful and clear diagnosis, including end-result, causal, and changing variables, improvement of a problem situation is likely to be difficult, risky, and possibly temporary. Clear models for the effects of different kinds of survey information on hospital problems would appear to be a desirable feature in any project like H.I.C.

We shall return to the matter of clarity later, for our best knowledge about optimal levels of clarity seems to indicate that it is also a matter of the timing and sequencing of clarity as well as absolute levels of clarity and structure throughout a change project.

## MORE EMPHASIS ON EMOTIONS, SUBJECTIVITY, AND CENTRAL-TEAM INFLUENCE

Near the end of the H.I.C. Project the central team initiated an activity that demonstrated the value of an emphasis on emotions, subjective orientations, and influence by the central team. During the Project, central-team members had been discussing the hospital projects in their weekly team meetings and had more or less reached agreement among themselves on outcomes and the factors determining these outcomes. But in order to complete a report on H.I.C. Project activity, they felt that they should check accounts of hospital project activity – accounts that were sometimes critical of the roles of particular hospital-team members – by showing them to hospital-team members and asking for their reactions and modifications.

In these accounts of hospital project activity, the central team indicated the roles of the various hospital-team members – particularly the degree of commitment to the Project by the supporting-team members and the extent of their facilitation of the work of operational-team members. Included were some of the tensions and other difficulties between team members, especially members of different professional groups. Another emotional aspect, namely about authority and one's autonomy to take action in certain areas, was also detailed. By and large, these emotional aspects of projects had not been discussed with the hospital teams before.

In detailing these emotional aspects of projects, central-team members were indicating some of their subjective views of project activities; that is to say, they were providing an account that was more or less internal to the central-team system. In addition, the project accounts included the central team's view of their own role and how it was handled by the hospital team. In a sense, the central team's 'own work' was being made a part of the H.I.C. Project. In this way, the central team and the hospital team were both taking a subjective orientation to the Project – they were both looking at their own activities.

Finally, in taking the initiative to present an account of hospital projects (and this was something central-team members had hoped hospital-team members would do themselves) the central team were being directive and using some of the potential influence they had not used during the course of the Project. This activity was more or less forced upon them, since they could not obtain accounts of the projects from hospital-team members detailing these emotional and subjective views, and they had to bring their own accounts to the attention of hospital-team members.

Central-team members were only able to meet a few of the hospital teams in order to discuss their mutual views of the projects, but this activity seemed to prove rather successful. They learned a number of things about each other, some misunderstandings were clarified, and they were given insights into a number of problems. Furthermore, central-team members felt that they could now work more easily with some hospital-team members. A series of matters not discussed earlier were out in the open, and there was some agreement about these matters, which enabled some work to be done on them. It was unfortunate that this happened at such a late stage in the Project, but it did demonstrate the value of placing a greater emphasis in H.I.C. on emotions, subjective orientations, and influence on the part of the central team.

We shall discuss below whether this kind of activity would have been either desirable or feasible at a much earlier point in the Project. However, it seems fairly clear that at this point the open discussion with each other of the commitments, conflicts, and differing views of the Project was of benefit beyond the task of writing a report of the Project. It was of therapeutic benefit in changing the views of both central and hospital teams and making it possible for them to work better together. Furthermore, for the evaluator (and potentially also for the central team) this kind of confrontation provided further diagnostic information. By linking one system with another and observing the effects of attempts at influence, a considerable amount might be learned about both systems and their internal dynamics, matters that are not very clear when systems are not fully in contact or attempting to influence (or to 'direct') one another.

There is one final point about this example. Not only does it illustrate the usefulness of the relatively neglected emphases in the Project, but it also suggests that it may be a matter of dual emphases – linking between cognitions and emotions, and between subjective and objective orientations, as well as a linking of influence attempts from both systems – that is useful. Thus, for example, some of the emotional aspects of relationships between hospital-team members were presented by the central team, but in a rational, cognitive fashion; and the discussion of these matters was also essentially in cognitive terms – team members thought about what they could write down that would accurately describe to non-participants what happened (including emotion-laden events). Similarly, it was the matching of subjective (views internal to the central-team system) and objective (hospital-team views including views of the central team) orientations that provided feedback to the central team and made the discussion useful. Presumably the linking of internal hospital-team views with the central team's account was of benefit to the internal system of the hospital team also. Finally, we shall argue below that a situation in which both parties have high and relatively equal influence over one another is more desirable than allocating influence to one side or the other. The important characteristic of these meetings was not that the central team had more influence, but that both parties to the meetings were in relatively highly influential positions.

## MUTUAL, LINKED EMPHASIS ON COGNITIONS AND EMOTIONS

Above we have indicated advantages and disadvantages of emphasizing the cognitive or emotional aspects of people, subjective and objective orientations, and so on. At this point we shall examine some arguments for emphasizing both aspects of what have been introduced as alternatives. If work on cognitions, for example, is linked to work on emotions so that the changes in the former go hand in hand with changes in the latter, the results are likely to be more than the mere sum of the separate efforts. We are suggesting that there must be not only a dual emphasis but rather an active linking of the alternative emphases we have described. There must be a mutuality or interaction between the dual emphases.

Making individuals aware of previously unexperienced emotions is desirable since it makes them potentially able to deal with these emotions. However, emotional experiences are diffuse, and we have no ready language to deal with emotions in all their great complexity. To the extent that experiences are unique, one cannot use the increased awareness in subsequent situations; one has not learned. Therefore the linking of emotional experiences to cognitions – to various ways of conceptualizing and describing the emotions – is a way of facilitating generalization and the application of learning and change. By working through emotional experiences and then also understanding – as well as feeling – differently, the individual has a way of dealing with the same emotions in other situations. Cognitive linkages make emotional learning transferable or of more general value.

In addition, the cognitions are now linked to emotions so that the thoughts are more 'real'. Looking from the other emphasis therefore, cognitions that are linked to emotional states are now more meaningful. However, because conceptual or cognitive learning is relatively readily acquired, there may also be a conflict with subsequently learned, 'newer' concepts, and the earlier learning may be confused, distorted, or 'forgotten'. This linkage and this meaningfulness also give cognitive changes greater stability (just as, as learning psychologists have shown, there is better retention of nonsense syllables when they are related to known and meaningful words).

In summary, linking cognitions and emotions on the one hand gives the cognitions meaning and greater stability (the learning is more durable). Linking also gives emotions meaning in a sense – meanings which are more communicable than the emotions themselves – thus facilitating the transfer and generalization of the learning outside the particular situations in which the emotions were experienced.[6]

## MUTUAL, LINKED OBJECTIVE AND SUBJECTIVE ORIENTATIONS

To focus on either internal or external system characteristics provides one with greater control over the respective systems. A subjective orientation allows one to analyse one's thoughts and feelings – to examine and to think through, and perhaps to learn and to change internally. The same holds for the external system. But change is the result of internal and external system forces together. To be aware of the opportunities and problems in the external environment, together with the internal situation, including internal resources as well as problems, is to be able to choose a rather better strategy for change. This greater awareness, obtained by linking the internal and external systems, allows one greater choice.

To think both subjectively and objectively simultaneously is perhaps not theoretically feasible. However, in practice, the juxtaposition of these modes of thought in fairly rapid sequence is to be aware of 'process'.[7]

Similarly, the focusing on a group's internal system in relation to its external system, and the internal and external systems of other larger units, allows one to analyse the flow and transactions between groups. Open-system theory as applied to organizations (Katz and Kahn, 1966) is one example of this approach. For ease of thinking and analysis one must at times restrict one's view to a closed system despite reality, but at some point the closed system approach must be replaced by another more inclusive approach – perhaps by simplifying the internal nature of the formerly closed system, so as to be able to examine transactions across the boundaries of that system.

Perhaps not as useful as the observation of 'process' or boundary exchange, but also of high value, is to make comparisons between one's own group or organization and other groups or organizations. Such a comparison entails a matching of subjective views of one's own unit with the objective data obtained about both units. We saw in Chapter 18 that hospital project data were infrequently the subject of comparisons, perhaps because hospital teams in each hospital often decided independently what problems and respondents to study and this precluded interhospital comparisons. However, the extent to which comparisons were made between one unit and another (usually within the same hospital) is highly positively associated with hospital-team members reporting improvements in their own work as a result of the project (see *Table 18-2*).

It is our tentative conclusion that the H.I.C. Project should focus more attention on internal relationships, but in the context of an objective orientation. The central team should be considered part of a system including themselves and the hospital teams, and they should study themselves as part of this system. That is to say, they might examine their values and how these compare with the values of hospital people, and so on. From an examination of forces in their mutual situations, there should come a better understanding of the change process. Hospital-team members should be encouraged where feasible to take an internal view of others, and to try to empathize with them. Even more desirable is the ability to view themselves from the standpoint of the other, and to develop from this a view of their own behaviour and that of others as making up a system that will lead to a 'human resources' approach instead of a 'human relations' approach (Miles, 1966) – that is to say, paying attention not to what one can do for others but to how one can interact and become involved with the other, so as to facilitate effectiveness. This kind of transactional view of change relationships is most useful in understanding the dynamics and outcomes of change efforts in the field of organizational development (Chin, 1961).[8]

## MUTUAL INFLUENCE RELATIONSHIPS

We have suggested that central-team members should be accorded more influence in order to make the H.I.C. Project more effective in terms of various outcomes. It is not merely a matter of equal influence relationships between the change-agent and client as advocated by Bennis (1961), but rather a mutual influence system. Each party brings to the relationship his own special competency, skills, and resources, but because these and the objects of their attention overlap, each will influence the others to some degree.

Thus, for example, central-team members will be able to contribute to the organizational diagnoses and the selection of problems for study by referring to their knowledge of the literature on organizations, as well as whatever experience and practical background they possess. On the other hand, hospital-team members will be able to provide their own views from day-to-day contact with problems in their work, as well as their years of experience with different problems and ways of solving them.

The central-team cum hospital-team system is temporary, but during its life it can be organized much as any other highly cohesive group. We here mean cohesiveness not in the sense of attraction between members of a group, but in the sense of group power over the members of the group (see Thibaut and Kelly, 1959). This kind of group power is derived from the high power of each member over the others, and vice versa. Such highly cohesive groups are able to organize their members and to use norms and group standards in the organization to obtain high performance from them towards the aims of the group. This results in highly effective groups, which are productive in terms of whatever goals they may have (Cartwright and Zander, 1968).[9]

Thus, if the goals of a group are, for example, projects, then more projects should be carried out by such highly cohesive groups with high mutual influence. If the goals are solving communication problems or other kinds of problem in the hospital, then more should again be accomplished by a highly cohesive group. If, in fact, a goal of the group is to change or improve communication behaviour, then this also can be accomplished.[10]

We have argued so far that high mutual influence in the central-team cum hospital-team system could be expected to lead to higher effectiveness. High mutual influence in an organization, or as Tannenbaum (1968) terms it, 'high total control', also leads to effectiveness in that organizational system. Applied to an organization, high total control means that staff at all levels and in all parts of the organization have considerable control or influence. Thus, if 'other' hospital personnel (item F137, Chapter 15) are given more influence over H.I.C. matters, then H.I.C. outcomes might be improved. Similarly, the argument by organizational theorists is that organizations characterized by high total control are more effective in terms of their organizational goals (in the case of the hospital, patient-care) than are organizations characterized by relatively low levels of influence across the boundaries between various echelons, departments, or segments.[11]

## CLARITY

We have indicated above that, in general, greater clarity or structure would have no doubt enhanced H.I.C. outcomes. By this we mean clarity of the goals of the Project, namely 'communication', and clarity about the means by which such communication improvements would be obtained, and about the models for alternative effects from various Project efforts. On the other hand there may have been too much clarity or too much structure about one element of the Project, namely the survey methodology as a means to improving communication.

This is by way of indicating that clarity and obscurity cannot be viewed simply as either desirable or undesirable. Neither is there any simple way of extending the foregoing discussion about the linking or mutuality of different orientations. It would seem, however, that overall goals cannot be entirely structured and definite; in fact, there are advantages in their being diffuse to some extent. Furthermore, the relationships between means and ends (or at least some hypotheses about them) as well as the means, probably should be clearer and, in some cases, measurable (capable of being operationally defined). Working towards measurable means or sub-goals gives the change programme some feedback on its progress, as well as structuring and limiting the focus of change efforts so that they are more readily achieved and at least some impact is made. But there should be a continual comparison between the achievement of means and the achievement of ends, and vice versa. Have the right means been chosen according to the character of the ends, or has there been some implied shift in ends, or is there perhaps better knowledge of the relations between means and ends? Similarly, should the ends be modified in the light of the preliminary achievements that are means to the ends? The ends, because of their diffuse nature, will be less readily modified, as they should be, and the means, with their measurable indications of achievement, will provide better feedback and quicker and easier opportunities for deciding on modifications.[12] We shall return below to the character of clarity in a project, for we shall see that clarity is also differentially important according to the sequential relations in a project.

## ORGANIZATIONAL STRATEGY IN DIFFUSING H.I.C. TECHNOLOGY

An organizational change project requires a strategy for changing the organization as a whole.[13] However, large and complex organizations are not easily changed by an individual or a small team, with the consequence that many change procedures are a matter of starting with relations between change-agents and individuals, or between change-agents and small groups (see Schein, 1969). In addition, the skills of change-agents are often limited (because the education of change-agents is usually discipline-based) to changes in technology or structure or people, but not all three. Thus there must be an explicit strategy so that the change-agents, either directly or indirectly, 'cover' much of the organization, if organizational change is to be achieved and maintained.

A comprehensive organizational approach to change would best include an organizational diagnosis.[14] This would cover organizational goal attainment, as well as the human, structural, and technological characteristics of the organization as a whole. Such an organizational diagnosis should examine the various pressures and forces for change and stability throughout the organization contemporaneously as well as prospectively. As we indicated in Chapter 3, a starting-point or sub-system should be selected, taking into account how the rest of the organization (other sub-systems) will react subsequently to initial change efforts and accomplishments. In other words, the change-agent must decide whether starting at any particular point will facilitate subsequent moves – so as eventually to cover important structural parts as well as the technological and human aspects of organizations.

In fact, as we have noted, the efforts and effects of the H.I.C. Project tended to be relatively limited in organizational terms, despite the period of three to four years in which the Project was in operation. It seems that there was no systematic diffusion process to cover the organization as a whole, the main emphasis being on the use of surveys by a small group, the hospital team.

It does appear, however, that the initial focus for changes in technology from the H.I.C. Project was relatively strategic in terms of organizational structure. To start at the 'top' is to take a potentially organizational approach to change, since one expects the 'top' to be extremely important in influencing the activities of the organization as a whole. Any increments or improvements in the information reaching this centre may have a pervasive, organization-wide effect. Ordinarily, this would be true of most organizations, but the top staff in a hospital typically do not have a broad scope of influence because of horizontal and vertical segmentation (Stanton and Schwartz, 1954) – because of barriers between the professional groups and the different status levels.[15]

These barriers are a problem in hospitals; and, in a sense, in an organization with such a basic communication and integration problem, the choice of a central focus for change efforts could not have been as effective as in some other more integrated organization. But considering hospitals alone, perhaps no point other than the top could provide a good starting-point. In any event, the H.I.C. Project started at the top, a relatively central focus in terms of the organization as a whole, and there is good, although not universal, evidence that such an approach is associated with success in organizational change efforts (see Greiner, 1965; Schein, 1969).[16]

While an apparently desirable organizational approach was made at the top, the composition of the starting group – the hospital team – left something to be desired in terms of an integrated approach. The creation of hospital teams in order to operate the survey technology did not, as is pointed out in Chapter 6, utilize individuals who were functionally related and who could thereby disseminate and reinforce the effects of acquired information within the team. Neither did they have much opportunity to support one another. Had they been given more time, and perhaps more support by their superiors, the temporary system of the operational-team members might have become a potent force for change.[17, 18]

In the event, hospital-team activity on any particular project was limited primarily to one or two individuals. Furthermore, on subsequent projects these active individuals tended to be different, and thus the effects of the project over time were certainly diffused, and were not integrated and reinforced in any systematic manner.

Sometimes a few hospital-team members continued to be active in projects over a relatively long period of time. This may well have been due in part to the existence of student help and the relationship created between the students and the hospital-team members. Activity, particularly by the nurse members of the operational teams, was reinforced by students – for the nurses, especially, saw students more or less as 'experts', and they accepted influence from them. A number of nurses reported that they were obtaining very useful management experience. This was in contrast to the administrators who were obtaining nothing very 'new'.

While the operational-team nurses were apparently impressed by both the technology and the expertise of the change-agents, the administrators seemed to be affected only by the latter, and to a lesser extent than the nurses. The whole of the hospital was the normal purview of the administrator, and thus hospital projects outside their sphere of working – providing much in the way of new learning – were rare. The technology was not such a valuable help to them as were the central-team members themselves, who viewed 'old' information in a somewhat different fashion.

Doctors on the hospital teams tended to be relatively uninvolved almost from the start (see *Figure 15-5*), or they studied problems of special concern to themselves (Chapter 18, note 4). Whatever the degree of participation by doctors, however, there was little likelihood of the H.I.C. Project and the effects of the doctors' work being diffused to many other doctors, because of the highly segmented nature of the medical side of the hospital. Doctors belonging to the same firm would be able to influence one another, but the relative autonomy of firms would hinder diffusion of the project between firms.[19]

Some nurses and some administrators did find the survey technology useful, and they participated in surveys to varying degrees (see Chapter 15). But for the survey technology to be accepted into the organization requires that other members find it of value, and that they support and encourage its use. Not all hospital staff were surveyed systematically by the evaluator, but informal contacts provided some information indicating that non-team members were not wholeheartedly supporting project and survey efforts by the teams.[20] We have already seen that 'other' hospital personnel (item F137) did not play much of a role in the H.I.C. work of the hospital teams. Failing to involve others probably did not facilitate support and diffusion.

Even more important, however, is the fact that hospital-team members failed to involve certain hospital staff who were important colleagues or significant members of their 'role set' (Kahn *et al.*, 1964) and who were subjected to possible threat by the use of surveys. A department head whose department was surveyed, but who did not have an opportunity to participate in designing the questionnaires or methods, was bound to feel that his superior (the administrative member of the hospital team) was checking up on him. In one hospital, in fact, an administrator said that the survey could provide a good opportunity to 'sack' an apparently poorly performing departmental head. This seemed to be the exception rather than the rule, but nevertheless the threat could still be imagined by the departmental head, untrue as it generally was. Even if relations with his superior were good, a departmental head might well wonder why a new mechanism of communication was being set up between top hospital staff and his own subordinates, by-passing himself. In a somewhat similar fashion on the nursing side, surveys tended to focus on the ward situation, by-passing the assistant matrons in the nursing office.[21]

Thus the organizational diffusion and consolidation of the H.I.C. Project, its survey technology, and its effects, were hindered by the choice of team members (in the case of diffusion and integration across professional barriers) and by the omission of intermediate levels of staff in the nursing and administrative hierarchies (in the case of diffusion and integration across status barriers existing within professional divisions). The latter failure, particularly, could have been rectified during the course of the Project, since it was the ways in which hospital-team members carried out projects that was at fault, not the initial decision by H.I.C. to begin the change projects by training certain top staff.

## INTEGRATED, STRATEGIC EFFORTS IN SURVEYS OF TECHNOLOGY, STRUCTURE, AND PEOPLE

So far we have emphasized the technological focus of the H.I.C. Project – its attempt to create functioning survey teams in the hospital – and the difficulties in diffusing survey participation and use of results across the structure of the organization. Despite this limited approach to organizational change, there is still the question of the substantive nature of the surveys conducted, and the degree of organizational relevance of the information gathered. Even if use of the survey technology was limited to several people at the top, it could still be directed to quite important objects of study with relevance to the organization as a whole. One may ask if the use of the survey technology and the resulting information was aimed at the study of important structural, technological, or 'people' factors, especially factors with potential effects on the task of the hospital – effects on patient-care.

In terms of the technology of patient-care – the procedures for caring for patients (Perrow, 1965) – the hospital projects would have done well to look at the doctors and patients rather closely. There were, of course, some ward studies, but they tended to exclude doctors and patients from direct participation. Nurses received the most attention (as one H.I.C. participant asked, 'Why are nurses always picked on?'). If doctors were studied, it was in terms of their role in the organizational structure, or of their attitudes, and not of the technological procedures for patient-care. Projects that did focus on the technology of patient-care, such as the usage of drugs at Severalls and the usage of surgical theatres at West Middlesex, were the exception rather than the rule.[22]

What of the focuses of surveys within the structural and 'people' systems of the organizations? Primarily because of the influence of hospital-team members on the selection of problems for study, as well as their influence in selecting most of the content of studies, the surveys did not touch on either structure or people in any systematic or strategic fashion. We have indicated above that in some hospitals different members with different interests made up the team at different points in time, thus hindering programmatic survey efforts. Perhaps even more importantly, there was almost no study of the nature of the hospital organization *qua* organization (as opposed to individuals or groups in organizations). A psychological approach, emphasizing aggregated data, predominated over an organizational and structural approach. Observations of organization-level phenomena, such as formalization and centralization, were not made. The key structural elements of programmed and non-programmed co-ordination were not systematically investigated (see Georgopoulos and Mann, 1962). These latter organizational factors have been shown to be highly related to the quality of patient-care obtained in hospitals. On the human side, there was no systematic effort to uncover pressures or anxieties, which are also key elements in understanding hospital functioning (Menzies, 1960).[23] Furthermore, the variables relating to people that were studied tended to be connected with satisfaction rather than with motivation, which is unfortunate in terms of the more central relationship of the latter to work effectiveness and productivity (see, e.g., March and Simon, 1958).

In other words, the H.I.C. Project focused away from organizational issues that are central in relation to patient-care outcomes, at least in terms of some of the organizational models now available for understanding the determinants of effectiveness. It was information that was the prime focus – a common feature of all the hospital projects being the technology that would facilitate information exchange in the organization. But the information itself was generally not crucial or central to organizational functioning. Neither was it systematically patterned over the course of various projects, so that more difficult, but central, information was approached in an indirect, less threatening manner (Harrison, 1970).

It is our expectation that using the H.I.C. survey technology to obtain information systematically about the different organizational systems (technology, structure, and people) to support diagnosis and change in them would have been more beneficial than the dispersed and non-programmatic efforts that were made. As we indicated in Chapter 3, technology, structure, and people tend to be interdependent, and integrated change in all three, rather than in one alone, is more likely to result in change in the goal attainment of the organization. The possible nature of such an integrated approach to organizational change may be inferred from an examination of a project on the surgical theatres at West Middlesex hospital (see also Chapter 9). This project was an attempt to focus change efforts around patient-care in the theatres. The information system was improved by setting up new ways of keeping records of theatre use. The student central-team member was able to talk to a number of people at length in order to reduce their anxieties and help them work through their personal situation with respect to this project. In terms of structure, the student served as a link between different groups and tried to facilitate greater communication and co-ordination by means of meetings and informal contacts between the groups. In short, the improved communication structure dovetailed with the new information technology, as well as the 'people' changes (these were less evident, but probably facilitated changes in the other two systems in the long run).

Several other projects used a survey or some other mechanism of information exchange so as to integrate some strategic technological, structural, and 'people' approaches to changing and improving patient-care. However this integrated strategic approach was relatively rare and appears to have been due to rather special circumstances. For one thing, the theatre project at West Middlesex placed a great deal of emphasis on change (as opposed to diagnosis) because, in fact, two students worked in sequence on the same project, thus providing considerable time for change as well as for data collection and diagnosis. To expect data collection, analysis, reporting, and change efforts on an important problem, all to happen during the six-month sojourn of a student in a hospital, is somewhat unrealistic. Not only was there more time for changing in this project, there were also considerable resources for these efforts, since the project had a relatively experienced student who was able to spend almost his entire time with the H.I.C. Project located in the hospital at the site of change. Attachment to the hospital gave the change-agent the very necessary extended period to work on changes in people and gave him the opportunity to use himself as a temporary structure in day-to-day functioning of the hospital so as to facilitate co-ordination, in addition to enabling him to work on the technological system for data collection.[24]

In summary, we are suggesting that if the efforts of the central team and hospital teams had been better organized in terms of an integrated focus on the strategic variables of technology, structure, and people in the hospital, then perhaps the H.I.C. Project might have achieved some major and extensive permanent organization-level changes, including changes in patient-care.

## A POTENTIAL ORGANIZATIONAL APPROACH: TECHNOLOGY TO PEOPLE OR STRUCTURE

We have described how the H.I.C. Project concentrated on the use of surveys to change the information system in the hospital, and how such changes in the technology of the typical hospital were not diffused and made general. Some suggestions were made regarding the potential benefits of integrated changes in technology, structure, and people. Here we shall describe an alternative or supplementary strategy of organizational change – a changing strategy over time. Such a strategy would be to move from an attempt to create survey teams, and the use of survey data in the hospital organizations, to an attempt at the more usual kind of organizational development programme, focusing primarily on changes in structure and people rather than technological changes (Beckhard, 1969).

This kind of approach might be termed a 'red-herring' approach. Change by means of the more readily accepted and less threatening emphasis on the use of survey technology in hospitals would be replaced – after sufficient data had been gathered showing the need for changes in structure and people, and after the change-agents had demonstrated interest and competence in these areas. However, it was not possible to discard the technological apparatus in H.I.C. Throughout the Project, surveys provided the basic framework for the projects in the hospitals.

The point in the Project at which hospital-team members indicated that lack of time hindered their using the technology to gather data – often after the first project had been done in a hospital – might have been an opportune moment to move to a more active consideration of structural and, particularly, 'people' focuses of change. Another point at which the transition could have been made was when the central-team director and another member resigned, leaving, in fact, two senior central-team members who were relatively more people-oriented in their change philosophies.

However, at the earlier point in time it seemed too soon for any radical change, and internal politics in the central team also failed to provide an opportunity for the proponents of a change of strategy to influence the matter. In any event, the use of students to facilitate continued work with survey technology proved a solution to hospital-team members' lack of time and also provided a number of positive benefits to the Project, as is evident above (see Chapters 5 and 17). At the second point in time, the central team's disorganization, together with the acceptance of the initial basic philosophy of the Project (that no 'directiveness' should be used by central-team members), ensured a continuation of the emphasis on improving information technology by means of surveys in the hospitals.

At a still later time, there was an explicit consideration of moving in the direction of change efforts oriented towards people and structure by adding to the central-team staff a person experienced in this field. Again, internal differences in the central team, together with the structure provided by the original philosophy, served to prevent implementation of this change in strategy.

The central team had begun to realize by this point, however, the need for some operation in terms of change strategies directed at people and structure as well as technology. It was decided to emphasize feedback and discussion in the current hospital projects, but because the survey technology given at the courses and practised subsequently was limited primarily to questionnaire instruments and to various data analysis techniques, and was not a feedback technology (i.e. instruments and procedures for feedback questions such as those used by Holloway and Lonergan, 1968), hospital projects throughout the H.I.C. Project continued to emphasize the diagnostic stage of change. Without a programme of feedback, either taught at the month-long course, or available in some documented and persuasive form, central-team members had little opportunity to initiate feedback meetings and discussion that would facilitate changes in people.

So it was that, for a number of reasons, the use of survey technology continued to be the prime focus of change efforts. It is perhaps unfair to be critical of the H.I.C. Project's inflexibility preventing movement from technology to change efforts oriented more towards people or structure. It is generally true that the training of experts or change-agents in these areas tends to be discipline-oriented and rather one-sided, thus providing an almost exclusive emphasis either on technology or on structure and people. If the lessons of this Project are to be utilized in further projects, it would appear that some way must be found to combine these approaches, whether simultaneously or sequentially, or both, so as to have a comprehensive organization-level change programme.

## A SEQUENTIAL VIEW OF THE H.I.C. PROJECT

Lewin's (1952) unfreezing-changing-refreezing model for describing change was introduced in Chapter 3 as a possible aid to understanding the H.I.C. Project. Let us use this model in viewing H.I.C. changes in the organizational information system.[25] 'Unfreezing' of the hospital-team members occurred in part by virtue of the pressures to which most top hospital staff are currently subjected – pressures from lack of resources, both human and material, and pressures from the ever increasing demands made upon hospitals. Revans was able to make the top hospital staff aware of their need for more information and more learning, and he was able to make them aware that there were ways of solving these problems – that they themselves might be able to do something about them, with the help of others conversant with the new means of solving problems (surveys).

'Changing' of the hospital-team members was obtained by means of the month-long training course and the subsequent use of the survey methods, both in the week-long practice project and in the hospital with central-team assistance. However, difficulties ensued especially because of time constraints (see Chapters 5 and 6). Furthermore, because the appropriate information was not obtained (team members said they learned relatively little that was 'new') or because the diagnostic information could not be translated into solutions to problems, there was insufficient reinforcement of the use of this technology. The result was that there was no permanent 'refreezing' or internalization of the behavioural patterns associated with the use of the survey technology by the hospital teams.

The Lewin model may be applied to the use of the survey technology and its effects on others in the hospital, the survey respondents. The use of surveys apparently served to 'unfreeze' the respondents (see Chapter 13 on the apparent increases in turnover immediately before survey activity occurred). The survey was a new event creating expectations of change. But delays inevitably occurred before feedback was possible, and the readiness to change tended to fade away. Even more important, the data obtained were primarily 'end-result' data (Likert, 1967), which did not provide a means for ascertaining the causes of difficulties and problems (Foundation for Research on Human Behaviour, 1964). Hospital-team members could 'set right' minor matters, but the sources of basic problems did not emerge in the surveys, nor, since intensive feedback programmes were rare, did any solutions emerge subsequently through the participation and involvement of other staff in feedback programmes. Thus, reinforcement for participating in surveys could not be obtained. Little cumulative 'changing' of respondents was in fact possible.

Lewin's unfreezing-changing-refreezing model helps to provide a generalized interpretation of the change process in H.I.C., but two process models (Parsons *et al.*, 1952; Parsons and Bales, 1955) help us to detail the sequences in the change process. Parsons has used these models in different ways and has elaborated their components considerably. Here we shall make use of what seem to be the most relevant components for our purposes.

One of the most basic distinctions made by Parsons is the dilemma of internal-external orientation. All systems are made up of a number of units and at any one point in time there is, as Hills (1968) puts it, a dilemma 'whether to give priority to the solution of the problems of co-existence of the units, or to the problem of optimizing the relation to the environment' (p. 19).

As we see Parsons's two process models, one (the LIGA model) gives initial priority to internal problems, or to the relations among units within the system. According to Parsons, socialization and psychotherapy (and in our view 'people' change processes generally) may be viewed as conforming to this LIGA sequence.[26] In this model of change, the change-agent and client relate to each other, with the change-agent initially concerned with establishing the relationship, diagnosing the client's need for change, and then – by responding in various ways to the actions of the client – helping him to change his patterns of action.

In the second (AGIL) model, initial priority is given to the problem of improving relations between the unit and the environment. Only subsequently in the change sequence is attention put on the relations among components within the unit. After solving external problems, and as a consequence of ignoring internal difficulties in favour of external achievements, attention is then put on repairing the internal relational problems that have arisen. But the main thrust of the change activities depicted by this model is change in the relations between the unit and the environment. In the light of the external emphasis, this might be termed a task-achievement model or a problem-solving model.

Let us return to the LIGA or internal change model – the model most appropriate for changing people and their attitudes, beliefs, emotional responses, etc. In the first, 'latency' (L), stage of this LIGA sequence the change-agent establishes a relationship with the internal system of the client. The change-agent and client decide they will work together, they commit themselves to each other, to form a unit for some purpose. Parsons (1951) sees this stage in psychotherapy (or in the social control of deviants) as characterized by the 'permissiveness' of the therapist (change-agent) towards the client.

In the second, 'integration' (I), stage of the LIGA sequence, the change-agent is concerned with the various responses of the client. By being 'supportive' the change-agent creates a solidary relationship and shows acceptance of the client and his problems, whatever the client wants to do or whatever his responses. Diagnosis by the change-agent of the needs for change of the clients' system may also be concentrated at this stage.

The third, 'goal-gratification' (G), stage is characterized by differential reinforcement of the clients' responses by the change-agent. The change-agent 'uses' the relationship (Lippitt *et al.*, 1958), to discourage certain responses or aspects of the client, thereby channelling them in other directions. This point in the psychotherapeutic process is characterized by the 'denial of reciprocity', or, in more traditional terms, the refusal of the therapist to form a counter-transference – a refusal to reward the patient's distorted image of the therapist.

In the fourth, 'adaptation' (A), stage the client 'changes' or learns the proper responses by adapting to the rewards (approval, esteem, etc.) given by the change-agent. The psychotherapeutic process finds the therapist using 'manipulation of rewards' at this point. Generally, at this last stage of the LIGA sequence, the client is helped to articulate and stabilize his newly learned responses so that they may be used subsequently in dealing with the external environment.

The second model, in contrast to the foregoing model for internal system changes, is concerned initially and primarily with changes in the client's relation to the external system – with what we might term task-performance or problem-solving changes. This model has been applied primarily to so-called problem-solving groups, or discussion groups given a problem that they are to solve. In this AGIL or problem-solving sequence, 'adaptation' (A), relating to the environment or problem, characterizes the first phase of change. The group members consider the problem, they offer information to each other regarding possible solutions and they evaluate the alternatives. In the next, 'goal-gratification' (G), stage, they achieve a solution for dealing with the external problem. This in turn leads to the 'integration' (I) stage or the dealing with the internal problems and tensions that have been created by task activity. There is gratification of unmet internal needs so as to maintain the solidarity of the group. The 'latency' (L) stage follows, during which there are no actions and the system merely continues to exist as a unit, before starting with the A-stage again.

Revans's approach in the early conferences was seen by participants and observers as especially effective and persuasive in creating a relationship for working together. Loomis's (1959) description of a charismatic leader entering the internal system of certain disorganized systems having an internal focus, seems to fit the available data on these early conferences. Participants at the conferences were 'unfrozen', and a relationship between Revans and the participants was established – at least with those who decided to remain with the Project. Evidently Revans was effective in convincing the participants of the importance of 'communication' and the value of the kind of project he wished to initiate, a study and improvement of their hospitals by means of surveys.

In terms of the LIGA sequence above, the early H.I.C. conferences apparently served to create L-stage conditions for participants. A change-agent and client relationship was created in preparation for change activity. There was unfreezing and readiness for internal changes – readiness to look at things differently and to feel differently. The permissiveness of Revans, especially regarding the efforts to be required of participants (length of course, proportion of time devoted to the Project, etc.) was highly effective in creating a relationship between change-agent and client.

An alternative approach in the conferences would have been for Revans and the hospital participants jointly to work through the general nature of hospital problems and the alternative approaches of possible value for their solution. This would have corresponded to the A-stage in the AGIL sequence. But on the contrary, the sessions were limited primarily to a presentation of Revans's ideas – that (a) communication should be studied, (b) by hospital staff themselves and under hospital direction, and (c) by means of projects or survey technology to be learned at a course. There was disagreement and discussion about alternative dispositions of time and about other specific topics such as which staff should participate in courses; concerning these, Revans was, as indicated above, quite permissive in relation to hospital desires. But there was no consideration of major alternative approaches to hospital problems – changing the influence structure of hospitals or changing the arrangement by which the hospital was structured around the medical staff, etc. The main thrust was the presentation by Revans of the above-mentioned major points regarding communication.

These points were, in fact, accepted by hospital participants, apparently as a result of the conference presentations and discussion by Revans. There were no demonstration projects or other activities in the hospitals ('external system' activities), either by Revans or by other H.I.C. staff. In short, the initial activities seem best described by the L-stage of a LIGA sequence.

The training courses and especially the practice project seem to have provided operational-team members with I-stage and also G-stage work in the LIGA sequence – trying out different ideas and responses and changing them in response to the directions indicated by the course. Probably very important was the initial great uncertainty of operational-team members about why they were at the courses, and the diffuse reactions they got from central-team members in response to requests for specific guidelines or directions to be taken by the Project. Only later did they get answers in the form of the very specific survey technology. The operational-team members spent two weeks in this kind of learning about the need to study 'communication' as well as how to do surveys. An additional week was spent implementing their new commitment and practising their skills, in a hospital environment. The return to the course for one week provided some evaluation of their efforts and reinforcement of the appropriate responses.

In other words, the I- and G-stages, basically corresponding to Lewin's 'changing' (especially the G-stage), consisted of learning the survey skills. But it would appear that there was only a limited amount of learning, during the I- and G-stages, of non-survey techniques addressed to changing people, such as the use of discussion groups in feedback.

The nature of the cognitive-emotional links provided in the I- and G-stages of the LIGA sequence are potentially valuable in explaining the subsequent outcomes at the A-stage. Exposure to 'group dynamics' and to the attitudes of H.I.C. staff (and of invited researchers) was a limited but potentially useful part of the courses. However, without the linking of these experiences to the goals of the Project and to specific behaviour, one would expect difficulty in subsequently transferring any learning out of the course situation back into the hospital. This is important, since the hospital does not, by virtue of its institutional nature, provide a permissive and supportive environment for such new learning. Neither did the particular participating hospitals have a great deal of 'organizational slack' (Rosner, 1968) to provide some leeway for further learning and its consolidation. In addition, the apparent lack of clarity of supporting-team members about the ultimate aims and nature of the H.I.C. Project prevented the provision of needed support from this quarter.

The relatively great clarity and the measurability of surveys, together with the conflicting pressures described, probably contributed to the hospital teams' emphasis, upon return to the hospitals, on practising survey skills, rather than any of the communications skills touched upon during the training courses. Some team members reported that they were subsequently able to approach another team member more openly as a result of attending a course together, but for others, without functional opportunities for this activity and without sufficient supports to ward off the pressures towards the resumption of previous habits, this new pattern could not persist to any major degree. To behave differently in the hospital, and to behave in line with the attitudes advocated by some during the courses – to 'cast off' authority and to encourage participation, was difficult when no specific behavioural responses were learned, and there was no cognitive linkage between the various attitudes towards 'people' and the aims of the H.I.C. Project.

Perhaps most important, there was no provision or time in the month courses for giving either a cognitive framework for understanding, or an opportunity for practising, feedback skills. Feedback can be taught in a relatively highly programmed fashion, just as was done for survey administration (see Holloway and Lonergan, 1968), and such feedback activity might have enabled H.I.C. to move from technology to 'people' change. In any event, neither 'people' changes, nor skills relevant to the change of others, were learned or applied subsequently. Learning was slight, primarily because these matters were simply not fully covered in the courses. Application of any learning was difficult, furthermore, because there was apparently insufficient cognitive-emotional linkage.

On the other hand, transfer of survey administration skills into the hospital was relatively successful, perhaps because of the usual stressful situation in hospitals, providing almost 'premature' refreezing of learning. The training course was constructed around survey techniques – and Revans himself was the strongest advocate of these techniques – so that in all likelihood the emotional commitment to the Project engendered earlier was linked to survey research and the functioning of the team in this mode, once back in the hospital.

Once transferred to the hospital, the survey activity could be reinforced by a number of factors. It was *avant-garde* and therefore produced esteem among hospital personnel. The central team, of course, reinforced the survey activity. In addition, some 'new' information was provided as a result of the activity – information that was an intrinsic reinforcement. Participation in hospital projects and other H.I.C. Project activity was also seen by some hospital-team members as a means to establishing contacts and favourable relations with staff from other hospitals and with people from hospital management committees, the Ministry, or the Hospital Centre.

When pressure of time and lack of support from the top caused some hospital-team members to give up direct participation in surveys, their basic commitment to H.I.C. was demonstrated by their support of central-team survey work, under hospital-team direction. But as one might expect, when all the various extrinsic rewards were no longer available – when activities were no longer new, when the central team had gone – then the intrinsic rewards of a (relatively) small amount of 'new' (and not so useful) information were insufficient. A new commitment can be maintained only so long in the absence of additional supportive factors.[27]

Thus, it seems that the adaptation or A-stage – during which newly learned responses were stabilized and made available for subsequent direction at the external environment (for possible external rewards in addition to the internal rewards) – was not brought to a successful conclusion. Sufficient external rewards were not obtained to bring the new pattern of response to a stable state.

Starting with the basic commitment to H.I.C. and its techniques in the L-stage, and then learning the proper responses in the I- and G-stages, prepared team members for carrying out surveys in the hospitals – using the learned responses in the external environment, as we have described the A-stage. This scheme was at first quite successful, especially with the help (reinforcement of responses) of the central team, but some immediate problems plus the subsequent loss of certain reinforcements apparently led eventually to a failure in the A-stage. Use of the survey technology was not consolidated, and teams gave up this activity sooner or later.

The central team unfortunately could do relatively little to modify the course of the Project. First of all, it seems clear that the central team could not operate in a LIGA mode as Revans had. The central-team members were unknown quantities as far as the hospital teams were concerned, they were mostly 'junior' and had 'academic' rather than practical qualifications or capabilities. The central-team members had little of the influence necessary to set up the diffuse relationship of the L- and I-stages. Even an experienced change-agent has relatively little influence when confronted with a change problem within the structure of an organization (Harrison, 1970). Finally, the central team was for the most part absent from the early conferences and the training courses, and they could not share the emotional relationship created between Revans and the hospital-team members (compare Dyer *et al.*, 1970). Thus, there was little possibility of a relationship between the change-agents and the internal system of the clients. The central team could not have done much in the way of L- and I-stage work even if they were unanimous about the desirability of such efforts. By and large, relationships with the external systems of hospital-team members were pursued instead (i.e. G- and A-stage work).

Probably the most important factor in determining the course of the Project was that the viewpoints of the hospital teams seemed to facilitate mostly G- and A-stage work by the central team. To backtrack and reinforce L- or I-stage work was not desirable even if it had been feasible. The hospital teams wanted to use their survey skills in the hospitals; they had no desire to go back and reconsider their learning – to go back and learn more about skills in changing people, about feedback or discussion groups. It was too late and too difficult for the hospital teams to worry about the basic nature of the H.I.C. Project and the nature of their commitment to it (L- and I-stage skills). It was 'easy' merely to continue with surveys.

The central team, in fact, did operate mostly in the G- and A-stage modes. They reacted to and reinforced different behaviour by the hospital members in relation to their external system – the change-agents themselves or the rest of the hospital. But these aspects of hospital team behaviour were often not the ones emphasized or 'changed' by Revans and the courses (in the L- and I-modes). The central-team members did generally find the hospital teams in the A-stage, applying the survey learning from the course, but they often tried to orientate the hospital teams towards projects that were relevant to changes in people (see Chapter 17) – towards projects with emotional and subjective orientations.

As we see it, the central team tried to create changes in people, but in an unusual way – using the AGIL change sequence. The central team for the most part entered the Project when hospital-team members were practising their new skills, but, instead of the usual initial concerns of forming a relationship and making a diagnosis (L and I in LIGA), they concentrated on reinforcing and differentially rewarding client responses (G and A in LIGA) learned beforehand. In our view, the central-team members eventually came to the realization that the survey aspects of hospital projects were not nearly as important as the 'people'-changing elements. Thus they reinforced hospital-team activity in looking at 'people' variables – hospital projects that examined the team member's own work, that involved other hospital staff in discussions, that considered the anxieties about authority and other emotional features of the hospital. One might view the central team as trying to facilitate adaptive project activity (A-stage) that had a goal (G-stage) of changing people – both hospital-team members and others in the hospital. The rest of this change sequence (AGIL) would consist of repairing tensions and difficulties (I-stage) that arose during the problem-solving activities, and maintaining the system (L-stage) for subsequent problem-solving.

It should be noted, however, that the reinforcement activities of the central team at the A- and G-stages in this AGIL sequence could never be very extensive, because the client responses available for utilization in these stages were strictly limited. The survey activities of the hospital-team members were inappropriate in a number of ways if they were to obtain new, useful, information facilitating the solution of the major 'people' problems of hospitals and if they were to obtain the reinforcement that would be provided by the solution of such major problems.

The central team could not really effect an AGIL sequence because their goal was not that of the hospital-team members. As we saw in Chapter 17, hospital-team members did not really want 'training' as a means to changes in people. In a sense, hospital-team members had learned their lessons in the course too well. The goal of the hospital teams was use of survey technology, which would solve various objective problems in the hospital. Thus, in all their A-stage work with the hospital teams, the central team continually had to fight the very seductive nature of the survey technology, learned so ably by the hospital teams at the courses and prematurely refrozen upon their return to the hospital situation. The refreezing of this behaviour, together with the ineffectual influence position of the central team, made it difficult to modify the original survey emphasis of H.I.C., until it was more or less too late to change back to a more people-oriented emphasis on communication. Such an emphasis, without any links with the basic H.I.C. commitment that Revans had elicited (during the L- and I-stages) and without a relatively secure place to experiment (so as to recreate an important aspect of the I-stage), was insufficient in magnitude to encourage new learning attempts by hospital-team members. The correlations in Chapter 17 between central-team activity and 'communications' (people) changes would seem to be due in part to the central team facilitating an AGIL change sequence on the part of the hospital teams.

Thus, we suggest that the highly successful L- and I-stage work by Revans (development of commitment to H.I.C.) followed by more I-stage and then G-stage work at the courses (in teaching survey work as a cognitive, objective exercise) led to the initially successful A-stage of implanting survey work in hospitals as a means of their improvement. This success, ensured in part by the early emphasis and commitment to self-direction, in fact prevented a shift away from the technological emphasis of the Project. Because of the situation of the central team, a shift of emphasis to 'people' in H.I.C. had to start with an A-stage in the external AGIL sequence. Lacking much influence, the central team could make relatively little progress against the direction already imposed on the hospital-team efforts.[28]

## H.I.C. SEQUENTIAL DEVELOPMENT IN RELATION TO DIFFERENT PROJECT EMPHASES

In our earlier analysis we have emphasized the need for combined cognitive/emotional, objective/subjective approach, together with a mutual influence system. Let us try to indicate how these points are relevant at various stages of a change project, and we will thereby indicate why central-team success in overcoming the structured situation found might not have been entirely desirable and could have had some negative effects.

In making L- and I-stage links with a client, the change-agent creates a diffuse integrative relationship based on feelings of trust and competence.[29] There is an emotional orientation in the change-agent/client relationship. Similarly, the change-agent creates a subjective focus for the client. The client asks: what can the change-agent do for me, what does he want of me, what does he think of me? In short, in the L-stage there is an emotional commitment to change oneself. The client develops a diffuse readiness to alter his own behaviour along the lines suggested by the change-agent.

We have said that the H.I.C. Project was essentially cognitive and objective in orientation. It is true that Revans implored hospital-team members to cast aside authoritarian relationships and to examine the anxieties and blockages in the hospital. But aside from these prescriptions, the continuing major efforts of the H.I.C. Project, in the G- and A-stages of the work begun by Revans, were in the cognitive and objective terms we have described. The emphasis was on obtaining information about others, by means of surveys. That is to say, the changes created in hospital-team members by means of the LIGA sequence were in their external capabilities. They came to use survey technology instrumentally on others.[30]

For a change-agent possessing the requisite power, use of the LIGA sequence of change is much more productive of internal or 'people' change than the alternative AGIL or problem-solving sequence.[31] Revans's use of the LIGA sequence was very appropriate in getting a commitment to, and subsequent use of, survey technology. The point is, however, that the potent LIGA sequence could have been used to obtain a commitment from hospital-team members to change themselves, and could have been used, in fact, to change hospital-team members. The question is whether the very effective use of the LIGA change sequence was for the wrong purpose. Should the change programme have been aimed at, for example, hospital-team members' views and feelings about their authority position in the hospital? For example, should T-groups have been used to make hospital team members more 'sensitive' to their own feelings and behaviour?

In retrospect, we would surmise that the technological emphasis by Revans was probably best in terms of staying within the competencies of hospital-team members as well as their desires and norms regarding the examination of 'private' feelings, and, finally, best in terms of the change-agents being responsible for the outcomes of a major change effort along deeper emotional lines. But we would add that the potential for change created by successful I-stage work was to some extent ineffectively dissipated by dealing rather too exclusively with less 'deep', cognitive and objective changes in the G-stage.[32]

Harrison's (1970) experience (with American clients) indicates that change activities that are 'performance' oriented (cognitive and also basically objective) or 'instrumentally'-oriented (cognitive, but subjective in terms of a 'process' orientation) are at about the right level, in terms of staying within client norms regarding invasion of privacy, and are probably most effective in terms of avoiding resistance to psychological probing. The instrumental approach, typified by Blake and Mouton's (1968) Managerial Grid, may arouse resistance in some cases, but the performance approach, typified by management by objectives, seems to arouse significant resistance quite infrequently. If Harrison's experience is any guide, and the evidence in the H.I.C. Project seems to suggest that his analysis is valid, then there was some, but not much leeway for the Project to move 'deeper' – to move more in the direction of an initial emphasis on people – without encountering significant resistance. There are a number of ways in which the Project could have moved towards 'deeper' changes or changes in people. The training courses apparently did elicit experiences that were emotionally satisfying. Some hospital-team members, for example, reported new-found ease in dealing with colleagues from other professions. These positive emotional experiences could perhaps have been more thoroughly interpreted. The cognitive meaning of these experiences could have been articulated without much danger and with some benefit for subsequent behaviour upon return to the hospital.

More importantly, the behavioural skills learned were limited primarily to those of both a cognitive and an objective orientation – how, for example, to administer a survey to others. Somewhat more threatening, but still apparently within the competence of hospital-team members, would have been more practice in skills that were partly subjective in orientation but also essentially cognitive – skills such as handling oneself as a discussion leader and encouraging participation from different discussion group members.

Another tactic of potential usefulness would have been practice in skills with a relatively emotional orientation, but focusing on other people – skills such as determining anxieties in discussion group members about authority relationships. The point is that the cognitive/emotional and objective/subjective dimensions are just that – dimensions. Movement in one may be balanced by movement in the other, so that the client's competence (in terms of readiness and ability to handle anxiety and to look at oneself) is not exceeded, but is pushed far enough for learning or change to be as effective as possible at a given time.

If these two points are followed – (1) balanced learning so as to attain, but not exceed, the most effective levels of emotional and subjective functioning and (2) integrated or linked cognitive/emotional and objective/subjective change experiences, providing effective but also transferable change – then the likelihood of the learned responses being successful and being reinforced in the A-stage and afterwards is bound to be relatively high.

Let us now examine change-agent and client influence in our sequential study of the H.I.C. Project. For problem-solving in relation to the external environment (the AGIL sequence) the client must perceive a problem or an opportunity, a discrepancy between what exists and what might be, with respect to his environmental position.[33] Seeing such discrepancies is a skill that must be learned, but if one assumes, as did those setting up the Project, that hospital-team members can see their problems,[34] then relatively little authoritative influence on the part of the change-agents (the central team) is needed to facilitate the change or problem-solving process. The discrepancy generates needs to solve the problem, and appropriate information from a change-agent is utilized accordingly. It is expert influence or the influence of the information itself that is necessary for such problem-solving. Of course, if clients cannot perceive their problems or do not have the appropriate problem-solving skills, then an influential change-agent is required. Such a change-agent must have expertise about the client's problems, their causes, and the means of solving them, and he must have some authoritative influence, so as to change the client himself and give him some of the necessary problem-solving skills.

If we accept that the problem in the H.I.C. hospitals was a matter of information, then the central team's lack of influence would appear to matter relatively little, since the hospital teams would get on with their problem-solving, and, with the help of information provided by the survey technology, their skills would enable them to solve their various external-system problems. The picture is quite different if the problem is a matter of internal-system change and a LIGA sequence is required. For it is usually the change-agent who supplies the skills in moving the client in the I- and G-stages of the LIGA sequence. The deeper the problem within the internal psychological system of the client, the less likely it is that the client himself can supply the skills to produce change. He must be dependent on the change-agent, and, contrariwise, the change-agent must have influence over him.[35] Self-directed change within the internal system – in creating 'people' changes rather than external, problem-solving changes – would not seem to be very likely.

We have described Revans's work in changing hospital-team members – in creating a commitment in hospital-team members to technology as a means of obtaining information. Revans's success in this matter was due to the great influence he had with hospital-team members, and to his use of the LIGA sequence for change. In contrast, the central-team members had aims that depended even more upon having influence – they wanted 'people' changes such as decreased 'authoritarianism', more openness, etc. – but the influence was lacking. Thus, the use of an LIGA sequence, which is so effective in obtaining internal-system or 'people' changes, was essentially denied them. Only the AGIL sequence – effective in creating the cognitive or technological changes of relatively little interest to them – was generally feasible. In other words, influence differences explain why Revans was successful in changing hospital-team members with regard to the use of the survey technology, and why the central team was relatively unsuccessful in creating 'people' change of any great magnitude.

The reader should not draw from this a conclusion that strong influence of the central team over the hospital team would have been desirable. We have argued above for a mutual influence approach to change in which both change-agent and client have great influence over each other. Our subsequent discussion of the dangers involved in the careless use of change-agents' influence to obtain 'deep' changes in people (in an LIGA sequence) provided additional support for a mutual influence approach. The strong influence of the client in such a situation allows him to protect himself, but also allows a collaborative determination and movement by change-agent and client to the best available level for change. This is not to deny the dilemma that necessary changes may lie too deep for mutually agreed-change activity to occur, but we have already indicated some good reasons why the best procedural solution may rest at the agreed level, within the desires and normative constraints of the client.

It is difficult to make any definite statement about the desirability and appropriateness of the change sequencing used in the H.I.C. Project, since it depends very much on the Project's ultimate aims, resources available, and the change situation itself. Given sufficient time, there will usually be a number of different ways of reaching essentially the same end, and thus a number of different sequence configurations might be useful. In addition, our usage of the change sequence model is not as well articulated, nor as well supported by systematic, objective observations, as the previous analyses we have pursued.

It is our basic assumption that the H.I.C. hospital needs for change lay essentially in the areas of people and structure, not in technology. A basic problem in the H.I.C. Project and in many projects is that comparative diagnosis was not made to ascertain the most pressing needs for changes. In this case, as in many change programmes, the available tools for change seem to receive the most attention and usage, whatever the actual needs. But we shall assume, on the basis of our own observations as well as Revans's assertion about parataxis and anxiety being endemic in hospitals, that some changes in people and structure were, and are, needed.

This still leaves the question of what specific changes in people or structure are needed. Our own view is that the authority and influence structures, as well as attitudes regarding authority, are the key elements in need for change, although Revans's linking of the lack of information and attendant anxiety also seems important. But in the light of these uncertainties regarding change needs, adequate diagnosis during the early stages of the LIGA sequence would have been most desirable.[36]

If we assume that changes in people (and perhaps structure) are needed, then we are able to narrow down the alternative routes by which such change may be obtained. They seem to fall into a single rather general configuration, namely, some linking of change efforts that rely on LIGA cognitive (and non-threatening) changes together with AGIL problem-solving and external change of others in the hospital. Greater central-team influence (in the context of a high mutual influence relationship with hospital-team members) would have facilitated further LIGA work following Revans's initial change activity, while greater central-team competence in organizational diagnosis and problem-solving would have greatly facilitated operation in AGIL sequences after the hospital teams returned from the courses.

Clearly, we do not see a potent central-team effort at change in people by means of the LIGA sequence as either feasible or desirable. Such an operation would have undoubtedly run into the dilemma that Harrison describes, that 'deep' change efforts may get at problems, but are also liable to be risky and counter-productive in terms of clients' desires or normative structure. Clients having relatively 'deep' problems are probably also unwilling to engage in changes at that level. The change-agent must consider whether he values solving clients' problems more than respecting clients' desires about what is done to them. To put it bluntly, is client improvement worth manipulation?[37]

One answer seems to be that over time the client may come to trust the change-agent, and a better and deeper relationship may develop. Then as the change-agent moves closer to the source of problems, the client becomes more able to collaborate with the change-agent in the work, and he becomes more tolerant of formerly 'external' threats to the self. In addition, with time the client would be helped to become more aware of various opportunities and options, including value options, and he should be more able to collaborate with the change-agent in planning further steps. Not covered by this optimistic view, of course, is the possibility that real value differences with the change-agent may still remain – either to be acknowledged or to be altered by the change-agent.

Increasing trust, closer relationship, and increasing competence, or cumulative changes in the client, may possibly come from an appropriate patterning of change sequences as well as from choosing the appropriate level of intervention. By describing the H.I.C. Project in terms of AGIL or LIGA sequences we have greatly simplified events. Within the overall movement according to the described phases, there were in fact movements by individuals, and sub-groups, through the phases in smaller or shorter cycles. One visit to a hospital could, in fact, start with the creation of a close relationship between central-team member and hospital-team member, and end with some reorientation by the hospital-team member with regard to some matter – i.e. a shift in attitude, if not a change. This was particularly true, of course, during the hospital project phase of H.I.C., when new projects brought new relationships between hospital team and central team into existence. We have alluded to the central team's efforts in these directions. It is our impression that several hospital-team members did, in fact, change in attitude or in communication behaviour as a result of central-team activity after the course, although the objective survey data do not permit one to pinpoint precisely when changes occurred.

While such change efforts could not be of very great magnitude, even cumulatively, owing to the lack of proper influence by central-team members, they do point to a way in which some change effects may be cumulated and the debilitating effects of conflicting phase sequences avoided. That is to say, a 'safer' change strategy may be to operate in one mode or the other in fairly short phase sequences or cycles. By evaluating the outcomes of such short cycles – by getting early 'feedback', the disastrous effects of too deep, too conflicting, or too superficial LIGA or AGIL cycles may be counteracted by changing the depth, the degree of linkage, or perhaps the type of phase sequence.

## CLARITY AND GOAL DISPLACEMENT IN PROJECT DEVELOPMENT

Our earlier discussions on the relative merits of clear and unclear Project goals and means may now be related to our discussion of the sequential development of the Project. We have suggested that generally a change project like the H.I.C. Project will have relatively diffuse ends. This is particularly true of a project aiming at changes in people, which are intangible because of our limited capabilities for systematically conceptualizing and measuring such changes. Technological ends (or sub-goals, if one takes a 'red-herring' view of H.I.C.) might be somewhat clearer.

The relative intangibility of ultimate ends in H.I.C. allowed individuals with a diversity of aims and intentions to participate in the Project, and also gave it some potential flexibility. We have seen, for example, how hospital-team members wanted relatively more in the way of diagnostic work done by the central team, while the latter wanted to emphasize training activities (see Chapter 17). We have also discussed above how there was some change in orientation from technology to people over the course of the Project.

However, our sequential study indicated why greater change in orientation of the Project did not occur. Central-team members had little power to reorientate the hospital teams once they had started their survey projects in the hospitals. But it is probably true for both central and hospital teams that the great clarity – or more precisely tangibility and measurability – of survey activities also contributed to a lack of eventual change in the 'people' and structural elements of the hospitals (and perhaps even in their information systems).

As Merton (1957) has indicated, structures, in the sense of means for various ends such as rules or procedures in a bureaucracy, may become ends in themselves. Such means are liable to be clear, and when the ends are not clear, the means may become the subjects of almost total attention whether or not they are in fact relevant to the ends. In other words, Project participants should have asked whether surveys were the best way to improve 'communication', whether in some cases the effects of a survey might not have the desired outcomes, and whether the ramifying effects might even include negative outcomes. Surveys became accepted as ends when in fact they were only a means to improvement in 'communication'.

It is very difficult to counter such effects of clearly specified means upon the efforts of project participants. In the H.I.C. Project, those carrying out surveys were rewarded in a number of ways. First of all, they were gathering a large volume of 'useful' information and they were making discernible progress along the clearly specified sequence a survey must follow (gather data, analyse data, issue report).[38] Knowledge of such progress makes any work easier and is also highly motivating. Furthermore, they were keeping busy and demonstrating the value of the Project to superiors, sponsors, or outsiders. Some would say they were being 'scientific'. Perhaps most important, they were not 'wasting time' arguing about 'communication' or what is the best way to change people. Most of all, these rewards had to do with the clearly specified nature of the survey activity.

Clearly structured situations, in which there is agreement about activities to be performed, are highly conducive to group as well as individual performance. Communication and attraction within a group are facilitated by having the same clear goals in mind. Such a group will become more cohesive, and because of the group's power over members derived from cohesiveness, the group will be more effective. In part this is also due to the facilitation of co-ordination among group members by the common perceptions, and by the knowledge of effects or feedback available from a clear goal.

The need for clarity at any one time, however, depends very much on the sequencing of a change project, which in turn depends on the ultimate ends as well as conditions obtaining in the change situation. A project to change people will need to begin with a diffuse situation so as to create the conditions for internal-system change. Ends are also relatively intangible and not known until diagnosis and changing are brought to a considerably advanced stage. There is increasing specificity over the LIGA phase sequence, although the end-point is still liable to be relatively intangible in terms of our ability to specify clearly the internal changes that will have taken place. In contrast, the problem-solving, external-system change sequence of AGIL is one of specific means in relation to more diffuse ends. The A-stage requires consideration of specific alternatives that, it is hoped, will lead to goal-attainment and a diffuse condition of success.

If this assessment is correct, it would suggest that the increasing clarity experienced by the hospital teams over the course of the Project could have denoted successful movement along the LIGA sequence.[39] If, in fact, the commitment of hospitals to the use of survey methods was the goal of H.I.C., the sequencing that took place seems quite appropriate. The team members moved from great obscurity regarding the Project to a specific conviction that surveys would help them in their work. We have suggested, however, that changes in people, including attitudes about authority and influence relationships, as well as related changes in influence structure, may have been desirable ends for H.I.C. If this was true, then the implanting of the survey technology served as an easy way out, a 'red-herring' as it were. This possible overemphasis on surveys could have been rectified by central-team activity, but as we indicated, they could not use a LIGA sequence. The clear operational survey activities added one more hindrance to such an approach.

In the alternative AGIL sequence pursued by some central-team members, the survey activities served as a useful starting-point towards solving problems, and central-team members took advantage of it. But the central team could only with great difficulty get hospital-team members to use surveys to move towards the more diffuse change in people. The problem was that the rewards encouraging surveys were great, and alternatives with clear, measurable sub-goals mediating means and ends were absent. In short, the clear ends of the LIGA sequence served as means for the AGIL sequence, but in the latter case the means tended to displace the ends.

There is no simple remedy for the apparent overemphasis on clearly specified means – survey activity – that took place in the H.I.C. Project, but several alterations might perhaps serve to lessen the intensity of the problem. Warner and Havens (1968) suggest that those at the top of a change programme, by virtue of their control of the reward system, may direct attention away from clearly specified means towards more diffuse ends by the rewarding of activities focused on the latter. Similarly, a project may be structured to begin with diffuse but 'easy' (rewarding) exercises with some bearing on the ends.[40] We have already indicated the great value in having a model for the relations between means and ends. Such a model is particularly important in this context.[41] If subsequent sub-goals are specified, then activity is drawn away from prior sub-goals by this very attraction,[42] which, in the absence of specified and measurable subsequent goals, can lead to overemphasis on the prior sub-goals. Finally, initial change activities should take place in relatively anxiety-free situations – or situations in which organizational maintenance needs are low, so as to remove one more force towards specified, limited change activity.[43]

## REASSESSMENT OF H.I.C. 'SUCCESS'

In the various sections above, we have discussed some of the problems within the H.I.C. Project. It is perhaps not clear from the at times critical discussion that the Project achieved considerable success in a number of ways. There were, in fact, changes in the communications behaviour of hospital-team members, and there were many technological and structural changes. All of this occurred in a very difficult situation, by which we mean not only that of the hospitals generally (including the authority and inter-professional difficulties that this Project in part set out to ameliorate) but also the major difficulties involved in experimenting with new kinds of change-agent and client roles (Chapter 5).

Moreover, this Project showed that hospitals are willing to attempt change and, when approached in the right way, are ready to use unorthodox methods for potential improvement. The hospitals participated in nearly forty different projects; they presented formal reports to specially convened audiences; they published reports in hospital or medical journals. There are certainly many other reasons for these activities, but the desire for improvement was important, and Revans wisely and successfully built upon this desire.

From a sequential analysis of the H.I.C. Project, it would appear that the shortcomings (especially in relation to organization-level changes and changes in people) in the long run were due to premature closure and to a disjunction in the sequencing from the initial course activity to later hospital-project and central-team activity. If this is correct, then Revans's early activity in establishing a commitment to H.I.C. and a relationship between himself and hospital-team members, together with the course activity in teaching survey methods, was even more successful than might appear in terms of final outcomes. In fact, the initial hospital-project activity by hospital-team members must be viewed as one of the successes of the H.I.C. Project.

The central team's efforts must also appear very successful in the light of the Project conditions at the time of their entrance – the fixation of hospital-team members on surveys as the means of hospital improvement, and, generally, the programming of hospital-team participation in terms of emphasizing cognitions, objective orientations, and self-direction. The central team's efforts towards changing people seem to have had some success in terms of questionnaire measures of outcomes, and correlations of these outcomes with central-team activities. It is the extent of these outcomes that falls short. Keeping in mind our observations about the situational imperatives that required the central team to operate in the AGIL or problem-solving mode, with its emphasis on external outcomes, it is somewhat remarkable that the central team was able to change the orientation of the Project to provide some of the desired internal-system changes or changes in people.

## SOME CONCLUSIONS

Several general conclusions are evident if we consider the H.I.C. Project less from the viewpoint of the particular different intentions of Project participants, and more from that of what new practical achievements in fact resulted.

We conclude that, first of all, it can be done.[44] Many managers are interested and willing to volunteer and use survey technology as a managerial tool in improving their effectiveness and that of their organizations. The Project demonstrates that the survey approach to change, as many investigators have found, is generally an acceptable, non-threatening technique for studying behaviour. This acceptability rests in the essentially rational, cognitive approach to change, in contrast to the more emotional focuses of 'deeper' change techniques such as sensitivity training. An additional consideration of interest to managers is that these change efforts based on surveys are relatively inexpensive and rely on resources that are not extremely scarce.

Second, despite the difficulties of both central-team and hospital-team members in developing and stabilizing roles towards each other and towards the others involved, this experimental project demonstrated that managers can learn enough about conducting surveys to be of some use. Data were obtained, with varying degrees of help from the central team, to permit a variety of actions modifying technical, procedural, and structural elements of the participating organizations.

Finally, we conclude that the self-survey method offers a means of obtaining behavioural changes in managers – the changes in attitudes, emotions, etc., that Leavitt (1965) has called 'people' changes. It is true that in the H.I.C. Project much of this kind of change was correlated with activity by the central team (rather than the survey work independently undertaken by the hospital teams), but the power (in terms of authority, rewards, and expertise) of these facilitators was generally minimal. The combination of minimal influence by the central-team helpers, together with the survey data produced by the managers, resulted in some tangible behavioural changes in the managers.

The major problem in these projects was the general absence of organization-level changes – that is to say, changes in the criteria of organizational effectiveness. For the self-survey method to be most effective at this level of change, it would appear (especially from several follow-up projects of a similar nature) that relatively small and simple organizations tend to promote the effectiveness of the method. In the next section we shall consider some possible further general directions for projects like H.I.C.

## RECOMMENDATIONS

It would be unrealistic to make specific recommendations regarding such a complex project as the H.I.C. Project. The problem in making recommendations is compounded by uncertainty about the situation of hospitals generally. Not only is there a lack of sufficient scientific diagnostic information, but there are also a number of policy questions that must first be answered – some of which in fact are currently being considered. Furthermore, there is the question of the amount of resources available for improvement efforts of various kinds.

Any kind of action research must depend for its directions, in the final analysis, on the task of the hospital in relation to other components of the health system. Policy decisions regarding this task made in conjunction with a thorough diagnosis of the present situation should yield a design for the future, including a design for further action research. Neither policy considerations nor diagnostic information on the situation of the hospital and the health system were significant inputs for the H.I.C. Project.[45]

Another potentially useful, but absent, input was scientific information about the determinants of organizational effectiveness in hospitals. Efforts to obtain such information would be of great value for further action-research projects of this nature. In the United States, for example, comparative survey data now exist for a nationwide probability sample of hospitals (Wieland, 1965; Georgopoulos and Wieland, 1968) as well as a smaller, but more intensively studied group of ten hospitals in one state (Georgopoulos and Mann, 1962). To such data should be added an in-depth analysis of the situation within hospitals,[46] as well as further research and development work on criteria of effectiveness in the hospital, a most difficult problem.

Thus programmatic research and development in the hospital field would proceed from two standpoints. Survey data on existing conditions would be used to design change experiments modifying the current status. On the other hand, policy considerations would suggest experimental work or action – research for examining the efficacy of various new ventures, not yet existing and therefore not amenable to survey analysis. The research must create the organization to be studied and evaluated.

All of this, of course, must be supported by research on change and on the diffusion of innovations. We need to know more particularly about inexpensive kinds of change programme. Such change studies need to compare different kinds of change-agents and change-agent efforts – just as organizational studies have moved from the case study to comparisons of organizations – and they should be studies of the change process over time, so that the process of changing is understood as well as the relationships between the change-agent and client at any one point in time. A very important component of such studies, as we have indicated above, is examination of the normative structure of client systems with respect to the permissibility of different kinds of interventions and change efforts.

An apparently desirable strategy for success in action research is to make sure that feedback loops on projects are relatively small. In addition, relatively small research investments spread over a number of innovative projects would seem better at this early stage in the development of knowledge on changing organizations. An emphasis on less costly, more flexible survey evaluations, as opposed to experimental evaluations, should be included (Rossi, 1967; Wieland, 1969b).

Because we know so little about how to change, and because it is very likely that there are a number of different ways of reaching a similar end-point, it is difficult to make recommendations for modifications in the H.I.C. Project.[47] If we assume that the aim of the H.I.C. Project is in the realm of change in people and structure, and if we assume changes are required in the area of more participatory and flexible organizational functioning, then many of the general points above would seem relevant. A technological approach to change might be quite useful as a starting-point, subsequently moving towards more structural and 'people' changes, but maintaining a balance between cognitive/objective and emotional/subjective approaches, together with the mutual influence relationship that we have described above. However, great care must be taken to observe the dynamics of sequential relationships and especially the clarity and operationality of the means in relation to sub-goals and goals.

Perhaps the strongest recommendations should be made with respect to the nature of the organizations to be used for further action research of this nature. In the H.I.C. Project, there seemed to be no extensive or pervasive changes extending beyond the hospital teams into the hospital organizations (although we do report some structural and other changes). This suggests that much needs to be done about the organizational strategy to be used in such a project. The resources available in the central team, and perhaps also in the hospital teams, were inadequate (see especially Chapter 5). Clearly more resources must be provided, but probably it would be even better to work with smaller and less complex organizations.

The hospital is probably an undesirable choice for an initial experiment with a change programme such as the H.I.C. Project. The high levels of anxiety in the hospital (Menzies, 1960; Revans, 1964b) probably predispose change projects towards the displacement of goals by project means, as we have seen in the H.I.C. Project. Such anxiety probably prevents project participants from wholeheartedly making their jobs part of the project or from involving other staff in collaborative work on it. In addition, the status and professional (tripartite) barriers to communication and value differences (Stanton and Schwartz, 1954) make diffusion difficult and thus indicate the need for large resources in order to attempt change in a number of sub-systems either simultaneously or in a closely articulated fashion. Finally, hospitals are probably among the most complex existing organizations – in terms of the heterogeneity of their make-up and the functional interdependencies and needs for co-ordination. This is not to say that hospitals should not be studied in change projects, but only to suggest that care should be taken to select the least defensive and most open organizations possible (see also Chapter 1), and to make sure that sufficient resources are available to make some organization-level changes feasible.[48]

In addition, a more truncated version of the H.I.C. Project should not be overlooked. Too many of the methods of obtaining organizational change are dependent on massive change efforts demanding major resources from both client and change-agent. Self-survey teams in organizations, without necessarily directly changing people or structure, should receive some consideration. Many organizations in the United States have such internal survey capabilities. While some have found relatively little value in survey activity, the state of the art has progressed to the point where surveys can be very useful tools for obtaining much information for administrative action (Foundation, 1964).

Holloway and Lonergan (1968) have developed a programmed, instrumented survey capability for hospitals which, with some small degree of appropriate consultant help, may be of value in effecting changes in terms of problem-solving of various kinds, including some 'people' problems. If the training of the hospitals' own change-agents (leaders for the feedback discussion groups) in this programme can be made routine and achieved with minimal external help,[49] then an effective and inexpensive survey and change programme may be within reach of hospitals. There are tremendous difficulties in making the survey and change-programme materials suitable for those with minimal education (such as porters and the like), yet still interesting and challenging for those with higher qualifications. While no systematic evaluation of 'people' changes in this programme has been made, the problem-solving outcomes are apparently sufficiently evident to encourage further development of the method.

The great virtue of Holloway's programme is that once this development work has been 'packaged', diffusion will be relatively easy. Given our limited resources for organizational improvement, it would seem that only such a package is sufficiently inexpensive and easily communicated to have a possible impact on more than a few select hospitals.[50]

A recent experiment initiated by Revans in five small industrial firms in Milwaukee, Wisconsin (Knapp and Larson, n.d.) seems to indicate the value of proceeding with further development of the survey approach to change in the information technology of organizations. The apparent success of this experiment indicates the value of a number of points we have made, as well as suggesting some further points for improvement. Each of the organizations was small, having about 100 employees; this probably reduced the effects of impediments to change found in a larger organization.[51, 52] There was evidently a close relationship between the university 'central team' and the survey trainees ('hospital teams') in the organizations. There were five university staff connected with the project, one for each organization, providing the opportunity for ample change-agent assistance. The training was short so that there was apparently no overemphasis on the information side of the project. The emphasis was put on action. These five organizations had already co-operated on other ventures before, and so the study of each other's organizations and the making of comparative assessments were easily done. One can more readily admit, and act on, problems in this kind of co-operative atmosphere. Again, no assessment of 'people' changes was made in this project, but apparent problem-solving outcomes of various kinds indicate the value of further developmental work on the self-survey method of organizational improvement.

## SUMMARY

The measured results of the H.I.C. Project were modest in terms of organization-level outcomes. Achievements were primarily in terms of problem-solving – scattered changes in 'technology' and 'structure' – and in terms of 'people' changes. Changes in organization-level outcomes, such as patient-care, were not discernible with the evaluation methods used.

Correlational analyses suggest that possible improvements in outcomes may flow from more involvement and active influence by the central team, including emphasis on feedback meetings and other methods for the examination by hospital-team members of their own work and their own feelings about various matters, as well as emphasis on involving in the Project work some of the other staff in the hospital. In an attempt to assess the meaning of these correlational findings for the H.I.C. Project, an examination is made of the Project in terms of the dimensions introduced in Chapter 3.

The Project was essentially technological in orientation, being an attempt to improve the technology of the hospital information system by importing the use of survey methods. Characteristic of this technological focus was the emphasis on cognitive and objective orientations by members of the central and hospital teams. Emotional and subjective orientations were present, but to a rather more limited degree. The influence relationship between the hospital team and the central team may be characterized as essentially high influence by the hospital team over the central team, but not the reverse. The central team had little influence, generally having to limit their concern to the peripheral matters of the methods used in surveys.

Another noticeable characteristic of the Project was its great lack of clarity for participants. While the means – the use of survey methods – was clear, and perhaps even too clear or overemphasized in an inflexible way, a model linking the means to the desired ends was lacking.

It seems that more emphasis by H.I.C. on emotional and subjective orientations and on greater central-team influence would have been beneficial. However, the increased emphases should be by way of a dual, linked emphasis on cognitions and emotions, on objective and subjective orientations, and on mutual influence between central team and hospital team.

Linking cognitions and emotions gives the former meaning and stability and the latter transferability. A dual objective/subjective orientation provides a balanced comparative perspective, and, more important, a dual orientation facilitates a process or transactional perspective. A mutual influence relationship is demonstrably more effective in many situations than a one-way influence relationship.

Perhaps the most serious barriers to organization-level achievements in the H.I.C. Project sprang from the lack of an organizational strategy. Choice of functionally unrelated hospital-team members and the failure to involve other significant hospital staff hindered diffusion of the survey technology both within the team and through the hospital. Major efforts to move from technology to a people- or structure-oriented change programme – a 'red herring' approach – encountered problems. However, this indirect approach seems to offer a hope for true organization-level change, in terms of integrated changes in technology, people, and structure having ultimate effects on goal attainment.

But even within any one of these three foci, there are possible modifications that could lead to improvements in organization-level outcomes. Change efforts must be aimed at strategic variables that have a direct impact on the task of the organization – an impact on patient-care, in the case of the hospital.

In terms of sequential analysis, the Project seems to have had some success in unfreezing and changing hospital-team members, and in creating a commitment to the use of survey technology. Parsons's LIGA model for internal change helps to explain the success obtained by Revans's early influence in setting up the Project (L-stage), and in terms of training-course and practice-project emphasis on the appropriate survey skills (I- and G-stages). However, subsequent use of the surveys on the external system (A-stage) met with insufficient success to maintain the changed behaviour in the face of time pressures.

Hospital-team members apparently did not transfer their relatively limited 'people' learning (i.e. learning about how to behave differently, to be more sensitive to other people) from the courses to the hospital situation because of a lack of emotional/cognitive linkage as well as difficulties in the hospital situation itself. Survey procedures, however, were relatively easily transferred and reinforced, at least for a time.

Most of the central team joined the Project during the A-stage of the LIGA sequence. The central team was unable to operate in the LIGA mode, however, because they had little influence, nor could they do anything immediate about changing the survey learning used by the hospital team in the A-stage of the sequence. In other words, the central team could not operate in the earlier L- or I-stages of a LIGA sequence, but instead they began work in the A-stage mode, reinforcing the behaviour of the hospital team towards their external system (the rest of the hospital). To the extent of their ability, the central team reinforced and encouraged the study of 'people' variables and, most of all, tried to get hospital-team members to involve themselves and others in collaborative study.

Because the central team had little influence for reinforcement purposes, the hospital teams tended to continue the cognitive, objective studies learned so well during the courses. Another reason for the central team's relative lack of success in obtaining changes of any magnitude in people is, of course, the fact that the AGIL change sequence with which they had to start was not the most suitable for some of the required internal-system changes (i.e. the 'people' changes in the hospital team). The clarity (concreteness and measurability) of survey procedures was also especially rewarding to hospital-team members, drawing attention away from, and displacing, the more diffuse ends.

In retrospect, the failure of the central team to obtain greater movement by the hospital teams towards people changes is perhaps not wholly undesirable. Efforts at changing people can be risky, and possibly counter-productive if not carefully attuned to the desires and normative structures of the client. The mutual influence and integrated cognitive/emotional and objective/subjective emphases cited earlier provide some guidance to the selection of the proper 'depth' of change efforts. Phase movement in terms of both AGIL and LIGA sequences may facilitate change work at the appropriate level of intervention, also. All this assumes, of course, that the H.I.C. hospitals and similar organizations require changes in people, but only appropriate diagnostic and analytical work can confirm this.

One implication of the sequential analysis of the H.I.C. Project is that both Revans's initial change efforts towards implementation of the survey technology (by means of the LIGA internal change sequence) and the central team's subsequent efforts at change in people (by means of the AGIL external change sequence) were relatively effective, but in different ways. Revans's success in obtaining use of the survey technology is amply confirmed by the many projects done. The central team's success is not so apparent to the outside observer, because their aim of changing people was made difficult by the necessity of beginning with an inappropriate AGIL sequence. Nevertheless, the evidence from evaluation questionnaire data strongly suggests that the central team was effective within the constraints binding their operation.

Despite the various shortcomings described above, it seems clear that the self-survey approach to change devised by Revans is eminently acceptable and capable of implementation by managers. They can learn useful information about their organizations, and can use it to improve their organizations; moreover, their own behaviour may benefit.

No explicit recommendations are made for further projects other than emphasising the need for linked cognitive/emotional and objective/subjective orientations, for a mutual influence approach, and the need to be aware of the organizational strategy and the dynamics of sequencing and means-ends relations. Without carefully examining policy considerations as well as the state of existing hospital functioning, one cannot do more than advocate a cautious continuation of programmatic change efforts that emphasize organizational-level projects, in suitable organizations (especially in terms of organizational complexity), and with adequate resources.

## NOTES

[1] The importance of involving central-team and other, non-team, hospital staff in projects was also demonstrated in the separate analysis conducted with hospital project data in Chapter 18. That analysis further suggested that discussions among these individuals, together with hospital-team members, would facilitate comparisons between one organizational unit and another, leading to improvements in the work of hospital-team members.

[2] For details, see Chapter 6 and Appendix 6B.

[3] The reader interested in recent work in this area should consult the *Journal of Applied Behavioral Science*.

[4] For a general listing of these approaches see Bennis *et al.* (1969, pp. 58-59) and for details see Harrison (1970).

[5] Dalton (1970) sees the provision of a new cognitive structure as integral to the process of change:

> '... the individual is given a new means for reordering the information he has about himself and his environment. Implicit in the framework are relationships of acts to outcomes so that certain ends call for certain behavior' (p. 98).

[6] For an example of the linkage of cognitive/emotional and objective/subjective orientations, see Harrison and Hopkins (1967) on experiential training in the Peace Corps.

> '... the educator should help the learner reflect about his experience. The process of linking thought and feeling is as difficult when one begins with a concrete problem and moves toward conceptualization of the experience as it is when one starts with ideas and facts and tries to move toward action based upon an intellectual analysis ...
>
> 'The purpose of experience-based cross-cultural training is to inculcate somehow in the learner the ability to see and know what he is learning and has learned, so that he can articulate it afterwards and act on his learning consciously. The role prescribed for the teacher ... [is to help] ... the learner to verbalize his feelings, perceptions, and experiences and to draw conclusions and generalizations from them' (pp. 445-446).

Also see Argyris (1967) on the seeming overemphasis in some encounter groups upon emotional learning at the expense of cognitive learning and linkages with emotions.

[7] One often finds a very real dilemma in choosing between subjective or objective orientations because of time pressures. A T-group, for example, at times devotes attention to the personal problems of particular members and helps them work through these problems, delaying work on other tasks concerning the group as a whole, or vice versa. This movement back and forth between orientations internal and external to the individual is paralleled by the movement back and forth between orientations internal and external to the group found in 'inter-group' exercises. In these exercises, groups find that they need to devote attention to internal structure and functioning, but the need to deal with the impingement of external stimuli and to maintain and develop relationships with other groups requires a turning away from internal problems until they once again come to demand attention.

While there are advantages in both internal and external (or subjective and objective) approaches, unfortunately it is not always possible to combine both even in a sequential fashion, and some hard choices must be made. In running training groups for doctors to improve their relationships with patients, for example, the trainers found that two kinds of doctors came to the courses (Balint *et al.*, 1966). Some doctors came because they had personal or internal problems and were consequently ineffective. Other doctors were relatively free from these internal problems and came because they wanted to improve their external behaviour or relationships with patients. The trainers felt it would be hard to do both kinds of work, and so only the latter were selected to participate.

[8] In her recent evaluation of relationships between researchers and clients, Klein (1969) highlights the need for a closer examination of the researcher's needs and rewards in the relationship.

[9] High mutual influence is not, however, an unmitigated blessing. The costs involved are in part psychological. Not all individuals like to participate fully and involve themselves completely in their work (Vroom, 1969). Furthermore, a high mutual influence system produces a lot of wasted effort. There are

many more attempts at influence than there are successes, and the clash of attempts produces, at times, high levels of conflict among participants. Studies of cohesiveness in groups have shown that highly cohesive groups, with high mutual influence among participants, display more conflict than groups with low cohesiveness (Thibaut and Kelly, 1959). For a general review of the possible costs and shortcomings of equal influence, or 'participation' as it has been termed by some 'human relations' advocates, the reader might refer to Strauss (1963).

[10] One way of disseminating H.I.C. effects throughout a hospital is by means of groups arranged in an overlapping fashion so that some members of one group are members of the next group, and some of that group are members of a still further group (Likert, 1961).

[11] It has been argued (Dessler *et al.*, 1969) on the basis of research by Lawrence and Lorsch (1967) that participation, corresponding to high total control, is more desirable in organizations facing uncertain environments, while 'autocracy', with power and influence concentrated at the top, is more desirable in organizations with more certain environments. The environments of different hospitals are bound to vary according to their catchment areas, their relations with general practitioners, regional boards, etc., but to the extent that hospitals must meet community needs and respond to emergencies, epidemics, etc., they would seem to have a more uncertain environment than many other organizations.

[12] The procedure of moving back and forth between means and ends may be viewed as somewhat analogous to the procedure used by scientists in moving back and forth between theory-language and data-language – or being deductive and inductive.

[13] Using Chin's (1962) terminology, there should be a change-agent cum organization 'inter-system'. The organizational system as a whole must be effectively related in some fashion to the change-agent system.

[14] Barnes (1967), in reporting Greiner's survey of organizational change efforts, cites as one condition differentiating successful from less successful efforts that the change-agent engages 'many parts of the organization in a collaborative, fact-finding, problem-solving diagnosis of organizational problems'.

[15] In one hospital project, for example, hospital-team members communicated data on a hospital-wide survey to department heads, assuming that communication would continue on down from that level to the next one and so on. In point of fact, a number of blockages occurred, and members of some departments learned nothing of the survey results.

[16] We use the term 'top' somewhat loosely in speaking of the H.I.C. Project. The main focus of attention was on operational-team members, not strictly speaking the 'top'. Revans (Chapter 1) suggests that more effort should have been given to gaining the support of the very top. This seems reasonable in the light of the often rather tenuous support subsequently given to the operational team. However, the absence of evaluation-team members from the early conferences prevents any comment here on the feasibility of a better 'selling job' at that time, or any comments on its desirability. For an alternative view on the importance of top support, see Beckhard (1969).

[17] Instead of choosing hospital-team members by office (or in the case of some operational-team members, by the various desires of the supporting-team members) an alternative strategy would have central-team members first making a preliminary diagnosis of the top staff, and then selecting the team members (with varying degrees of participation by hospital staff in the decision) on the basis of qualifications for the role of change-agent. This would include not only

organizational position – and many positions, both formal and informal may have considerable influence depending on local situations – but also the personal characteristics of the individual. Most important would be the ability to see opportunities for change – being a 'variance sensor' as Bennis (1969) terms it. See, for example, Beckhard (1969) for details of the various internal positions and the various personal characteristics desirable in a change-agent collaborator in the organization.

[18] In the terms used by Miller and Rice (1967), the hospital teams were neither 'task' nor 'sentient' systems.

[19] For a somewhat contrasting view of the influence relations among doctors in American hospitals, see Goss (1961). For a view of European doctors in relation to American doctors, see Glaser (1963).

[20] The evaluator's observations indicated, more often than not, that lower-level contacts in the hospitals did not know that the H.I.C. Project even existed.

[21] By-passing hierarchical levels is especially threatening in a hospital or any other organization that is status-conscious. See Mann and Likert (1952) for further rationales for using hierarchical structure fully, especially in the feedback of survey results.

[22] For a general presentation on technology in organizations, see Leavitt (1965) and Perrow (1969), and in hospitals, see Perrow (1965).

[23] Variables related to anxiety and similar deep constructs were rarely studied. This is understandable, of course, in terms of the relative emphasis on questionnaire technology as opposed to less structured and more 'open' types of assessment that allow flexibility for probing in depth (see, e.g., Sofer, 1964).

[24] One of the most effective learning situations for people is by means of a coach-trainer (see Dyer *et al.*, 1970). Being in the hospital gave the student change-agent the opportunity to function with hospital staff members in a one-to-one situation. Students could act as coach-trainers providing psychological support and security, and providing immediate feedback on efforts. Similarly, structure cannot be diagnosed without day-to-day observation of structure in relation to the changing influences, without time to seek out leverage points, and without time to organize groups and create means of leverage.

[25] This series of analyses is very tentative not only because of observational limitations of the evaluation study, but also because our theory of changing is so deficient – we know so little about which of the many possible relevant factors to look at, and about the proper ways to conceptualize and systematize observations. As Lewin said, 'there is nothing so practical as a good theory', and a good theory is just what we lack. This difficulty is no less applicable to successful change projects. Our lack of knowledge, together with related methodological limitations, requires a change-agent to do as much as is possible in the way of change efforts, and success often only tells the investigator that a rather large array of change efforts is successful, but not which efforts in relation to which situations or (most difficult of all) at what times. It appears that a survey-correlational approach to evaluation, obtaining multiple-time-series data, in connection with an action-research change mode (i.e. different actions or changes phased over time), would do much in the way of providing data suitable for theory-building, especially the developmental theory of change that is now lacking.

[26] We are assuming sufficient similarity between psychotherapy and other kinds of 'people' changes (such as the attempts in H.I.C. to modify attitudes) so that applying some of the more general aspects of Parsons's LIGA model to H.I.C. is not inappropriate (see, for example, Lippitt *et al.*, 1958, on

similarities between psychotherapy and organizational change efforts).

[27] See also Dalton (1970) on the need for a 'heightened sense of self-esteem' as part of the change process.

[28] Even where the central team had enough influence to create the L- and I-stage conditions for a LIGA sequence, there would most likely be problems in relation to the remaining A-stage orientations of the hospital-team members. Starting with both internally (L and I) and externally (A and G) oriented stages simultaneously is probably difficult, unless the two efforts are very finely articulated. The I-stage requires an internal or subjective point of view, while the A-stage requires a focus primarily on external problems and opportunities. The I-stage requires a major focus on emotions, so that these may be changed along with cognitions, while the A-stage requires feelings to be held in abeyance, for they are not handled till later when the goal is achieved. Finally, the I-stage requires internal flexibility made possible by a protective environment, by a barrier between internal systems, while the A-stage requires information from the external system in order to diagnose the situation accurately – the A-stage requires permeable boundaries and information from outside.

[29] L. B. Barnes (1967) cites 'successful' change studies as characterized by 'a newcomer with experience and a reputation for improving organizations [who] enters the picture'.

[30] It is somewhat ironical that Revans seemingly used the diffuse, emotional relationship part of the LIGA sequence to form a commitment in the hospital-team members to a cognitive approach to change. However, as we have seen, an attempt at a deeper, more emotional, change early in the Project could have encountered a number of problems subsequently.

[31] Dalton (1970), in discussing organizational development, argues that 'prestige and power on the part of the initiator seems to be a necessary, if not sufficient, condition for introducing large-scale change in any system' (p. 86).

[32] This is, of course, to assume that at least some changes in people were required in H.I.C. hospitals.

[33] See Zollschan and Hirsch (1964) on 'exigencies'.

[34] Hospital-team members often reported that they knew their problems and that what they needed was a way of solving them.

[35] For the inverse relationship between influence and dependency, see Emerson (1962). For details regarding client dependence on different kinds of change-agents, see Harrison (1970).

[36] See Lippitt *et al.* (1958) on the important place of diagnosis early in the formation of the relationship between change-agent and client.

[37] See also Lakin (1969).

[38] Several surveys, for example, were explicitly done not to change matters or solve problems, but 'to see how it is we are doing so well' or, in another case, as a matter of curiosity about interests, attitudes, typical working patterns, and so on. Use of the survey method and the acquisition of information could, for a number of reasons, take precedence over solving problems.

[39] See items R219 and R220 in Chapter 15, showing increasing levels of clarity over time in the Project. In addition some inferential evidence on the efficacy of the initially diffuse LIGA sequence in creating changes in people is provided by the relationship between *unclear* data and changes in the work of hospital-team members (*Table 18-2*). *Clear* data is related to objectives achieved, which in most cases was solving others' problems. An example of unclear data leading to discussion and (inferentially) to changes in people, rather than administrative action to solve 'external' problems, is provided by Hillier in Chapter 5.

[40] This is not to say a change programme with an 'easy' target is undesirable. Experience of success helps build momentum in a programme, if not for the client (because of the lack of integration between sub-systems), then, because of increased morale, for the change-agents. Dykens *et al.* (1964), in their programme of improvement in a mental hospital, advocate doing low-risk and low-gain projects as well as low-risk and high-gain ones.

Low-risk projects are also especially suitable at the beginning of a project, such as H.I.C. with its relatively inexperienced central team, because the team is able to cope with most contingencies, and they ensure a good beginning. While an 'easy' project is most commonly advocated because of its positive effects on the client, in this case the success experience (completion of the project) would be most useful in providing reinforcement for the initially uncertain central-team organization.

[41] One of the advantages of the Blake and Mouton (1968) Managerial Grid approach to organizational change is the linking of some quite clear instrumented concepts for new managerial behaviour with similarly clear and instrumented examination of organizational goals. However, where the organizational goals are less clear, as in the case of the university compared to industry, such a change programme may still encounter difficulty (Jackson Greyson, personal communication).

[42] March and Simon (1958) describe the tendency for daily routine (with its clear goals) to drive out planning activity (with its diffuse goals) as the 'Gresham's Law' of planning. Programmed activities tend to replace unprogrammed activities.

[43] In this respect, the choice of hospitals as organizations to change was perhaps unfortunate for the H.I.C. Project. Changing requires effort, and if the change programme is to be held in abeyance for some reason (such as limited resources for operating continuously over all change focuses), then the system must be moved to a relatively stable state. In other words, there must be refreezing (see, for example, Seashore and Bowers (1970) on 'locking in' change). This is especially true of systems that are accustomed to or require structure, such as hospital systems. Systems that must deal with emergencies and with life-or-death matters tend to have an especially high degree of structure (Menzies, 1960).

Thus in the hospital one must expect movement towards closure and towards restructuring if change efforts are halted or are not pursued vigorously. Furthermore, there must be continuous support when the system is unfrozen, because of the competing demands on it, and because of the traditional culture of the system that requires such structure. Organizational slack is most desirable for these purposes. This enables resources to be devoted to holding the system in an open and fluid state as well as supplying resources to support the comparatively costly change efforts.

[44] These general conclusions are also supported by work on similar self-survey projects recently completed in Milwaukee, U.S.A. (Knapp and Larson, n.d.) and currently under way in West Flanders, Belgium (under the direction of F. Musschoot). Both projects were prompted by the ideas of Revans.

[45] For example, many of the current policy questions concern the interface between the hospital and the community – relations between the hospital service, the local authorities, and general practitioners – but the H.I.C. Project was primarily concerned with the hospital as a closed system. The H.I.C. Project was a study of hospital 'internal' communications. Almost without exception, hospital teams studied their own hospitals and problems falling within it. However, an exception, a study of another smaller hospital in a hospital group, indicated, by the difficulties encountered, that the H.I.C. Project, at least in

terms of existing resources and operational capabilities, was probably right in limiting projects to an 'internal' focus.

[46] See Kahn *et al.* (1964) for an example of a study incorporating a nation-wide survey – to provide population parameters for some key selected variables – together with an intensive study of selected organizations – to provide a full dynamic picture of the area under study.

[47] For some detailed recommendations see Chapters 4-6 above.

[48] There is general consensus among change-agents (see, e.g., Barnes, 1967; Beckhard, 1969) that pressures upon the client, and difficulty on his part in coping with them, are prerequisites to successful change efforts. However, the client must also have the resources for the change efforts and for organizational development. Many of those in the field of organizational development, in fact, see the change-agent as helping the client to use his own resources. It is not the change-agent who solves problems, it is the client who has had his already existing resources made operational by the help of the change-agent.

[49] To programme this may be somewhat difficult. See Chestler and Flanders (1967) for an account of the complexity of forces operating in the feedback situation.

[50] A simple inexpensive self-survey programme along these lines for use by hospitals in studying patient satisfactions has been developed by Raphael (1969). In the U.S.A., computerized versions of patient questionnaires have also been devised (Eisenberg, 1969).

As Revans indicates (Chapter 1), patients, also, have a need for information. This and many other needs of patients are all too easily ignored. As Duff and Hollingshead (1968) found in their study of an American medical centre, doctors may be ignoring the social side of patients' disorders and treating only the physical side. The self-survey could make a real contribution to informing doctors in this area, although the problems here are so great that more than objective, survey-type instruments are needed.

[51] See also Schmuck and Runkel (1970) for an apparently successful change project in a school comprising 54 staff members. The organizations involved in the West Flanders study (cited in Note 44) range from 100 to 200 members. These are all in contrast to the organizations involved in H.I.C. – which ranged from 500 to 2000 staff.

[52] It is, of course, not so much the small size itself that seems to be important, but rather the concomitants of small size. We make the following assumptions about the value of small organizations for further experiments with the H.I.C. approach to change:

First of all, the top members of a smaller organization tend to have a greater concern with, and awareness of, internal organizational functioning, while top members of larger organizations fill primarily an environmental-linking function. Greater internal awareness and concern tends to insure that the participation of an organization is based on intrinsic reasons. There is sometimes the danger that top members of large organizations will volunteer the participation of their organization in a project for political reasons or other reasons having to do with external relationships. On this account, the matching between the values and style of the change programme and the nature of the organization at middle and lower levels may not be so close as when the head of an organization with only two or three levels volunteers to participate.

Smaller organizations are likely to facilitate the diffusion of project changes. The change efforts – both in terms of the effect of the (central-team) change-agents on the survey teams and the survey team's effect on their subordinates and junior colleagues - are more likely to receive support and to diffuse widely and thoroughly in a relatively small organization having less heterogeneity, and often higher morale and better social relations (see, e.g., Georgopoulos and Wieland, 1968).

Finally, the relationship between the change-agents and the survey team in a smaller organization is likely to be on a more nearly equal basis. As we have indicated, those doing survey training and consultation are likely to need to influence organization members regarding various aspects of the project – explaining technical matters, providing psychological support, or focusing survey activity on certain substantive matters – and the status and influence of any given change-agent is likely to be more nearly equal to members of smaller organizations than to those of larger organizations, at any given rank.

PART FIVE

# *Appendices*

# APPENDIX 6A

FIGURE 6A-i *Hospital projects, 1965-1968*

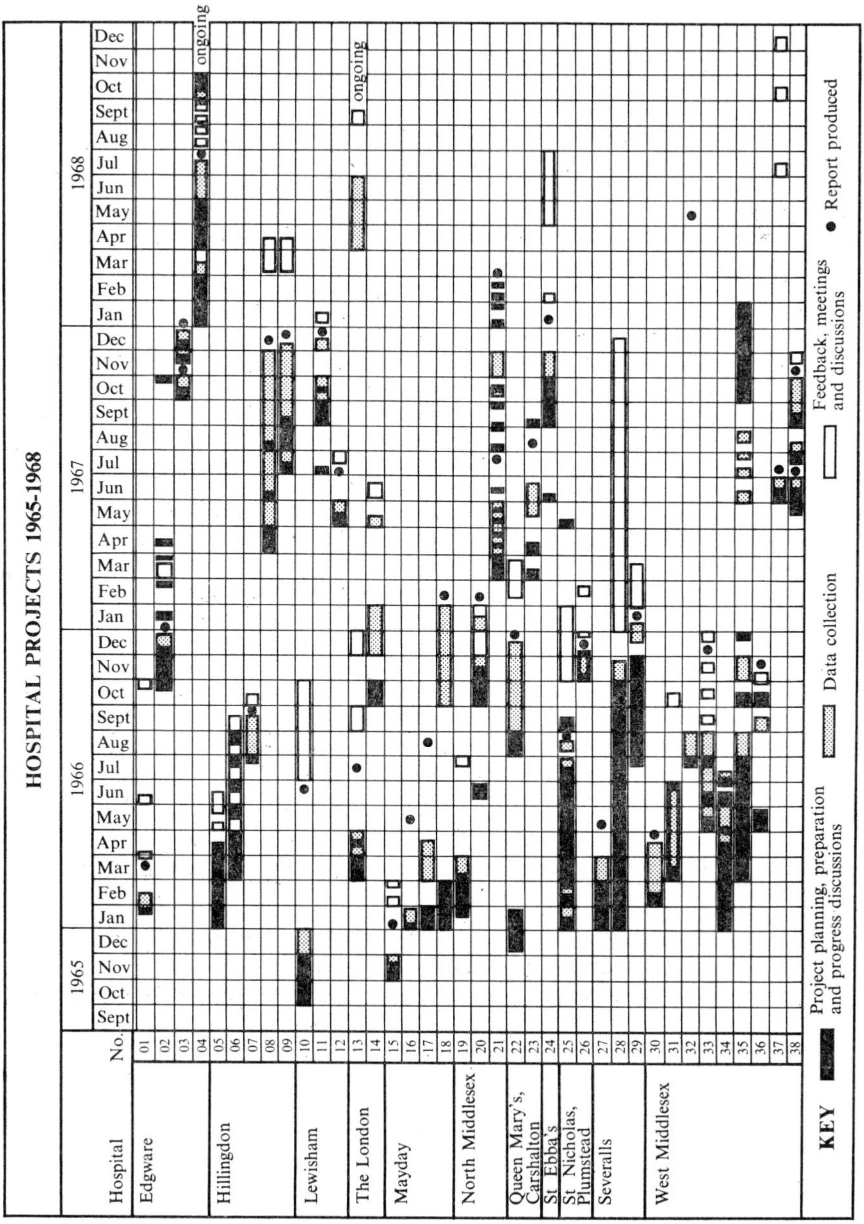

## APPENDIX 6B

# *Further examples of project outcomes*

1. Allocation of room in nurses' home to provide additional library facilities for resident students.
2. Introduction of name badges for ward staff.
3. Introduction of regular meetings for heads of departments.
4. Rationalization of workloads among medical social workers; joint appointment of an additional medical social worker by the local authority and the hospital.
5. Drastic change in advertisements for nursing staff; commencement of study days for nursing assistants.
6. Institution of post-registration management course for nurses; student nurses instructed about the role of social workers through practical work and lectures.
7. Setting up of a catering consumers' committee; hospital orientation programme for newly appointed ward and departmental sisters.
8. Introduction of appointment system for casualty reattendances; practical course in casualty nursing for post-registration nurses now includes lectures and demonstrations; improvements in nurses' off-duty rotas.
9. Collection of data on surgical theatre usage adopted as part of normal administrative practice; provision of more satisfactory work rotas for theatre technicians and porters.
10. Changes in filing system and procedures in X-ray department and procedural changes in medical records and in pathological laboratory to speed up the flow of information to out-patient clinics.
11. Introduction of a system of seven-day prediction of the bed state, covering most of the hospital (this resulted from an operational research study and an attitude survey on the problems created by emergency admissions; only the attitude survey was an H.I.C. project).
12. Introduction of messenger system covering all wards and clinical service departments.

## APPENDIX 7A

# *Notes on the second series of inter-team meetings (compiled at the time by the convener and the participant observer)*

### FIRST MEETING

After introductions, conversation settled down easily with an even spread and no silences. An administrator spoke at length about his team's project and came in for some searching questions, from two nurses on two other teams, which he tried to dodge. The group got angry with a doctor who believed that 'research objectivity' and the managerial role could not be combined. One of the nurses and another administrator both began to describe their projects, in which they were trying to combine the two roles.

The group felt easy to be in and the convener had little to do. Speakers followed up each other's comments and seemed ready to listen. It may have been too good for a first session. No one expressed any doubts about the group's purpose. Everyone felt they were having a rough time but were understanding each other's difficulties and were able to compare and identify with them.

Towards the end, the convener asked for feedback on how the session went and if the group should continue on the same lines. The members liked the small size of the group and felt this eased communication, but they wanted more structure to the discussion. The convener asked how and of what kind. The group decided that each member should give a report of his team's project, which would then be discussed. The second administrator offered to give a report next time.

### SECOND MEETING

The second administrator and his nurse colleagues gave an account of their project, which was now in the reporting stage. The group took up the question of discussing the report with respondents. The administrator felt that junior staff expected direction and were not accustomed to contributing to decisions or to sharing opinions with seniors: they wanted only practical and observable results. The group rose with hostility and accused him of being authoritarian. He then asked the convener for advice.

(*from the transcript*)

ADMINISTRATOR. We thought when we came here that this was the idea of the meeting, that you were going to tell us how to carry out feedback at this stage. This is really why we attended, to see whether what we had in mind was in line with the dogma of the central team.

CONVENER. I'm not sure we have any dogma ...

NURSE. You've got it all wrong. The idea is that we pool ideas, teach each other, therefore we gain a little from everyone else.

ADMINISTRATOR. Having taken us to a month's course to learn how to use these techniques, it would be reasonable to suppose that the next step would also be known to our teachers.

CONVENER. What does the group feel?

NURSE. I didn't expect you to. I don't think the central team knows any more than we do.

(Later the convener linked the administrator's comment on the expectations of junior staff to his own expectations of the central team, that both they and he wanted direction. A short silence. Then the group decided to abandon the plan for reporting projects and, at the suggestion of a nurse, to talk about how to change people's attitudes.)

(*from the transcript*)

DOCTOR. Presumably the people at Hastings (at the training course) thought the courses would change our attitudes. I expect some of us did and others didn't, but we went through an experience there together, and I don't think people's attitudes change unless they experience something together.

NURSE. Yes, but how do you gain this experience? I mean how do people get this experience whereby their attitudes do change?

The convener felt the group's simply and directly expressed need to know more about attitudes and behaviour could best be met by directing discussion back to the actual problems the teams were having in their own projects.

The participant observer noted:

'Quite clearly an "in-group" feeling occurred when the administrator said he thought the idea of the meeting was that the central team would tell the teams how to do feedback. The "in-group" against him was the more significant in that he represents a hospital that has worked very much on its own and is so far little known to the others. This has nothing to do with the validity of their research; he is paying for his team's isolation. The group reacted to his remarks and rejected him. This "in-group" feeling is important. It includes the feeling of being committed, which may carry the Project in the future when there is no central team.'

THIRD MEETING

The administrator who was admonished by the group last time and his nurse colleague were absent;[1] so was another administrator who telephoned earlier to say he did not feel the group was of any use to him,[2] and another nurse.[3]

It seemed obvious that the group was shedding its more vulnerable members, and making no attempt to retain them. The group now has twelve members, eight from hospital teams, three from the central team, plus the evaluator, who, together with the information officer had asked for, and received, permission from the group to attend from then on.

Discussion centred on the problem of changing attitudes, the group taking its cue from the nurse who had suggested this as a topic. Hostility to the convener now became more open, especially when she commented that the group was talking only about other people, as if these were the only ones whose attitudes needed to be changed. The group showed a two-way split: on one side the members with psychiatric training who presented a liberal viewpoint and believed themselves to be more in line with 'H.I.C. philosophy', on the other a sub-group who were accused of being authoritarian and of 'missing the whole point'. An attempt was made to heal the split by avoiding examination of the immediate situation and moving discussion out to the hospitals. Members drew closer as they commiserated on common problems, particularly on the inadequate help they were getting from the supporting members of their teams. The convenor took this as a reference to their feelings about the kind of support she was giving, but avoided direct comment on this point and decided to let the group continue in its own way. She asked how members felt the central team could help in the problem of the supporting members, but no one took this up.

NOTES

[1] They did not attend any further meetings for over a year.

[2] See first meeting, in which he was questioned by the group.

[3] She had said nothing in the previous two meetings and always sat slightly outside the circle.

APPENDIX 7B

## *Assessment of third series of inter-team meetings*[1]

| | Meeting | | | | |
|---|---|---|---|---|---|
| | *3rd* | *4th* | *5th* | *6th* | *7th* |
| A. QUALITY OF COMMUNICATION | | | | | |
| (i) How did the group communicate? | | | | | |
| 1 much misunderstanding throughout | 0 | 1 | 0 | 0 | 0 |
| 2 some misunderstanding: none cleared up | 0 | 0 | 1 | 0 | 0 |
| 3 some misunderstanding: some cleared up | 18 | 10 | 12 | 8 | 7 |
| 4 some misunderstanding: all cleared up | 6 | 4 | 3 | 3 | 7 |
| 5 full understanding throughout | 3 | 1 | 0 | 3 | 2 |
| (ii) How trusting and open was the group? | | | | | |
| 1 much distrust: close and inhibited | 0 | 0 | 0 | 0 | 0 |
| 2 little trust: much defensiveness | 6 | 0 | 1 | 0 | 0 |
| 3 fairly trusting and comfortable | 6 | 5 | 8 | 5 | 7 |
| 4 considerable trust and openness | 11 | 7 | 7 | 6 | 8 |
| 5 very trustful and open | 4 | 4 | 0 | 3 | 1 |
| (iii) How sensitive were group members towards each other? | | | | | |
| 1 insensitive: no listening: all self-absorbed | 0 | 0 | 0 | 0 | 0 |
| 2 most members self-absorbed and not listening | 0 | 1 | 1 | 0 | 1 |
| 3 group fairly sensitive | 8 | 5 | 5 | 5 | 7 |
| 4 group sensitive and able to listen | 17 | 10 | 10 | 8 | 8 |
| 5 remarkable sensitivity | 2 | 0 | 0 | 1 | 0 |
| (iv) How cohesive was the group? | | | | | |
| 1 disintegrated most of the time | 0 | 0 | 0 | 0 | 0 |
| 2 some disintegration: not dealt with | 3 | 1 | 3 | 3 | 1 |
| 3 some disintegration: some dealt with | 7 | 5 | 6 | 1 | 2 |
| 4 fairly cohesive: disintegration dealt with | 12 | 5 | 7 | 7 | 9 |
| 5 cohesion maintained throughout | 5 | 5 | 0 | 3 | 4 |
| B. USE OF GROUP RESOURCES | | | | | |
| (i) How interested was the group in the material presented and the content of discussion? | | | | | |
| 1 not interested: bored | | | | | |

| | *Meeting* 3rd | 4th | 5th | 6th | 7th |
|---|---|---|---|---|---|
| 2 some interest: frequent change of topic | 1 | 1 | 1 | 0 | 0 |
| 3 fairly interested most of the time | 11 | 9 | 10 | 6 | 11 |
| 4 interested all the time | 12 | 4 | 5 | 6 | 5 |
| 5 great interest throughout | 3 | 2 | 0 | 2 | 0 |
| (ii) How far did the group draw on and use its own knowledge and experience? | | | | | |
| 1 not at all | 0 | 1 | 0 | 0 | 0 |
| 2 some attempts: usually discouraged | 1 | 0 | 1 | 0 | 0 |
| 3 fair use generally: encouraged | 11 | 8 | 8 | 2 | 5 |
| 4 good use | 12 | 6 | 7 | 10 | 11 |
| 5 fully effective use | 3 | 1 | 0 | 3 | 0 |
| (iii) How dependent was the group on the convener (or 'expert', if any)? | | | | | |
| 1 very: needed advice and direction | 1 | 0 | 0 | 1 | 0 |
| 2 dependent most of the time | 0 | 1 | 0 | 1 | 0 |
| 3 somewhat dependent sometimes | 7 | 4 | 4 | 3 | 4 |
| 4 mostly independent | 14 | 9 | 10 | 6 | 11 |
| 5 independent throughout | 5 | 2 | 2 | 3 | 1 |

C. PERSONAL ASSESSMENT

| | 3rd | 4th | 5th | 6th | 7th |
|---|---|---|---|---|---|
| (i) How do you rate your own contribution? | | | | | |
| 1 did not contribute | 6 | 5 | 4 | 0 | 3 |
| 2 poor: was dissatisfied | 5 | 1 | 2 | 4 | 1 |
| 3 fairly satisfied | 15 | 10 | 8 | 9 | 10 |
| 4 good | 1 | 0 | 2 | 0 | 0 |
| 5 very good | 0 | 0 | 0 | 1 | 0 |
| (ii) Do you personally feel you learned something of practical value to your work? | | | | | |
| 1 nothing: not worth coming | 0 | 1 | 1 | 0 | 0 |
| 2 a little perhaps | 11 | 4 | 4 | 2 | 7 |
| 3 something: enough | 5 | 1 | 2 | 3 | 1 |
| 4 something: would like to learn more | 10 | 8 | 9 | 8 | 8 |
| 5 a great deal | 1 | 2 | 0 | 0 | 0 |
| (iii) Do you personally feel you learned something about yourself and the way you communicate? | | | | | |
| 1 nothing: not worth coming | 5 | 2 | 1 | 0 | 1 |
| 2 a little perhaps | 15 | 6 | 7 | 8 | 9 |
| 3 something: enough | 1 | 0 | 3 | 0 | 1 |
| 4 something: would like to learn more | 6 | 7 | 4 | 6 | 4 |
| 5 a great deal | 0 | 1 | 1 | 0 | 0 |

(iv) Do you personally feel you learned something about group processes and dynamics?

| | Meeting | | | | |
|---|---|---|---|---|---|
| | *3rd* | *4th* | *5th* | *6th* | *7th* |
| 1 nothing: not worth coming | 3 | 4 | 0 | 0 | 1 |
| 2 a little perhaps | 12 | 5 | 8 | 5 | 9 |
| 3 something: enough | 1 | 2 | 2 | 1 | 0 |
| 4 something: would like to learn more | 11 | 5 | 6 | 7 | 5 |
| 5 a great deal | 0 | 0 | 0 | 1 | 0 |
| Total number of respondents* | 27 | 16 | 16 | 14 | 16 |
| Total attendance at meeting** | 33 | 28 | 30 | 34 | 39 |

* Including central team and evaluation team.
** Evaluation team and some members of the central team did not take part.

NOTE

[1] Questions in A (Quality of Communication) were borrowed, much revised, from a similar form used by management training groups in Europe, supplied by Professor Revans. Those in **B** (Personal Assessment) were taken from an assessment form used in staff training groups at the Psychiatric Department, Ulleval Hospital, Oslo, where the writer also worked as nurse consultant.

# APPENDIX 7C

## *Notes by Professor Revans on formal presentations (circulated with invitations)*

What we badly need, and what the teams alone can supply, are some professional accounts of how these attempts at management therapy have actually worked out.... We must develop the approach of the pathologist and ask why it is that some conditions persist and others treated by the same methods seem to show improvement.

We can develop such evaluations only if we discuss our separate projects in a scientific manner. We need to meet in the same spirit that any group of research workers in any science would meet, listen to a professional presentation of an experiment and then discuss it as objectively as possible. In such presentations and discussions our first interest is not primarily the internal content of the experiments ... but in such facts as:

(a) how each hospital chose its particular project (to what extent and on what evidence it judged between this and other projects; who were involved in the decision and what arguments for and against it they brought),

(b) how the decision was made known (what initial efforts, if any, were made to engage the interest both of those whose work would be directly affected and of others more remote),

(c) how the project, and any survey on which it was based, was actually organized (who was asked to interview whom, to observe or analyse what; what meetings were held to keep those concerned in touch with what was being done; how far ideas that came from those who got involved contributed to progress and what obstructions were introduced by those who saw the project as a threat or a waste of time),

(d) when the problem at the heart of the project had been defined, what efforts were made to get action taken (how any report was presented to those concerned – management committee, senior staff and staff whose work would be affected – what the upshot of such presentations was and how they formed a learning process for those involved),

(e) what follow-up action was taken and what problems this raised (how far this action suggested further studies; how far it proved impossible to take any action at all).

This may read as a formidable list of detailed implications. What, at first sight, seems to be an obvious or even trivial exercise, turns out in practice to be more than a little complicated. But one of the most difficult tasks is to learn from experience, and it is a task which some persons rarely master. We need to spend some time and effort on its detailed analysis.

---

*Key to Categories in Table 7D-i*

| | | |
|---|---|---|
| A = supporting admin<br>B = supporting nurse<br>C = supporting doctor<br>D = operational admin<br>E = operational nurse<br>F = operational doctor<br>G = new members<br>H = other admins<br>I = other nurses<br>J = other doctors<br>K = management committee | ten participating hospitals | O = social scientists<br>P = management tutors<br>Q = management students<br>R = regional hospital board officers<br>S = Ministry of Health officers<br>T = H.I.C. advisory committee<br>U = professional organizations<br>V = Hospital Centre staff<br>W = H.I.C. central and evaluation teams (including ex-members)<br>X = others |
| L = admins<br>M = nurses<br>N = doctors | other hospitals | |

## APPENDIX 7D

# *Audience composition and participation in formal presentations*

TABLE 7D-i *Numbers and Composition of Audience at Formal Meetings*

| | *1st meeting The London* | *2nd meeting Severalls* | *3rd meeting Lewisham* | *4th meeting Q. Marys* | *5th meeting W. Midd.* | *6th meeting St Nicholas* | *7th meeting Mayday* | *8th meeting Edgware* |
|---|---|---|---|---|---|---|---|---|
| A* | 1 (10)** | – (10) | 1 (9) | – (9) | – (9) | 1 (10) | 1 (10) | – (9) |
| B | 2 (9) | 3 (9) | 3 (9) | 1 (9) | – (9) | 1 (9) | 2 (10) | – (7) |
| C | 1 (10) | 2 (10) | 1 (10) | – (9) | – (10) | 1 (10) | – (9) | – (9) |
| D | 2 (9) | 3 (10) | – (10) | 2 (10) | 3 (10) | 1 (9) | – (10) | 1 (9) |
| E | 2 (9) | 3 (8) | 1 (9) | 2 (9) | 3 (9) | – (9) | 2 (9) | 2 (9) |
| F | 1 (9) | 3 (7) | 1 (9) | 1 (8) | – (8) | – (7) | 2 (7) | 1 (7) |
| G | 1 (7) | 6 (14) | 4 (16) | 3 (17) | 6 (21) | 5 (21) | 4 (22) | 2 (23) |
| H | 1 (2) | – – | – – | 4 (4) | 3 (4) | 1 (3) | 1 (4) | 3 (7) |
| I | 4 (5) | 3 (4) | – (1) | – (1) | 11 (12) | – (1) | – (1) | – (1) |
| J | – (3) | – (1) | – (1) | – (2) | – (1) | – (2) | 1 (2) | 3 (5) |
| K | – (1) | – – | 1 (1) | 1 (1) | – (1) | – (1) | 1 (1) | 1 (1) |
| L | 2 (2) | 2 (2) | – (1) | – (1) | 1 (3) | – (3) | – (3) | – (3) |
| M | 3 (5) | 9 (13) | 1 (4) | 1 (6) | 1 (7) | 1 (7) | 1 (7) | 1 (8) |
| N | – – | 1 (4) | – (2) | – (2) | – (3) | – (2) | – (2) | – (2) |
| O | 10 (18) | 15 (20) | 8 (22) | 10 (21) | 6 (24) | 13 (28) | 11 (32) | 9 (33) |
| P | 1 (5) | 5 (7) | 2 (8) | 4 (10) | 3 (9) | – (9) | 3 (9) | 2 (8) |
| Q | – – | – – | – – | – – | 2 (3) | – (2) | 5 (5) | 1 (2) |
| R | 3 (10) | 5 (21) | 6 (26) | 4 (26) | 3 (28) | 6 (29) | 4 (30) | 7 (31) |
| S | 3 (3) | 2 (5) | – (1) | – (1) | – (2) | 2 (2) | 1 (2) | – (2) |
| T | 3 (6) | 2 (6) | 1 (7) | 3 (7) | 3 (7) | 2 (6) | – (7) | 2 (7) |
| U | – – | 1 (1) | – (1) | 1 (2) | 2 (3) | 1 (3) | 2 (4) | 6 (7) |
| V | 1 (2) | 1 (2) | 1 (2) | 2 (4) | 1 (4) | 1 (4) | 2 (5) | 1 (5) |
| W | 11 (17) | 13 (20) | 12 (21) | 4 (21) | 10 (23) | 12 (24) | 10 (25) | 12 (24) |
| X | – – | 2 (3) | 2 (3) | 1 (2) | – (2) | 1 (2) | – (2) | 1 (3) |
| Total | 52 (142) | 81 (177) | 45 (173) | 44 (182) | 59 (212) | 49 (203) | 53 (218) | 56 (222) |
| Per cent | 37% | 46% | 26% | 24% | 28% | 24% | 24% | 25% |

* For key to categories see facing page.
** Numbers in parenthesis indicate members invited.

TABLE 7D-ii *Numbers and Composition of Audience at Formal Meetings (with percentages of larger categories)*

| *Audience composition* | *Meeting* 1st | 2nd | 3rd | 4th | 5th | 6th | 7th | 8th |
|---|---|---|---|---|---|---|---|---|
| H.I.C. hospitals | | | | | | | | |
| original members | 9 | 14 | 7 | 6 | 7 | 4 | 7 | 4 |
| new members | 1 (29%) | 6 (28%) | 4 (26·5%) | 3 (32%) | 6 (47%) | 5 (20%) | 4 (26%) | 2 (23%) |
| other staff | 5 | 3 | 1 | 5 | 14 | 1 | 3 | 7 |
| Staff from other hospitals | 5 (9·5%) | 12 (15%) | 1 | 1 | 2 (3·5%) | 1 | 1 | 2 (3·5%) |
| Social scientists | 10 (19%) | 15 (18·5%) | 8 (18%) | 10 (23%) | 6 (10%) | 13 (27%) | 11 (21%) | 9 (16·5%) |
| Management tutors and students | 1 | 5 (6%) | 2 (4·5%) | 4 (9%) | 5 (8·5%) | — | 8 (15%) | 3 (5·5%) |
| RHB and MOH officers | 6 (11·5%) | 7 (9%) | 6 (13%) | 4 (9%) | 3 (5%) | 8 (16%) | 5 (9·5%) | 7 (12·5%) |
| H.I.C. advisory committee, central and evaluation teams | 14 (27%) | 15 (18·5%) | 13 (29%) | 7 (16%) | 13 (22%) | 14 (28·5%) | 10 (19%) | 14 (25%) |
| Professional organizations and all others | 1 | 4 (5%) | 3 (6·5%) | 4 (9%) | 3 (5%) | 3 (6%) | 4 (7·5%) | 8 (14%) |
| Total numbers | 52 | 81 | 45 | 44 | 59 | 49 | 53 | 56 |

TABLE 7D-iii *Numbers of Attendances at Formal Meetings by Members of Different Audience Categories*

| *Audience category* | Number of times attended: *Once* | *Twice* | *Three* | *Four* | *Five* | *Six* | *Seven* | *Eight* |
|---|---|---|---|---|---|---|---|---|
| A* | 4 | | | | | | | |
| B | 3 | 4 | 1 | | | | | |
| C | 3 | 1 | | | | | | |
| D | 2 | 2 | 2 | | | | | |
| E | 3 | 1 | 3 | 1 | | | | |
| F | 1 | 1 | 2 | | 1 | | | |
| G | 13 | 5 | 1 | | 1 | | | |
| H | 7 | 3 | | | | | | |
| I | 12 | 3 | | | | | | |
| J | 4 | | | | | | | |
| K | | | | 1 | | | | |
| L | 3 | 1 | | | | | | |
| M | 13 | 1 | | 1 | | | | |
| N | 1 | | | | | | | |
| O | 17 | 6 | 6 | 5 | 2 | 1 | 1 | |
| P | 6 | 3 | 1 | | 1 | | | |
| Q | 8 | | | | | | | |
| R | 21 | 2 | 3 | 1 | | | | |
| S | 2 | 1 | 1 | | | | | |
| T | 2 | 1 | | | | 2 | | |
| U | 6 | 2 | 1 | | | | | |
| V | 4 | | 2 | | | | | |
| W | 9 | 8 | 12 | 24 | 10 | | 3 | |
| X | 1 | | | | | | | |

* For categories, see *Table 7D-i.*

TABLE 7D-iv *Presenters at Formal Meetings*

| *Presenter* | Meeting: *1st* | *2nd* | *3rd* | *4th* | *5th* | *6th* | *7th* | *8th* |
|---|---|---|---|---|---|---|---|---|
| Supporting administrator | | | x | x | x | | | x |
| Supporting nurse | | | x | | | x | | x |
| Supporting doctor | | | | x | | | | x |
| Operational administrator | x | | | | | x | | x |
| Operational nurse | | x | | | | x | | x |
| Operational doctor | | | | | | | x | x |
| Others: doctor | | | | | x | | | |
| nurse | | | | | x | | | |
| administrator | | | x | | | | | |
| student | x | | | | | | | |
| central team | | | | | | | | x |

TABLE 7D-V *Discussion Contributions at Formal Meetings by Audience Category**

| *Audience category*** | *Meeting* *First The London* | *Second Severalls* | *Third Lewisham* | *Fourth*† *Q. Mary's* |
|---|---|---|---|---|
| A | 2 (1)‡ | – | (1) | – |
| B | 5 (2) | 4 (3) | 1 (3) | (1) |
| C | 3 (1) | (2) | 4 (1) | – |
| D | (2) | (3) | – | 2 (2) |
| E | 8 (2) | (3) | (1) | 2 (2) |
| F | 5 (1) | 1 (3) | (1) | (1) |
| G | 4 (1) | (6) | 4 (4) | 4 (3) |
| H | (1) | – | – | (4) |
| I | (4) | (3) | – | – |
| J | – | – | – | – |
| K | – | – | (1) | (1) |
| L | (2) | (2) | – | – |
| M | (3) | 12 (9) | (1) | 1 (1) |
| N | – | 1 (1) | – | – |
| O | 9 (10) | 19 (15) | 4 (8) | 10 (10) |
| P | (1) | 1 (5) | 1 (2) | 5 (4) |
| Q | – | – | – | – |
| R | (3) | (5) | 4 (6) | (4) |
| S | 6 (3) | (2) | – | – |
| T | 6 (3) | (2) | (1) | (3) |
| U | – | (1) | – | (1) |
| V | (1) | (1) | (1) | (2) |
| W | 8 (11) | 14 (13) | 4 (12) | (4) |
| X | – | (2) | (2) | (1) |
| Total | 56 | 52 | 22 | 24 |

N.B. Figures indicate the number of comments or questions, not the number of times an individual spoke.

* Excluding presenters and chairmen.
** For categories, see *Table 7D-i*.
† Discussions taped at the last four meetings were not clear enough to be transcribed.
‡ Numbers in parenthesis indicate number of people in this category at meeting.

TABLE 7D-vi *Initiators of Discussion Topics*
(from first four meetings)

| *Topics* | *Initiator* | | | | |
|---|---|---|---|---|---|
| | *Hospital* staff* | *Research† workers* | *Central team and advisory committee* | *All others* | *Total* |
| A: Relating to material presented | | | | | |
| Preparing staff for project | 1 | 1 | | | 2 |
| Data-collecting methods | 1 | | | | 1 |
| Feedback methods | 3 | 1 | 2 | | 6 |
| General design and timing | 2 | | 1 | | 3 |
| Management committee involvement | | | | 1 | 1 |
| Effect of results on staff | 2 | 3 | 1 | | 6 |
| Future plans and follow-up | 4 | 2 | 2 | 1 | 9 |
| Students' role | | 1 | 2 | | 3 |
| Audience's interpretation of data | | 3 | | | 3 |
| Audience's solution to problem being studied | 2 | 3 | | | 5 |
| B: General | | | | | |
| Research questions | | 4 | 1 | | 5 |
| Hospital organization | 3 | 3 | 1 | 2 | 9 |
| Staff training | 1 | | 1 | | 2 |
| TOTAL | 19 | 21 | 11 | 4 | 55 |

* Including the ten participating hospitals.
† May also include chairman as initiator.

APPENDIX 8A

## *Questionnaire used at Severalls Hospital for Nurses' Survey*

| | |
|---|---|
| Serial No. | ☐ |
| Card No. | ☐ |
| Grade | ☐ |
| Full or Part-time | ☐ |
| Sex | ☐ |

CONFIDENTIAL *Do not put your name on this sheet*

Grade Full-time/Part-time Sex ☐

Unit or department ☐

Day or night duty ☐

Nursing qualifications ☐

Country of origin ☐

How long have you been nursing? ☐

How long at this hospital? ☐

Resident or non-resident ☐

In this document there are a number of statements. None are necessarily true, none are necessarily false. They contain no hidden meaning: there are no catches in them. ☐

You will agree or disagree with them to some extent. Will you please show under each item what your opinion is by putting a ring round the appropriate letters. ☐

SA means Strongly Agree
A means Agree or tend to Agree

U means Uncertain or Undecided
D means Disagree or tend to Disagree
SD means Strongly Disagree

The statements which do not have these letters underneath them contain the instructions for their completion.

1 The number of staff on my ward is adequate. 1 ☐
SA A U D SD

2 Old people have earned their rest and should be allowed to doze all day if they like. 2 ☐
SA A U D SD

3 Even when the consultant is in my ward/department he does not give me the opportunity to ask him anything. 3 ☐
SA A U D SD

4 Industrial therapy should be done in the wards as well as the industrial department. 4 ☐
SA A U D SD

5 Patients' case conferences are a waste of my time. 5 ☐
SA A U D SD

6 They tend to be a bit mean with patients' food here. 6 ☐
SA A U D SD

7 The various staff meetings held in this hospital benefit patients. 7 ☐
SA A U D SD

8 If there was no unit system nurses could be distributed more fairly. 8 ☐
SA A U D SD

9 Accompanying patients to the town shopping is nursing time well spent. 9 ☐
SA A U D SD

10 Domiciliary visiting is part of a ward nurse's work. 10 ☐
SA A U D SD

11 The social worker should confine her efforts to patients who have been discharged. 11 ☐
SA A U D SD

12 Senior nurses do not like junior nurses asking them questions. 12 ☐
SA A U D SD

13 The unit system has improved communications between the nurses and the matron/chief male nurse. 13 ☐

SA A U D SD

14 Patients benefit from having nurses of the opposite sex on the ward. 14 ☐

SA A U D SD

15 Because of the unit system doctors are more remote. 15 ☐

SA A U D SD

16 The quality of the patients' food here is good. 16 ☐

SA A U D SD

17 I prefer to nurse psychiatric patients who are also physically sick. 17 ☐

SA A U D SD

18 When the consultant is in my ward/department he gives me the chance to ask him questions. 18 ☐

SA A U D SD

19 There is no need for locked wards. 19 ☐

SA A U D SD

20 Doctors are not interested in what we have to tell them about patients. 20 ☐

SA A U D SD

21 I do not like the food we are expected to eat here. 21 ☐

SA A U D SD

22 Social work would be better done by registered mental nurses. 22 ☐

SA A U D SD

23 Male and female nurses should not work in the same ward team. 23 ☐

SA A U D SD

24 I am expected to talk to the patients about their problems. 24 ☐

SA A U D SD

25 Night staff cannot learn how to continue patients' rehabilitation into the evening unless they have regular experience of day duty. 25 ☐

SA A U D SD

26 Ward sisters / charge nurses should work from 8 a.m. to 5 p.m. | 26 ☐

SA A U D SD

27 The doctor does not spend enough time on my ward / department. | 27 ☐

SA A U D SD

28 Staff meetings contribute little to patient care. | 28 ☐

SA A U D SD

29 There should be as much activity in the ward at the weekend as during the rest of the week. | 29 ☐

SA A U D SD

30 Domiciliary visiting is not a ward nurse's job. | 30 ☐

SA A U D SD

31 When patients are occupied in departments outside the ward I think it is necessary to visit them. | 31 ☐

SA A U D SD

32 Senior nurses ignore my suggestions. | 32 ☐

SA A U D SD

33 It is difficult to get promotion in this hospital without an SRN qualification. | 33 ☐

SA A U D SD

34 Taking part in meetings does not help patients. | 34 ☐

SA A U D SD

35 I think I should attend patients' case conferences. | 35 ☐

SA A U D SD

36 The unit system makes the most of the limited number of nurses. | 36 ☐

SA A U D SD

37 People at the top keep us informed of what is going on in this hospital. | 37 ☐

SA A U D SD

38 It is a waste of nurses' time to accompany patients shopping in the town. | 38 ☐

SA A U D SD

39 It is good for patients to take part in meetings. | 39 ☐

SA A U D SD

40 Most geriatric wards need to be locked during the day. 40 ☐

SA A U D SD

41 Male and female nurses should work together on the ward as a team. 41 ☐

SA A U D SD

42 On my ward/department the nurse in charge does not explain what I have to do. 42 ☐

SA A U D SD

43 People look down on you if they know you are a psychiatric nurse. 43 ☐

SA A U D SD

44 It is not sufficient to have only one male and one female locked ward in this hospital. 44 ☐

SA A U D SD

45 Nursing patients of the opposite sex is not appropriate in a psychiatric hospital. 45 ☐

SA A U D SD

46 I do not learn much from the doctor when he/she visits my ward/department. 46 ☐

SA A U D SD

47 Doctors are grateful for any information about patients given them by the nursing staff. 47 ☐

SA A U D SD

48 I think the unit system should be abolished. 48 ☐

SA A U D SD

49 I am not encouraged to talk to the patients about their problems. 49 ☐

SA A U D SD

50 Please give a list of all meetings that take place in your *present* ward/department. If none held please enter 'NIL'. 50 ☐☐☐☐☐☐☐

______________________________

______________________________

______________________________

51 Who is in charge of the nursing staff in your unit? 51 ☐

______________________________

52 What is the work of the assistant matron/assistant chief male nurse in your unit? 52 ☐

______________________________________________

______________________________________________

53 What do you think his/her work should be? 53 ☐

______________________________________________

______________________________________________

54 What jobs does your assistant matron/assistant chief male nurse do that could be done by someone else? 54 ☐

______________________________________________

______________________________________________

55 With which unit would you prefer to work? 55 ☐

______________________________________________

56 Please list which meetings in your present ward/unit/department you attend when on duty. If none please state 'NIL'. 56 ☐☐☐☐☐☐

______________________________________________

______________________________________________

57 Please list which meetings in your present ward/unit/department you attend only sometimes when on duty. If none please state 'NIL'. 57 ☐☐☐☐☐

______________________________________________

______________________________________________

58 Do you think nurses should wear a badge on their uniform giving their name and grade? 58 ☐

Yes ☐ No ☐

Serial No. ☐

Card ☐

59 Do you think nurses should wear uniform? 59 ☐

Yes ☐ No ☐

60 Are the side-effects of their tablets made known to the patients before they leave hospital? 60 ☐

Yes ☐ No ☐

61 Do you think the patients should have a say in the running of the ward? 61 ☐

Yes ☐ No ☐

62 Please list meetings held in your present ward/unit/department which you *never* attend. 62 ☐☐

________________________________________

________________________________________

________________________________________

63 In which unit do you think patients receive the best psychiatric care? 63

________________________________________

*Please note*—the following statements require answers by *ticking* where appropriate.

64 Domestic work should be done by: (Please tick more than one if appropriate) 64

- Ward maids ☐
- Nurses ☐
- Patients ☐
- Nurses and patients together ☐
- Ward maids and patients together ☐

65 Which of the following groups of patients would benefit from living in wards with patients of the opposite sex? (Please tick more than one if appropriate) 65

- (a) Long stay ☐
- (b) Short stay ☐
- (c) Geriatric ☐
- (d) None ☐

66 Do you think meetings with your unit benefit: (Please tick more than one if appropriate) 66

- General Practitioners ☐
- Doctors ☐
- Nurses ☐
- Patients ☐
- Social workers ☐
- Administrative staff ☐

Management committee ☐

No one ☐

67 Domestic work in my ward/department is done by: (Please tick more than one if appropriate) — 67 ☐☐☐☐☐

Ward maids ☐

Porters ☐

Patients ☐

Nurses and patients together ☐

Ward maids and patients together ☐

68 Do you think the unit system helps: — 68 ☐☐☐☐☐☐☐☐

(Please tick more than one if appropriate)

General practitioners ☐

Doctors ☐

Nurses ☐

Patients ☐

Social workers ☐

Administrative staff ☐

Management committee ☐

No one ☐

69 If we are to change wards at regular intervals I think it should be every: (Please place a tick in the appropriate space) — 69 ☐

6 months ☐

1 year ☐

18 months ☐

2 years ☐

3 years ☐

5 years ☐

8 years ☐

12 years ☐

*Please Note* The following statements require answers by *numbering*. 70

70 As far as psychiatric nursing is concerned, I feel I can do most good on the following wards. Please number in order of importance, i.e. 1, 2, 3, 4, 5.

- Admission wards ☐
- Geriatric wards ☐
- Long-stay wards ☐
- Physically sick wards ☐
- Locked wards ☐

71 The most rewarding nursing duties are on the following wards. Please number in order of importance, i.e. 1, 2, 3, 4, 5. 71

- Admission wards ☐
- Geriatric wards ☐
- Long-stay wards ☐
- Physically sick wards ☐
- Locked wards ☐

72 Put the following in order of importance by marking your choice, i.e. 1, 2, 3, 4, 5 and so on. 72

(a) The ward looking neat and tidy. ☐

(b) The patients being well cared for. ☐

(c) The clerical work being up to date. ☐

(d) Helping the patients individually. ☐

(e) Chasing up the administration over the repairs and replacements that want doing. ☐

(f) Keeping the doctors happy. ☐

(g) Keeping members of the ward team happy. ☐

(h) Seeing that the patients always have something to do. ☐

(i) Attending meetings. ☐

(j) Advising and instructing members of the team. ☐

To be answered ONLY by SISTERS AND CHARGE NURSES

75 I think a lay person could take responsibility for the paper work in my ward. 75 ☐

SA A U D SD

To be answered ONLY by DEPUTY SISTERS AND ALL GRADES BELOW

76 Sister/charge nurse is too busy to talk to us. 76 ☐

SA A U D SD

77 Sister/charge nurse on my ward/department tells us something about the patients. (Please place a tick against the one which applies) 77 ☐

Every day ☐

Twice a week ☐

Once a week ☐

Once a month ☐

Not at all ☐

To be answered ONLY BY STAFF NURSES, STATE ENROLLED NURSES, AND GRADES ABOVE

73 Trained staff require postgraduate courses. 73 ☐

SA A U D SD

74 I like working on the same ward/department. 74 ☐

SA A U D SD

APPENDIX 9A

# *Operating theatre studies carried out at West Middlesex Hospital, March – December 1966*

*K. D. EASON*

## INTRODUCTION AND BACKGROUND

The West Middlesex Hospital suffers from an acute pressure on beds and the large proportion of emergency admissions results in the frequent cancellation of waiting-list cases at short notice. In March 1966, shortly after the hospital had become involved in the H.I.C. Project, a meeting was held to consider this problem. At the meeting Professor Revans, members of the central H.I.C. team, members of the hospital's H.I.C. team, and some of the hospital's surgeons were present. It was proposed that a study be made of the surgical beds in the hospital to determine whether it is really underbedded or whether the existing services could be used more effectively. Professor Revans suggested that the most rewarding way of conducting such a study was on a comparative basis; to select two other hospitals comparable to the West Middlesex, one with a longer, and one with a shorter, length of patients' stay in various diagnostic categories and to conduct studies to ascertain why the variations existed.

However, it was felt that the time was inopportune for such a study in view of the effect that recent staff shortages were having on the operating theatres. In October 1965, and again in January 1966, these shortages made it necessary to curtail many of the scheduled lists and as a consequence the hospital was then suffering from a bottleneck in which it could not make the full use of its theatre facilities or, as a consequence, its surgical beds. In the circumstances the medical committee resolved that the proposed study be deferred until the theatre staffing situation improved and the theatres returned to full working.

It should be pointed out that the operating theatre facilities of the hospital had, for many years, been considered inadequate, and that future major development schemes make provision for the building of a new set of theatres in 1973/74. In the meantime all staff are asked to work in conditions far from ideal, a factor that was felt to be one of the roots of the present difficulties.

Following the medical committee's resolution, the hospital's H.I.C. team determined, with the help and co-operation of the theatre staff, to study the factors relevant to the staff shortage in an endeavour to assist the hospital to resolve these problems and return the theatres to full working. The investigations reported are the results of these efforts and constitute a series of studies with explicitly stated short-term objectives, commissioned and co-ordinated by the hospital secretary with the full support of the medical and nursing staff. This report is a consideration of the investigations carried out and the changes in the theatre situation that have either been implemented or are being considered.

In carrying out this project many hospital staff have been involved and I would like to thank them for their willing co-operation and invaluable advice.

## THEATRE USAGE DATA COLLECTION

Although it was generally known that the theatres had problems, about the exact nature and extent of the difficulties there was very little collective information available that those in authority could use to correct the situation. As a first step in the investigations, a central-team member collected from the operation registers of the theatres details of how the theatres were used throughout the month of March 1966.

The charts compiled from this information indicated clearly that the medical committee resolution issued at the time of the curtailment of lists, which asked that all afternoon theatre lists be completed by 5 p.m., was not being observed. Frequently, mostly in the general surgery theatres, the lists went on until 9 or 10 p.m., to be followed often by emergency work. This was having a detrimental effect on the morale of the theatre staff, who were often expected to stay on duty long after their off-duty times in order to complete these late lists.

It was clear that the collection of relevant data would yield useful information on theatre usage, which could be used to reconsider the staffing organization in an effort to deploy existing staff in a way that would avoid the working of long and irregular hours. Consequently, each of the theatre sisters was asked to complete weekly returns detailing how long her theatre had worked each day, which firm was working, and how many list and emergency operations were completed. These data have been collected for the months of July, August, September, and October, and have proved of considerable use in showing the relationship between theatre activity and staff deployment.

ANALYSIS OF USAGE DATA

The usage data were originally intended as an aid to optimum staff organization, and this has indeed proved their main function. However the data also provided much information about how the theatres work, and it was felt that this might be of interest and value if it was presented to demonstrate the work-load of the theatres and how it was handled. The data were presented to give a month-by-month picture of the different facets of the situation.

*A. Excess list hours*

The immediate result of the data collected for March 1966 was the recognition that the theatres worked a large number of list hours after the scheduled closing time of 5 p.m. It had been hoped that the reconstitution of lists would funnel this work back into normal list time, thus reducing the excess hours. *Table 9A-i* indicates what actually happened.

TABLE 9A-i *Excess Theatre List Hours per Month* (i.e. after 5 p.m.)

| *Months* | SURGICAL THEATRES | | | | | | |
|---|---|---|---|---|---|---|---|
| | *General* | | | *Ortho-paedic* | *ENT* | *Gynae-cology* | |
| | *G1* | *G2* | *Total* | *O* | *E* | *G* | *Total* |
| | *Hours* | *Hours* | *Hours* | *Hours* | *Hours* | *Hours* | *Hours* |
| March | 26·15 | 20·35 | 46·50 | — | 3·10 | 9·00 | 59·00 |
| July | 14·35 | 24·15 | 38·50 | — | 1·45 | 10·45 | 51·10 |
| August | 15·00 | 37·45 | 52·45 | — | 2·05 | 8·20 | 63·20 |
| September | 20·30 | 9·10 | 29·40 | — | 1·25 | 8·05 | 39·10 |
| October | 24·10 | 6·05 | 30·15 | — | 11·05 | 4·35 | 45·55 |
| Totals | 100·30 | 97·50 | 198·20 | — | 19·30 | 40·45 | 258·35 |
| Average | 20·06 | 19·34 | 39·40 | — | 3·54 | 8·09 | 51·43 |

Although the table does not show a smooth reduction in excess hours, it does indicate an overall drop of some twenty hours per month. Most of this drop was due to the two general surgery theatres that originally carried most of the excess hours gaining list hours in the reconstitution of sessions in September. A noticeable trend in October was the increase to significant proportions of excess hours in E theatre.

There was another change not revealed in the table. Comparing March and October, a breakdown of the lengths of over-running sessions showed the following:

| | *March* | *October* |
|---|---|---|
| No. of lists with excess hours | | |
| less than 1½ hours | 5 | 17 |
| between 1½ and 3 hours | 13 | 9 |
| greater than 3 hours | 8 | 1 |
| | 26 | 27 |

Thus although the total number of over-running sessions did not change those of October were of much shorter duration than those of March.

*B. List operations*

In reconstituting the lists (see part 5), the surgical firms were given more time in which to perform operations and one might expect a consequent increase in the numbers of operations performed. However, there was also the possibility that numbers of operations would remain the same because fewer excess hours were worked.

TABLE 9A-ii *Theatre List Hours per Month* (i.e. after 5 p.m.)

| *Months* | SURGICAL THEATRES | | | | | | |
|---|---|---|---|---|---|---|---|
| | *General* | | | *Ortho-paedic* | *ENT* | *Gynae-cology* | |
| | *G1* | *G2* | *Total* | *O* | *E* | *G* | *Total* |
| | *Hours* | *Hours* | *Hours* | *Hours* | *Hours* | *Hours* | *Hours* |
| March | 85·35 | 101·20 | 186·55 | 59·50 | 105·05 | 137·50 | 489·40 |
| July | 73·50 | 110·35 | 184·25 | 57·55 | 110·00 | 142·15 | 494·35 |
| August | 77·15 | 130·50 | 208·05 | 86·05 | 112·20 | 134·50 | 541·20 |
| September | 96·20 | 79·10 | 175·30 | 78·05 | 108·15 | 130·00 | 491·50 |
| October | 138·00 | 54·35 | 192·35 | 68·05 | 109·50 | 113·10 | 483·40 |
| Totals | 471·00 | 476·30 | 947·30 | 350·00 | 545·30 | 658·05 | 2501·05 |
| Average | 94·16 | 95·16 | 189·30 | 70·00 | 109·06 | 131·31 | 500·13 |

TABLE 9A-iii *Numbers of List Operations per Month*

| *Months* | SURGICAL THEATRES | | | | | | |
|---|---|---|---|---|---|---|---|
| | *General* | | | *Ortho-paedic* | *ENT* | *Gynae-cology* | |
| | *G1* | *G2* | *Total* | *O* | *E* | *G* | *Total* |
| | *No.* | *No.* | *No.* | *No.* | *No.* | *No.* | *No.* |
| March | 50 | 150 | 200 | 79 | 128 | 193 | 600 |
| July | 74 | 144 | 218 | 84 | 154 | 210 | 666 |
| August | 73 | 166 | 239 | 121 | 174 | 214 | 748 |
| September | 99 | 112 | 211 | 99 | 180 | 207 | 687 |
| October | 147 | 62 | 209 | 95 | 167 | 202 | 673 |
| Total | 443 | 634 | 1077 | 468 | 803 | 1026 | 3374 |
| Average | 89 | 127 | 216 | 94 | 161 | 205 | 675 |

*Tables 9A-ii* and *9A-iii* suggest that the latter was the case, there being no increase in the amount of work done by the theatres.
Features of interest include:

(i) The extra fifty operations conducted in August over and above the average at the expense of only an additional ten hours excess time.
(ii) Although the number of operations in E theatre each month varied considerably ($\pm$ 16 per cent) the hours used for operating remained unusually stable ($\pm$3 per cent).

*C. Emergency operations*

One of the difficulties about deploying staff within the theatres is the volume of unpredictable emergency operations that have to be performed. The following evaluation of frequency and distribution of emergency operations was carried out to show the extent of this problem.

TABLE 9A-iv *Hours Devoted to Emergency Theatre Work per Month*

| *Months* | SURGICAL THEATRES | | | | | | |
|---|---|---|---|---|---|---|---|
| | *General* | | | *Ortho-paedic* | *ENT* | | *Gynae-cology** |
| | *G1* | *G2* | *Total* | *O* | *E* | *Total* | *G* |
| | *Hours* | *Hours* | *Hours* | *Hours* | *Hours* | *Hours* | *Hours* |
| March | 37·45 | 34·35 | 72·20 | 8·00 | 3·45 | 84·05 | N/A** |
| July | 20·30 | 48·05 | 68·35 | 26·10 | 4·05 | 98·50 | 0·15 |
| August | 35·45 | 34·30 | 70·15 | 26·20 | 6·35 | 103·10 | 6·45 |
| September | 33·50 | 50·25 | 84·15 | 12·25 | 2·10 | 98·50 | 3·00 |
| October | 38·55 | 24·20 | 63·15 | 33·30 | 5·10 | 101·55 | 4·25 |
| Total | 166·45 | 191·55 | 358·40 | 106·25 | 21·45 | 486·50 | 14·25 |
| Average | 33·21 | 38·23 | 71·44 | 21·17 | 4·21 | 97·22 | 2·48 |

* Gynaecology hours not included in totals because of problems of defining an emergency.
** Not available.

TABLE 9A-v *Numbers of Emergency Operations per Month*

| *Months* | SURGICAL THEATRES | | | | | | |
|---|---|---|---|---|---|---|---|
| | *General* | | | *Ortho-paedic* | *ENT* | | *Gynae-cology** |
| | *G1* | *G2* | *Total* | *O* | *E* | *Total* | *G* |
| | *No.* | *No.* | *No.* | *No.* | *No.* | *No.* | *No.* |
| March | 29 | 42 | 71 | 10 | 3 | 84 | N/A** |
| July | 23 | 46 | 69 | 29 | 6 | 104 | 1 |
| August | 36 | 39 | 75 | 24 | 8 | 107 | 19 |
| September | 32 | 56 | 88 | 14 | 3 | 105 | 9 |
| October | 36 | 20 | 56 | 28 | 7 | 91 | 11 |
| Total | 156 | 203 | 359 | 105 | 27 | 491 | 40 |
| Average | 31 | 41 | 72 | 21 | 5 | 98 | 8 |

* Gynaecology operations not included in totals because of problems of defining an emergency.
** Not available.

The data tabulated in *Tables 9A-iv* and *9A-v* indicated the following:

(i) In the five months covered no seasonal fluctuations in emergency work were found, all monthly totals being within 11 per cent of the average.

(ii) The hospital averaged 98 emergency operations per month, which represented 12 per cent of the work-load. In terms of time the emergency operations represented 16 per cent of the total work-load.

(iii) The bulk of the emergency work was carried out by the general surgery theatres and the orthopaedic theatres. In order to appraise the weekly fluctuations of this load on these theatres, an examination of 22 weeks' working was made which indicated:

(a) In general surgery the average number of emergency operations per week was 17 (16·40 hours) with a maximum of 28 (33·05 hours) and a minimum of 9 (10·10 hours). The standard deviation was 6·35 hours, which implies that, in 68 per cent of weeks, emergency work will require $16{\cdot}40 \pm 6{\cdot}35$ hours or between 10·05 and 23·15 hours.

(b) In orthopaedics, the average number of emergency operations per week was 5 (5·25 hours) with a maximum of 16 (17·20 hours) and a minimum of nil. The standard deviation was 4·30 hours, i.e. 68 per cent of weeks will require between 0·30 and 9·30 hours for emergency work.

(iv) The data shown in *Tables 9A-iv* and *9A-v* were deficient in that the emergency work in the gynaecology theatre was not clearly defined and was not differentiated at all in March. Subsequently some part of what may be called emergency work was collected, but confusion still existed and much of what was termed list work here was, in fact, emergency.

(v) The distribution of emergency work through the week indicated quite clearly that as far as theatres were concerned *true* emergencies that had to be rushed straight into theatre were comparatively rare. The bulk of emergency work was conducted in the evening, when the lists had been completed, and at the weekend, with very little work done between 2 a.m. and 9 a.m., and only a few cases actually interrupting the flow of list cases during the day. This analysis suggested that emergency operations are not as unpredictable and disrupting as previously thought, and that deployment of staff can be made to take account of the likely volume of emergency work.

### *D. Average length of operations*

A factor of considerable relevance to staffing was the average length of operation in each theatre. The data tabulated in *Table 9A-vi* were a gross figure obtained by dividing the total number of operations by the total number of hours, and hence included not only the time between the incision and closure but all manner of waiting times that occur during theatre lists. It remains of interest to compare theatres and to note trends in individual theatres where, presumably, the nature of the operations performed remained approximately the same.

TABLE 9A-vi *Average Length of Operations in Minutes*

| *Months* | SURGICAL THEATRES | | | | | | |
|---|---|---|---|---|---|---|---|
| | *General* | | | *Ortho-paedic* | *ENT* | *Gynae-cology* | |
| | *G1* | *G2* | *Average* | *O* | *E* | *G* | *Overall* |
| | *Mins* | *Mins* | *Mins* | *Mins* | *Mins* | *Mins* | *Mins* |
| March | 95 | 43 | 79·0 | 46 | 50 | 44 | 55·6 |
| July | 58 | 50 | 54·0 | 45 | 42 | 40 | 48·0 |
| August | 57 | 48 | 52·5 | 46 | 38 | 36 | 45·0 |
| September | 60 | 46 | 53·0 | 48 | 36 | 38 | 45·6 |
| October | 58 | 57 | 57·5 | 50 | 38 | 34 | 48·4 |
| Total | 328 | 244 | — | 235 | 202 | 192 | 242·6 |
| Average | 65·6 | 48·8 | 57·2 | 47·0 | 40·4 | 38·8 | 48 6 |

It is worthy of note that:

(i) The overall average length of operations in all theatres decreased by some 7 minutes over this 8-month period.

(ii) Most of this decrease was brought about by decreases in G (10 minutes) and E (12 minutes).

(iii) The two general surgery theatres exhibited marked differences in speed of working, with G2 considerably faster than G1. This discrepancy narrowed in later months as the bulk of list work passed from G2 to G1.

(iv) Comparing the various theatres, general surgery exhibited the longest average length, followed by orthopaedics, ENT, and gynaecology.

While these data were very interesting, it was difficult to pinpoint the reasons for the trends with gross information of this kind. It seemed to indicate, however, that there were factors in the theatre situation that were variable and affected the efficiency and effectiveness with which work was carried out. Further detailed investigation is recommended to isolate these contributing factors.

## STAFFING STUDIES AND REORGANIZATIONS

In considering the current staffing organization and any modifications to be made, the following criteria were selected as being necessary for resolving short-term staffing problems.

(i) The limited number of staff available should be deployed to cover the work of the theatres (as indicated by the usage data) in the most effective way possible.

(ii) An attempt should be made to develop stable teams within each theatre. Theatre work depends very much on the close co-operation and understanding of the various team members, and preliminary study indicated that under the present organization staff were moved from theatre to theatre with a rapidity that did not facilitate the building of a 'team spirit' in individual theatres.

(iii) Provision should be made for regular and fair hours for all staff. The work rosters developed should enable staff to plan their off-duty hours well ahead and they should be able to rely on being able to go off duty at the time indicated.

Detailed examinations were undertaken of the organizational structures of three kinds of theatre staff – nurses, technicians, and porters. The findings and resultant changes are described below:

### THEATRE NURSING STAFF

Armed with the hours that the theatres worked (as shown by the usage study data) the matron and the theatre superintendent reviewed the organization of the theatre nursing staff, and concluded that none of the above criteria were being adequately implemented. They therefore developed a scheme for the gradual building-up of theatre nursing teams in each theatre.

In this scheme each of the theatres was to have two teams of nurses, each consisting of a sister, a staff nurse trained in theatre work, a graduate nurse training in theatre work, and a student nurse. One of the sisters was to be senior to the other and would have general responsibility for the theatre. The work of the theatre was to be covered by the two teams working shifts depending upon the scheduled list work. Basically, the first team would work from approximately 8 a.m. to 4 p.m. and the second from 1 p.m. to 9 p.m., the teams rotating at regular intervals to ensure that each team would do its share of early and late shifts. The considerable overlap in hours was included both to allow the nursing staff to take lunch while the theatre continued to work, and to enable lectures to be given to the nurses on the post-graduate training course. Each of the four members of the team was to work the same hours through the week and each of the teams would take it in turn to cover for emergency work at nights and weekends.

This system was first put into practice at the beginning of September 1966, when the theatres were so understaffed that only a few full teams, with several part-teams, could be formed. Since that time the recruitment of trained theatre staff has been a top priority and there has been an addition of two full-time and two part-time sisters, and the number of staff nurses has increased from two full-time and two part-time to seven full-time and four part-time. Most of the theatres now (December 1966) have two teams, but in a number of cases the second team is led by a senior staff nurse and has less than its complement of trained theatre nurses. Where this is so the senior team led by the theatre sister carries most of the theatre list work.

The postgraduate nurses' training course was reinstituted in September, 1966, and it was proposed that each course would last six months. It was hoped that this course would provide the hospital with a much needed supply of trained theatre staff, and it appeared to be one of the chief reasons, coupled with the hospital's ability to offer specified hours to nursing staff, for the improving staffing situation. Allied to these improvements in staffing, there were changes in the physical conditions in the theatres. The two general surgery theatres had their ancillary rooms reorganized to provide the nurses with a rest and shower room in each theatre. These facilities had already been made available before this investigation in the orthopaedic theatres, and there are plans in the rebuilding of the ENT theatre for similar facilities.

### THEATRE TECHNICIANS

A preliminary survey, conducted in August, of the technicians' rota and how it matched theatre hours revealed that none of our three staffing criteria was being realized. This was highlighted in September when a deputation from the technicians complained to the matron about their working conditions. In an effort to collect the full facts before attempting any reorganization, each of the technicians was given the opportunity, in a confidential interview, to air his grievances fully. The main areas of discontent revealed in these interviews are summarized below.

#### (*i*) *The work rota*

There were many complaints about this, including comments on the frequency with which it was changed without warning, and dissatisfaction with the way it caused the technician to be moved from theatre to theatre. The idea that they might stay in one theatre on a permanent basis was welcomed, except that some felt a three-month, six-month, or one-year period was long enough in one theatre.

#### (*ii*) *Authority*

The technicians are administratively controlled by the matron and organized by the theatre superintendent. When in the theatre they are controlled by the theatre sister, but most of their work during operations is done with and for the anaesthetist. The technicians reported that this situation led frequently to conflicting orders being given by the various 'bosses'.

(*iii*) *Status*

While the technicians were most enthusiastic and keen about their work in theatres, they complained that they were never allowed to be of maximum usefulness. The work they did for the anaesthetist required responsibility and know-how, but the other theatre staff treated them as 'everybody's dogsbody', as a sort of in-theatre porter. They were resentful of the fact that they had to wear the same short white coats as the porters when they were not in the theatre, that they had to change in the surgeon's rooms, where they felt like intruders, and that they had to walk the corridors when not in the theatres because they had no room of their own. (A scheme for the building of a technicians' room adjacent to the orthopaedic theatres was placed on the minor capital expenditure programme for 1967). Many of them reported that throughout the country the nursing profession was oppressing the theatre technicians because they were fearful of losing their position in the theatres. Theatre work was not nursing, and hence, for fear that non-nursing staff might become the theatre managers of the future, the nursing profession was keeping the technician in the theatre at the status level of a porter.

(*iv*) *Training course*

The technicians stated that on many occasions they had been promised by the hospital a training course that would enable them to pass the examinations of the Institute of Theatre Technicians and thus become qualified. This had never materialized, owing mostly, it was felt, to the apathy of the nursing profession. They were forced, if they wanted to better themselves, to try to take evening classes as best they could, working a twenty-four-hour rota. (The HMC had now approved the institution of such a course.)

Following the interview programme, a series of weekly meetings were held by the theatre superintendent, the senior consultant anaesthetist, the deputy hospital secretary, and myself to (a) design a new work rota for the technicians and (b) define the duties of the technicians both in and out of the theatres. The roster finally evolved allowed each of the theatres to retain its own permanent technician, with the surplus technicians covering the theatres whenever the residents were absent and otherwise performing duties outside the theatres. The hours worked by the resident technicians were matched with the hours of theatre usage, and it proved possible, making use of the days when the theatres were closed, to cover late-evening work by both float and resident technicians, with only minimum disturbance to the theatre team. Each of the technicians worked a standard

40-hour, 5-day week, and float and resident technicians alike worked a rota to cover the weekend work. At the time (1966) the hospital had only eight theatre technicians; two of these covered the night duties, leaving six to cover five theatres during the day. Consequently, the level of overtime per man arising from the weekend rota was high, the technicians being expected to work one weekend on duty and the next off; so some displacement of a man from his theatre was unavoidable. The hospital had an establishment for thirteen theatre technicians (plus two plaster technicians); it was expected that as the numbers employed were brought up to the full establishment the weekend rota would thin out, it would be possible to match residents with theatres exactly, and overtime per man would correspondingly fall.

In preparing this roster some effort was made to clarify the line of authority for supervising technicians. The roster identified two types of shift, one for residence in a specific theatre and one for float duty. When working the former kind of shift the technician was considered to be under the command of the theatre sister, providing his particular service for the anaesthetist and surgeons when the theatre was operating, and working through a list of weekly theatre maintenance tasks when it was closed. When the roster indicated a floating shift the technician joined a pool from which he might be deployed to any theatre requiring assistance, and which was responsible for the care and maintenance of anaesthetic equipment throughout the hospital. The hospital was at that time without a senior technician, but it was envisaged that the man appointed would command the pool of floating technicians, which would be increased in size from its present one man, plus occasional shifts by resident theatre staff, to six technicians at full establishment. In the restricted circumstances at that time the theatre superintendent continued to deploy the float technicians and endeavoured to leave resident theatre staff in their theatres as far as possible.

A two-year training course for the technicians was approved in principle by the HMC, the course to be run on the lines suggested by the Institute of Theatre Technicians and to lead to the award of their diploma. This course was aimed at attracting recruits straight from school, the years before they were of age to enter the theatre being spent in departments associated with the theatres, e.g. CSSD and pathology. When of age, the trainees would progress to maintenance of anaesthetic equipment, observation in theatres, acting as technician's assistant, and finally to full duty in the pool before the examination was taken. The organization and running of this course, which included a comprehensive series of lectures to provide the theoretical background of theatre work, was to be in the hands of the senior technician, working closely with the theatre superintendent and the senior consultant anaesthetist. Its inception awaits the appointment of the senior technician.

THEATRE PORTERS

A review of the theatre porters' rota and organization conducted in August 1966 revealed the following. There was an establishment for eleven theatre porters administratively controlled by the head porter for the hospital secretary, but deployed and co-ordinated in the theatres by the theatre superintendent. She endeavoured to provide each working theatre with a pair of porters whose principal function was to transport patients between the wards and the theatre. The porters worked through a ten-duty rota, each man changing duty each week. The rota covered the hours 8.30 a.m. to 9.30 p.m. and included two duties each for E (ENT) and G (gynaecology) theatres, because these theatres worked every weekday. Other theatres were covered, when in use, by the remaining six duties. The replacement of two men in each of E and G theatres for a week was only partly successful because the porters' hours did not match the theatre hours. Deployment of porters each day was carried out by the theatre superintendent as they came on duty in the morning, with reallocations continuing throughout the day as theatres opened and closed, as men came on and off duty, and as theatres working throughout the day required lunch-time reliefs.

Discussions with theatre staff revealed a number of problems with this system which, viewed from the vantage point of each type of staff involved, may be summarized as follows:

(i) *The porters* found they were moved from theatre to theatre without warning, sometimes several times a day, and were never able to achieve any identification with a theatre. They frequently found that the relief promised for lunch or going off duty was late in arriving and they were faced with either working on or breaking the rules and leaving the theatres unattended. In addition they were faced with conflicting orders from the theatre sister and members of her staff.

(ii) *The theatre sisters.* The porters were required at the end of the case to bring in the next and take the one completed back to the ward. They were also required to fetch blood, or carry specimens, at any time during the operations. To perform these duties the porters waited outside the theatre until called, and frequently the theatres could find no porters available when needed. In this situation the sister could either spend considerable time on the telephone trying to locate the porters or get her own staff to perform the necessary duties, which resulted in technicians, nurses, surgeons, and anaesthetists pushing trolleys around the hospital.

(iii) *The theatre superintendent*, in addition to her many other duties, was required to maintain an hour-by-hour check on where the porters were throughout each day. With the continually changing theatre situation, redeployment under the existing system was continuous, and took a great deal of time. The theatres are spread out along the north side of the hospital, and this does not make the passing of orders to the porters in person easy. The theatre superintendent frequently found it necessary to utilize a middleman, thus increasing the dangers of misunderstanding and conflict. As the theatres steadily reconstituted their lists, more theatres worked each day, and with the existing establishment of eleven men usually below strength, because of sickness or absenteeism, it became increasingly difficult to provide each theatre with a team of two porters. In this situation the theatre superintendent turned to the head porter for assistance.

(iv) *The head porter* found that the calls made for additional cover, particularly at lunch-time, became quite frequent and placed a strain on the general portering pool, which was considerably below full strength. The short notice given of such difficulties also complicated the situation, because makeshift arrangements were required and carefully laid plans went awry.

It was evident from this picture that the three staffing criteria were not being realized, and further investigations revealed that the situation was not one in which they could all be realized, because of the obstacles to the allocation of a pair of porters to a theatre permanently, which were:

(a) The theatres, from the porters' point of view, were not equivalent. In the gynaecology theatre, for example, portering would be frequently required when a succession of minor operations was being carried out, and work was very hard because patients had to be transported over long distances along open roads between the wards and the theatre. In contrast, the general surgery theatres performed longer operations and were fed by wards close to the theatres, which could be reached under cover. To allocate porters permanently to the gynaecology theatre would be putting them at a disadvantage compared to their colleagues.

(b) The chances that the porters would become integral parts of the theatre team were limited. Observations in theatres revealed that their contact with the other members of the theatre team was small, the porters spending most of their time waiting outside the theatre, orders being passed to them by the theatre technician.

Faced with these difficulties, the ideal of including the porters within a stable team structure was abandoned, and the proposals made, which were still under discussion at the time, retained the porters as a separate group providing overall theatre coverage rather than decentralizing them as was attempted with other theatre staff. In outline the proposals featured the appointment of a chargehand porter to take on the onerous duties of deployment and co-ordination that had been carried out by the theatre superintendent. The chargehand was to be administratively responsible to the head porter for the porters, and responsible to the theatre superintendent for providing adequate cover for the theatres. A new roster was designed for the same establishment of porters, which circulated a pair of porters through a week in each of the outpost theatres E and G, with hours matched with theatre hours, a week on late shifts and two weeks on pool duty. The pool provided for four porters working under the close supervision of the chargehand, to cover the orthopaedic theatre and the two general surgery theatres, which were located nearby. These three theatres worked simultaneously on Wednesdays and Fridays only, but research indicated that, even if this were the rule rather than the exception, a team of five would be able to manage, given an improved communications link between the theatres and the porters. To improve communications it was suggested that each theatre should be provided with a bell by which the theatre could summon the porters from outside the theatre in the case of the two outpost theatres, or from a small room located near one of the other three theatres; this room was to serve as a theatre-porter control centre. It was felt that, given such facilities, the chargehand could do much, by suitable planning ahead, to improve the service offered to the theatres. Provided with the theatre lists early in the morning, he would be able to pick out peak demands and plan accordingly and, if warranted, could notify the head porter well beforehand about when and where help would be required.

The new rota, like the old, provided for six-day cover each week between the hours of 8.30 a.m. and 9.30 p.m., with night and Sunday cover being provided by the north-side shift porters, with assistance on Sundays from a theatre porter on voluntary overtime. The principal duties of the north-side shift porters were surgical ward portering, and only one porter was available from this source at any one time. Investigations were then undertaken to determine the need, at the time and in the future, for a night theatre porter or an extra shift porter to provide a full team of two porters for the theatres at all times.

## THEATRE LIST REORGANIZATIONS

The improving staff situation on the nursing side and the increased flow of data from the theatres concerning specific problems led to a steady reconstitution of theatre lists and a redistribution of theatre hours among the surgeons, which was aimed at both restoring the theatres to full working and alleviating some of the specific problems.

In September 1966, one of the three consultants in general surgery retired and a reallocation of theatre lists was made before his succcessor took up his post in October. Before, the staff shortage had meant that the two general surgery theatres could not work simultaneously, but during this interim period, when two consultants were carrying the work of three, it became possible to open the theatres simultaneously on Wednesday and Friday mornings, representing an increase in sessions from ten to twelve per week. The RHB was requested to proceed with the appointment of a fourth general surgeon. The staff situation permitting, it was hoped that the upward trend in weekly sessions would be maintained until both theatres worked a full Monday-to-Friday week.

The orthopaedic theatre was in reality two theatres, one main theatre and a small one suitable for plaster and minor operations. Before October 1966, the two orthopaedic consultants worked lists in the theatre on only three mornings a week, both working at the same time, one using the large and the other the small theatre. These arrangements were changed in October, when the firms began to work separately and the theatre became open for list work six mornings of one week and five of the next. All major surgery was carried out in the main theatre, the minor theatre reverting to its intended use as a plaster theatre. The full-time working of the theatre meant that orthopaedic nursing teams could be fully employed throughout the week rather than being rushed off their feet three times a week.

The ENT theatre (E) had been working a full ten sessions, Monday to Friday each week, which included sessions devoted to dentistry and plastic surgery. It was hoped in the near future to transfer the plastic surgery sessions to one of the general surgery theatres, since this would obviate the need for patients to be transported across open roads between the wards and the theatre, which was detrimental to the patients' health as well as arduous for the porters. The ENT theatre was shortly to undergo rebuilding to provide better operating facilities (including improved ventilation), staff rest-room facilities, and a recovery room.

Other plans included the continued reorganization of theatre ancillary rooms as clinical secretaries were given rooms elsewhere and as the CSSD service to theatres, which began shortly after, obviated the need for theatres to incorporate large stock-rooms. Besides providing rest rooms for staff, the rooms vacated also provided space for recovery wards, which enabled patients to come out of the anaesthetic completely before returning to the ward and therefore represented a further advance in patient-care.

Future developments included a major theatre-building plan scheduled for 1973/74 incorporating a twin theatre suite. This would enable the gynaecology operations to be performed in one of the present general surgery theatres, which would again obviate the need for patients to be transported along open roads. The existing gynaecology theatre could then revert to purely obstetric work.

## SUMMARY

Since the staff shortage necessitated the curtailing of theatre sessions in October 1965, and again in January 1966, a number of improvements were made. The theatre nursing staff were reorganized, additional theatre staff were recruited, and a theatre course was started for postgraduate nurses which would lead to a further recruitment of trained theatre staff. The duties of the technicians were defined, their work roster revised, and a training course for them approved by the HMC. Proposals for the reorganization of theatre porters were prepared. In addition, improvements were made in theatre accommodation – rest rooms provided in the orthopaedic and the general surgery theatres, and schemes approved for improvements in the remaining theatres. Two of the curtailed sessions were reconstituted and it was hoped, with the improved staffing position, that all theatres would soon be back to normal working.

APPENDIX 9B

# *Summary of reasons given by eight students for withdrawing from nurse training*

| | | |
|---|---|---|
| *Home* | | |
| general | 4 | by 6 nurses |
| attachment to mother | 1 | |
| to be near home | 2 | |
| frequent travelling home | 1 | |
| *Nursing and hospital life* | | |
| work too hard; too tired | 2 | by 4 nurses |
| upsets on ward | 1 | |
| uninterested in nursing | 1 | |
| dislikes work | 1 | |
| hates death, disturbed by blood and bowel wash-out | 1 | |
| bad reports; and deferred promotion | 2 | by 5 nurses |
| resents trivial and unnecessary discipline and criticism | 4 | |
| efforts unappreciated and not treated as responsible person | 3 | |
| fear of 'cruel' sister | 2 | by 2 nurses |
| two weekends off in two years | 1 | |
| seniors unapproachable | 1 | by 3 nurses |
| frightened by size of hospital | 1 | |
| no one to discuss difficulties with | 2 | |
| lacking in self-confidence | 1 | |
| personal fear of bleeding to death | 1 | |
| *General* | | |
| to get married | 1 | by 3 nurses |
| low IQ | 1 | |
| poor pay | 2 | |

# APPENDIX 11A

## *The problem of evaluating H.I.C.*

There are many different ways in which one may evaluate the H.I.C. Project, and the reader is invited to decide for himself just how the present evaluation approaches his own views of a proper evaluation. While the great diversity of possible methods prevents one from spelling out any single 'correct' evaluation, there would appear to be a number of ways of looking at, and evaluating, the Project that are either unfair or invalid. This appendix describes some of these views.

One reaction of observers is that the H.I.C. Project is 'completely unique'. Nothing like it has been done before. To the extent this view is held, no evaluation would seem possible, since an evaluation implies a comparison. To evaluate is to place a value on something and to imply that alternatives, with alternative values, are possible. According to our thinking about the problems of evaluation, it is necessary to conceptualize the H.I.C. Project in terms amenable to comparison, and to think in terms of variables or characteristics that may have alternative values. The H.I.C. Project may be unique, but it can be divided up, or analysed, into different aspects, the presence or absence of which is more or less desirable. This, at least, is the conception of evaluation followed here. The basic assumption is that the H.I.C. Project can, in principle, be evaluated.

One extreme, negative reaction to the H.I.C. Project is to dismiss it out of hand because it is just 'poor research'. 'Research', it is said, can only be done by skilled professionals, by social scientists, not by hospital people or second-year university students. Again, it is probably most fruitful to think of 'research' as characterized by a number of variables or dimensions – the reproducibility of the methods used, the 'objectivity' of the researcher, etc. – and the H.I.C. Project or aspects of it would then be seen as falling somewhere along these dimensions.

There is, however, the danger that the observer of H.I.C. concerning himself with the research methods will neglect the *results* of the research. For example, even methodically superb research can provide a minimal contribution to knowledge. In other words, the evaluator of the 'research' in the H.I.C. Project ought to try to look at the results of the research, as well as how it was carried out. While there is a relationship between the quality of method and the value of results, the correspondence is not exact. In addition to the 'research' in the evaluation section of this report, the reader is reminded to examine what was learned by the H.I.C. participants and detailed in other sections of the report.

Besides whatever was learned in the H.I.C. Project, there are the practical, concrete actions that resulted. The H.I.C. Project, in my view, is an 'action-research' project, encompassing not only learning about organizations by acting or changing things, but also acting in ways that will lead to practical, concrete benefits (see Chapter 5; also compare Foundation for Research on Human Behavior, 1960; Sanford, 1969).

Many observers of the H.I.C. Project and its activities are struck by the lack of clear specification concerning its goals (for more details, see Chapters 11 and 19). Project participants themselves, including those on the central team as well as hospital-team members, often asserted that they did not know the 'real' purposes of the Project, or, if they did, their conceptions were contradicted by those of others. 'How can anything so unclear be evaluated?' observers ask. Certainly, one must evaluate an activity according to the extent to which it has reached its objectives, and if objectives are not specified one might be tempted to conclude 'objectives were not reached'. But a comprehensive evaluation also takes into account the effects of the project whether they were specified as objectives or not. Unintended effects, both negative and positive, are an important component of any evaluation.

More specifically, unclear objectives may be viewed by some individuals as usually being associated with, or leading to failure. But ambiguity can be useful for some purposes, too – one need only think of sensitivity training programmes. Rather than automatically assuming that unclarity of objectives is always 'bad' and ineffective, it is better to examine what actually comes out of the objectives and associated activity. The effect of clear (or unclear) goals can be a researchable question instead of a matter for dogmatic assertion (see Chapter 19).

One possible evaluation reaction on reading the accounts of various projects done by H.I.C. hospital teams is that the practical outcomes, or the concrete changes made, were sometimes negligible. How can one spend a great deal of time doing a survey merely in order, say, to move a desk from one side of a room to the other? Here one must be careful not to equate the results of the research activity with a particular physical action subsequent to a survey or similar project. In fact, the most important outcomes possible from participation in the H.I.C. Project are changes in people – in their behaviour and attitudes (e.g. in their 'insight', their emotional temper, or perhaps the extent to which they 'listen' to others). These changes in people are not always as visible as a new piece of equipment, or a change in the physical location or arrangement of a 'thing'. Changes in people are difficult to describe, even for social scientists, and it is quite possible that hospital members writing on their projects may underrate such outcomes. In fact, it is these outcomes – changes in 'people' and relations between people – that will be a primary focus of the evaluation.

This leads to the point, no doubt already clear, that the H.I.C. Project was extremely large and complex. The observer of such a project may succumb to selecting particular portions that are familiar to him, and then evaluating the project as a whole on this basis. For example, a particular training officer may criticize the courses given, pointing out how different and how deficient they were compared with the courses he is used to giving. Someone with experience in discussion groups might criticize some of the meetings. On the other hand, a nurse or a doctor might commend an especially relevant hospital project about nurses or doctors, respectively. A psychologist might praise the handling of certain ambiguous and highly anxiety-provoking situations. Each one of these possible evaluations could be well founded, but for any of these specialists to generalize, and to evaluate the bulk of the Project on the basis of certain delimited but familiar aspects, would be of rather doubtful validity.

Even less valid than taking a part of the Project and generalizing that particular evaluation, is to project solely one's own values and objectives into the rather ambiguous objectives of H.I.C. Mention was made above of the need to differentiate criteria into scientific learning, practical actions, etc., but these must be much more specific. This is also true for the means used in the Project. By clearly specifying one's criteria for evaluation – the goals and sub-goals which, when reached, are desirable or of value – one leaves room for intelligent and even profitable disagreement with others about the value of the H.I.C. Project.

The final point in this report on the problems of evaluating H.I.C. is that the observer of the Project must guard against his prejudices and his emotional reactions to aspects of the Project. The writer will be the first to admit he possesses prejudices and emotional reactions. Research in an applied or real-world setting will no doubt elicit such reactions in many of the people involved in the research and in observers of the research. The significant different value commitments among hospital staff are no help in this respect. The charisma of the doctor – especially on the British scene – is also a particular source of emotional reaction. Those who see doctors as 'akin to gods' will doubtless criticize the Project's failure to involve them, while those who see nurses as the important key to hospital functioning will probably praise the great reliance by the Project on their help. These kinds of emotional reactions by observers of the Project can greatly impede a clear understanding of what was done and what was accomplished.

Perhaps the greatest stimulus of bias and emotionality in viewers of the Project is Professor Revans, its originator and guiding force. His use of extreme statements ('only if . . .') and his habit of opposing views head-on seem often to polarize the attitudes of others towards him and his Project. Neither uncritical acceptance of Revans's views nor total opposition can be of service in evaluating the Project. My approach in the evaluation has been to try to deal with any emotion-provoking statement in the fashion described above. A statement, for example, that only hospitals themselves could cure their communications troubles (*Further Comm.*, 1964) is most properly analysed in terms of the various outcomes and the various circumstances, people, actions, etc., for which this could be true. What is the research evidence about self-involvement and the involvement of consultants, change-agents, etc., in relation to various change outcomes, and are there any circumstances in which those findings are relevant to the H.I.C. Project?

This kind of analysis may elicit a number of useful ideas and hypotheses for observing and testing. But even if one disagrees with any particular statement – or feels that it is not valid – it is an empirical fact that a member of the Project has made the statement to his staff or to Project participants. This fact of behaviour may have any number of positive consequences.

Experience in describing the H.I.C. Project to others suggests that these last points are most important, if one is to obtain a more or less objective and realistic understanding and assessment of the H.I.C. Project and its achievements. The philosophy and opinions of the H.I.C. Project and its participants can be seen primarily as means towards various ends. The outcomes are at least as important as the means, and it is not unknown for 'good' to come from those with whom one disagrees.

Finally, it should be noted that Project staff have been extremely forthcoming in describing the problems of the Project. It has been their fervent belief that the Project must be viewed as a learning experience – that mistakes, frustrations, etc. must be aired and analysed, if anything is to be learned. This self-critical perspective of Project staff should be taken into account in obtaining a balanced, relatively objective perspective of the Project and its accomplishments.

In summary, it is suggested that one may attempt to evaluate any kind of project or activities. Whether the activities seem to be like or unlike 'research', whether their goals are clear or unclear, the effects of these activities may be examined and weighed against alternative activities. Effects or outcomes in the social realm are difficult to measure, but this should not lead to their neglect in evaluating the effects of projects.

The evaluator of a large, complex project can easily fall into the trap of selecting only 'familiar' aspects for assessment. One may project solely one's own values as a framework for understanding the effects of activities. Similarly, emotional reactions to people or to portions of a programme should be guarded against if a comprehensive assessment, including a weighing of the outcomes of activity, is to be made. Finally, the Project staff have taken a self-critical view of the events and outcomes so as to make the Project a learning experience, and this, too, should be weighed in any assessment of the H.I.C. Project.

## APPENDIX 13A

# *Hospital project effects on turnover and absenteeism*

This analysis is concerned with specific hospital projects and project events, such as data collection, reporting, and feedback, pinpointed by particular quarters in a year. Because project activities occurred at different times over the course of nearly three years, the problem encountered in Chapter 13 – the effect of any contemporaneous major non-H.I.C. influence on absence or turnover – is mitigated. The high absence rates of February-March 1967, which distorted the measures of H.I.C. activity in 1966-67 to an unknown degree, affect only a small portion of any set of comparisons here. The distribution of projects over time similarly reduces other possible distorting effects. Data collection in the seventeen projects used here could have occurred as early as November 1965, and as late as November 1967. Similarly, the issuing of reports or feedback could have begun at any time from January 1966 to December 1968.

For the analysis, groups of staff connected with the project conducted (i.e. some of the group were respondents) and large enough in size to give stable absenteeism and turnover scores (i.e. 30 individuals or more) were chosen. Some 13 groups meet these requirements: 10 groups of sisters or charge nurses, 2 medical records departments, and 1 engineering department.

The 13 groups participated in 17 different projects. Others of the 38 projects are not represented because data are not available (e.g. data on doctors' absenteeism are not available, and turnover and absence data are not available over a sufficiently long period for some of the later projects), or the groups are too small (e.g. in studies of departmental heads) or too heterogeneous (departmental heads or casualty department nurses).

The analysis utilizes data from 8 hospitals with 17 projects, as follows: 1 hospital with 1 project, 5 hospitals with 2 projects each, and 2 hospitals with 3 projects each. Despite the fact that only 8 hospitals and 13 groups are used to provide data for 17 projects, the effective $N$ for statistical tests – if they were appropriate – would probably be quite close to 17. This is because different groups in a hospital show rather different quarterly graphs and especially because the difference scores and the difference-of-a-difference scores used below are not correlated when taken at different times from the same graphs (for typical graphs see *Figures 13A-i* and *13A-ii*).

Two major different kinds of comparisons are made – 'simple' comparisons or difference measurements, and 'complex' comparisons or difference-of-a-difference measurements. Both kinds of comparisons deal with turnover or absenteeism for a quarterly period encompassing, or following, a project activity – data collection or feedback. Because in some cases no feedback occurred – only reporting – some comparisons are based on reporting instead of feedback. The final activity, whether reporting or feedback, is always used.

In a 'simple' comparison, the turnover or absence rate during (or after) a project activity is compared with the quarter immediately prior to the activity. An increase or decrease in the turnover rate between the two compared quarters then provides some evidence for the effects of the particular project activities being examined. 'Simple' comparisons are also made for periods of one year. Instead of using an immediately prior quarter, a comparison with a quarter exactly one year (four quarters) earlier is made.

There is an important potential source of error in each of these simple comparisons. A change between one quarter and the next may reflect some seasonal effect, while a change between one year and the next may reflect some long-term trends, such as changes in staff composition or recruiting practices. In order to reduce the effects of both seasonal and long-term trends, one may make a simple comparison and then compare this change with the change between two corresponding quarters, each a year earlier than the two quarters used in the first comparison. In other words, is an increase or decrease between two periods before and after project activity more or less than the change between two periods, each exactly a year earlier? For example, if a simple comparison shows a decrease of 10 per cent and the same comparison a year earlier shows a decrease of 15 per cent, then the net movement before and after the project activity, but controlling for changes 'normally' occurring between these times of year, is an *increase* of 5 per cent. Any demonstration of H.I.C. effects by these 'complex' comparisons must be given great weight, for both seasonal and long-term distortions in the data are reduced to a relatively low level (for a discussion of these and other problems see Campbell and Stanley, 1963).

Before turning to the data, we should note one possible problem in this analysis, not found in the earlier turnover analysis. This is 'contamination' of turnover or absenteeism rates for one period of project activity because that period of project activity is contemporaneous, or nearly so, with a period of activity for another project. For example, a group of sisters might be involved in two projects. While feedback of the results of the first project was occurring, the data collection for a second project might be starting or about to start. This was not a problem in the year-by-year analysis in Chapter 13, since it concerned H.I.C. Project activity overall, or during

FIGURE 13A-i *Sample turnover graph for ward sisters, 1964-1968*

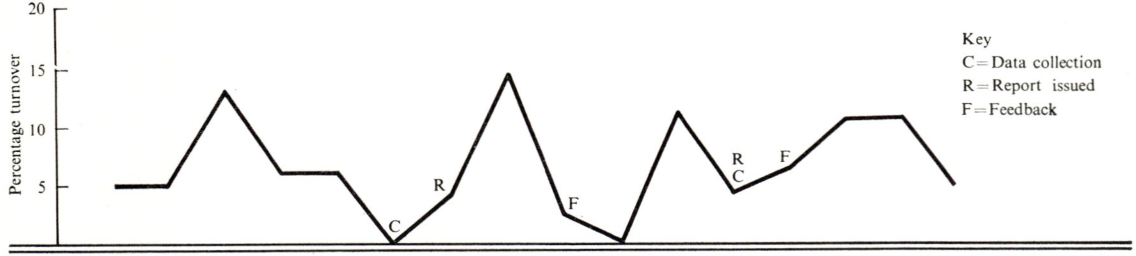


FIGURE 13A-ii *Sample absence graphs for ward sisters, 1964-1968*

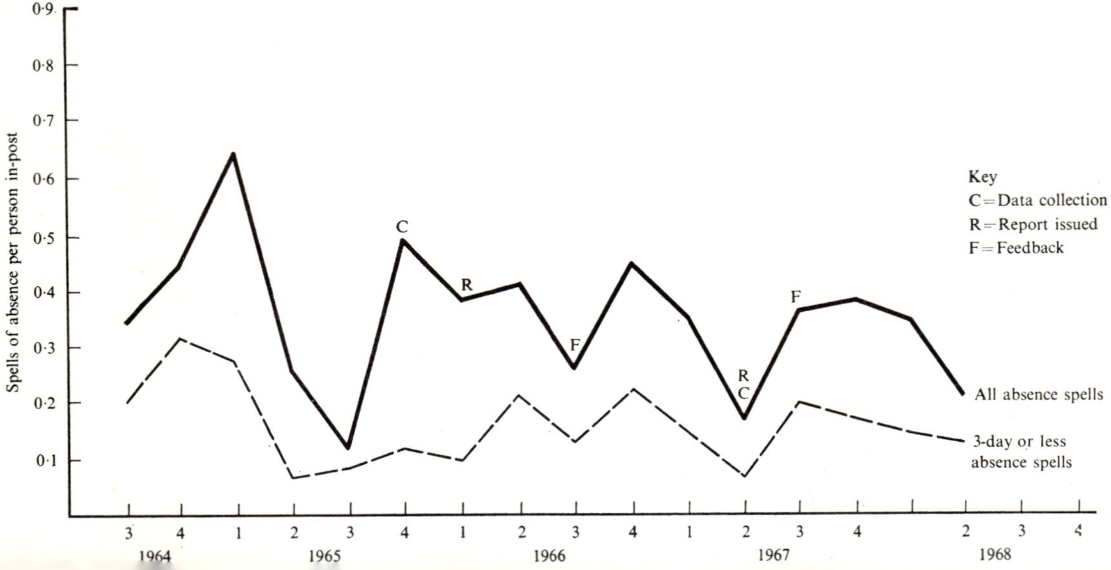

TABLE 13A-i *Turnover and Absenteeism Changes for Project Participants During and After Data Collection and Feedback*

($N$=17 projects)

| | | *Comparisons made* | | | | | |
|---|---|---|---|---|---|---|---|
| | | *'Simple' comparison* | | *'Complex' comparison* | *'Simple' comparison* | | *'Complex' comparison* |
| *Indicator and project period* | *Direction of change* | *During v. 'prior' quarter* | *During v. year earlier* | *During v. 'prior' quarter* | *One quarter after v. 'prior'* | *One quarter after v. year earlier* | *One quarter after v. 'prior'* |
| Turnover during and after data collection | Increase | 3 | 5 | 3 | 4 | 9 | 3 |
| | Decrease | 11** | 8 | 13** | 11* | 7 | 12** |
| | NA or no change | 3 | 4 | 1 | 2 | 1 | 2 |
| Turnover during and after feedback | Increase | 7 | 10 | 12** | 3 | 2 | 6 |
| | Decrease | 6 | 5 | 4 | 6 | 7* | 7 |
| | NA or no change | 4 | 2 | 1 | 8 | 8 | 4 |
| Absenteeism during and after data collection | Increase | 13** | 11 | 10 | 13** | 12** | 10 |
| | Decrease | 3 | 5 | 7 | 4 | 4 | 7 |
| | NA or no change | 1 | 1 | 0 | 0 | 1 | 0 |
| Absenteeism during and after feedback | Increase | 6 | 12** | 3 | 5 | 4 | 3 |
| | Decrease | 10 | 3 | 12** | 9 | 10* | 11** |
| | NA or no change | 1 | 2 | 2 | 3 | 3 | 3 |

* Significant at a probability less than 10 per cent, one-tailed test.
** Significant at a probability less than 5 per cent, one-tailed test.

the course of several years, without focusing on any particular project, and any effects could accumulate over time. However, while there is some contamination in the present analysis – only 10 of the 17 projects examined are 'first' projects – it is not very important for many of the projects or groups involved. This is because: (a) significant project activities were often separated by a year or more of time, and (b) even for some 'second' projects, the 'success' and contaminating effects of the previous project are minimal.

Let us turn first to the examination of changes in turnover in the 17 different projects. Comparisons for the quarter of data collection, or one quarter afterwards, with the quarter prior to collection, as well as the similar 'complex' comparisons, provide evidence that data collection activities in hospital projects apparently had beneficial effects on turnover (see *Table 13A-i*). However, the 'simple' comparison with one year earlier, as well as the 'complex' comparisons for two quarters after collection, do not show these effects. Furthermore, two of the 'complex' comparisons for the feedback stage of projects show increases in turnover.

One possible interpretation of this pattern of results is that the beneficial effects of data collection on turnover are only temporary, and that, by the time feedback occurs, the reverse trend has begun as a reaction. In point of fact, an examination of the change in turnover from two quarters before data collection to one quarter before collection also shows more groups with turnover increases than with turnover decreases. Thus the apparent beneficial effects during and immediately after data collection may be an artifact – due to the abnormally high turnover just before collection begins.

The best interpretation of these results seems to be that staff intending to leave anyway will leave a little earlier when they learn that there are to be investigations and surveys by top staff or outsiders. Most of these leavers are gone by the time collection occurs, and a subnormal rate of turnover gives the impression subsequently that feedback is having an adverse effect compared to the period immediately before feedback. Whether or not this interpretation of anticipatory leaving and consequent fluctuations in turnover is correct, it would seem fairly clear that the data do not show any general, overall positive effect on turnover from the H.I.C. Project.

The results for absence are also rather inconsistent, but if one gives more weight to the 'complex' comparisons, as is proper, then apparently there is some evidence for beneficial absence effects. The simple comparisons for the data collection period, or one quarter afterwards, compared with the previous quarter or compared with one year earlier, show increases in absence (see *Table 13A-i*). But the relevant 'complex' comparisons, controlling for seasonal or long-term distortions, are not significant. The distribution of times for data collection is one possible reason for the combination of (a) a significant increase between the previous quarter and the quarter during which collection occurred and (b) the absence of any such significant change for the appropriate 'complex' comparison. Of the

17 projects, 7 were characterized by data collection activity during the last quarter of the year, usually a period of increasing absenteeism compared with the previous quarter. The 'complex' comparison controls for this seasonal effect by using the same comparison a year earlier as a base-line. The same explanation may account for the significant increase between the previous quarter and the quarter after data collection.

FIGURE 13A-iii *Turnover and absence from three quarters before to four quarters after data collection*

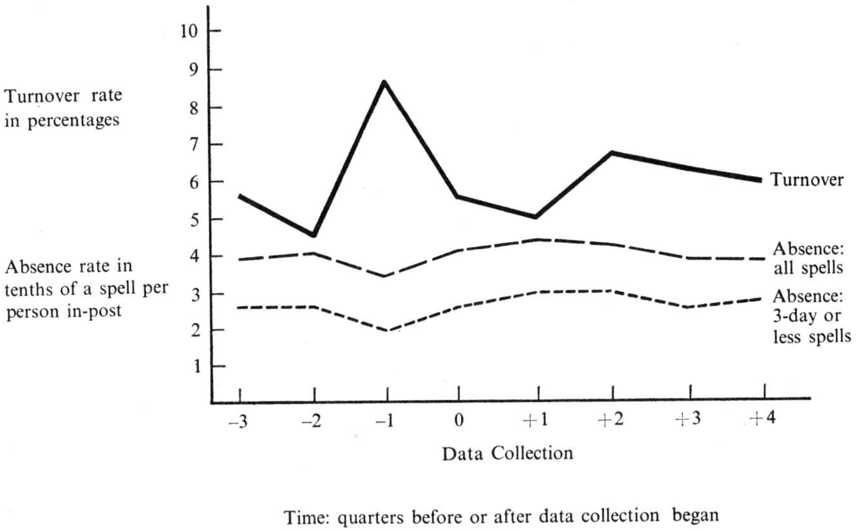


However, 'complex' comparisons for the period of feedback or for the following quarter show an apparent beneficial H.I.C. effect on absence. These positive findings are not balanced, as in the case of turnover, by findings in the opposite direction for data collection. None of these 'complex' comparisons is significant or suggestive. But it should be noted that the comparison for two quarters after feedback does not show any effects, so the apparent effects are perhaps limited to the period during and immediately after feedback. The other factor tempering any conclusions about absence is that the 'complex' comparisons for three-day absence (not shown in the table) are not significant either. Almost all of the significant comparisons for total absence are also significant for three-day absence, except for the 'complex' comparisons. The 'complex' comparisons show significant decreases in the case of total absence, but show increases and decreases in three-day absence almost equally divided among the projects.

*Figures 13A-iii* and *13A-iv* present the turnover and absence graphs averaged over the 17 projects. While rates of turnover and absence vary considerably from project to project and thus do not permit any great

FIGURE 13A-iv *Turnover and absence from three quarters before to three quarters after 'last' activity began*

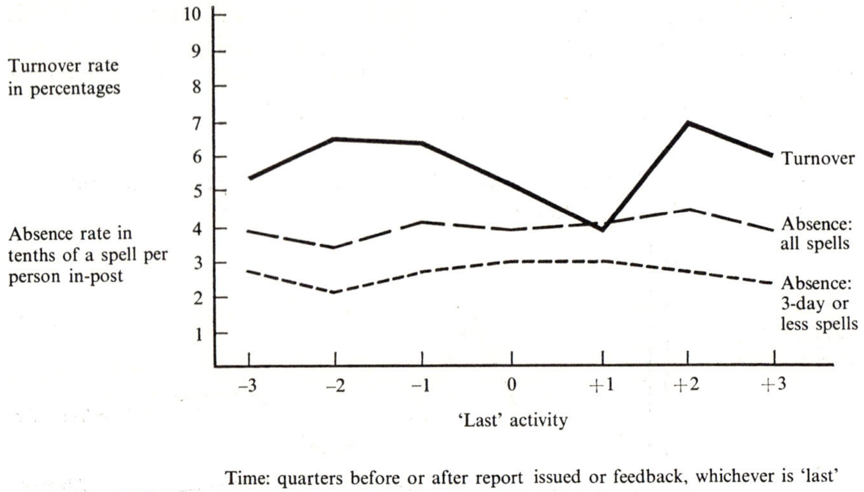


confidence in the averages, they do provide a supplementary illustration of the results from the analysis by quarters before and after project activities. The graphs clearly illustrate that project activities do not seem to have reduced, in any major way, turnover or absence rates among the staff groups studied.

# APPENDIX 14A

TABLE 14A *Percentages for Questionnaire Item Responses*

*(A table of percentages for alternative responses to questionnaire items with up to 7 alternatives)*

| *Item Number* | *0* | *1* | *2* | *3* | *4* | *5* | *6* | *7* | *DK** | *NA*** |
|---|---|---|---|---|---|---|---|---|---|---|
| | | | | *Response alternatives* | | | | | | |
| F27 | | 4 | 4 | 32 | 40 | 7 | | | 3 | 10 |
| F28 | | 7 | 6 | 31 | 35 | 8 | | | 6 | 8 |
| F29 | | 0 | 1 | 25 | 44 | 18 | | | 3 | 8 |
| F30 | | 0 | 18 | 68 | 1 | 0 | | | 3 | 10 |
| F31 | | 1 | 17 | 65 | 3 | 0 | | | 4 | 10 |
| F32 | | 1 | 22 | 62 | 1 | 0 | | | 3 | 10 |
| F33 | | 1 | 22 | 51 | 15 | 0 | | | 1 | 8 |
| F65 | | 14 | 25 | 19 | 12 | 19 | | | 1 | 8 |
| F66 | | 7 | 22 | 12 | 17 | 32 | | | 1 | 8 |
| F67 | | 6 | 18 | 8 | 6 | 53 | | | 1 | 8 |
| F68 | | 7 | 8 | 18 | 12 | 44 | | | 1 | 8 |
| F69 | | 7 | 7 | 8 | 12 | 54 | | | 3 | 8 |
| F70 | | 7 | 19 | 31 | 12 | 21 | | | 1 | 8 |
| F71 | | 6 | 15 | 42 | 12 | 12 | | | 3 | 10 |
| F72 | | 12 | 32 | 38 | 8 | 1 | | | 1 | 7 |
| F73 | | 7 | 25 | 40 | 17 | 1 | | | 1 | 8 |
| F76 | | 1 | 10 | 49 | 26 | 4 | | | 1 | 8 |
| F77 | | 1 | 33 | 43 | 7 | 1 | | | 1 | 12 |
| F78 | | 3 | 18 | 36 | 32 | 3 | | | 1 | 7 |
| F79 | | 1 | 14 | 43 | 21 | 8 | | | 3 | 10 |
| F82 | | 10 | 18 | 43 | 17 | 8 | | | 0 | 4 |
| F83 | | 6 | 10 | 33 | 26 | 19 | | | 0 | 6 |
| F85 | | 0 | 7 | 21 | 36 | 32 | | | 0 | 4 |
| F86 | | 0 | 1 | 19 | 32 | 43 | | | 0 | 4 |
| F87 | | 0 | 8 | 39 | 26 | 22 | | | 0 | 4 |
| F90 | | 7 | 15 | 12 | 6 | 0 | | | 31 | 29 |
| F91 | | 14 | 11 | 12 | 3 | 0 | | | 31 | 29 |
| F92 | | 11 | 17 | 6 | 4 | 1 | | | 32 | 29 |
| F93 | | 4 | 4 | 14 | 15 | 4 | | | 29 | 29 |
| F94 | | 9 | 14 | 20 | 2 | 0 | | | 42 | 13 |
| F95 | | 9 | 22 | 13 | 2 | 2 | | | 42 | 11 |
| F96 | | 4 | 18 | 43 | 11 | 6 | | | 12 | 6 |
| F97 | | 4 | 4 | 29 | 18 | 10 | | | 26 | 8 |
| F98 | | 11 | 24 | 32 | 12 | 6 | | | 8 | 7 |
| F99 | | 22 | 22 | 26 | 8 | 6 | | | 7 | 8 |
| F100 | | 21 | 15 | 6 | 4 | 7 | | | 31 | 17 |

| *Item Number* | *Response alternatives* *0* | *1* | *2* | *3* | *4* | *5* | *6* | *7* | *DK** | *NA*** |
|---|---|---|---|---|---|---|---|---|---|---|
| F101 | | 7 | 14 | 28 | 15 | 3 | | | 26 | 7 |
| F102 | | 1 | 15 | 17 | 6 | 14 | | | 32 | 15 |
| F136 | | 4 | 22 | 24 | 21 | 19 | | | 0 | 10 |
| F137 | | 3 | 12 | 43 | 14 | 17 | | | 0 | 11 |
| F139 | | 15 | 21 | 31 | 10 | 14 | | | 1 | 8 |
| F140 | | 10 | 18 | 22 | 17 | 18 | | | 1 | 14 |
| F141 | | 10 | 19 | 40 | 15 | 4 | | | 0 | 11 |
| F142 | | 25 | 40 | 14 | 0 | 1 | | | 0 | 19 |
| F143 | | 19 | 24 | 26 | 7 | 10 | | | 0 | 14 |
| F144 | | 22 | 29 | 17 | 3 | 7 | | | 0 | 22 |
| F145 | | 11 | 22 | 32 | 15 | 7 | | | 0 | 12 |
| F146 | | 1 | 4 | 31 | 21 | 29 | | | 1 | 12 |
| R26 | | 39 | 28 | 29 | 2 | 0 | | | 0 | 1 |
| R28 | | 19 | 23 | 18 | 7 | 1 | | | 1 | 31 |
| R29 | | 6 | 14 | 18 | 17 | 5 | | | 1 | 39 |
| R30 | | 6 | 21 | 21 | 6 | 1 | | | 1 | 43 |
| R31 | | 11 | 27 | 19 | 10 | 0 | | | 2 | 31 |
| R32 | | 6 | 12 | 18 | 19 | 10 | | | 1 | 35 |
| R33 | | 14 | 14 | 20 | 11 | 2 | | | 1 | 37 |
| R39 | | 6 | 20 | 11 | 24 | 4 | | | 1 | 35 |
| R40 | | 5 | 15 | 14 | 18 | 4 | | | 1 | 43 |
| R41 | | 7 | 23 | 10 | 12 | 2 | | | 1 | 45 |
| R42 | | 13 | 14 | 11 | 23 | 2 | | | 2 | 35 |
| R43 | | 5 | 14 | 15 | 23 | 5 | | | 1 | 37 |
| R44 | | 11 | 20 | 13 | 14 | 1 | | | 1 | 38 |
| R50 | | 26 | 21 | 14 | 5 | 1 | | | 1 | 31 |
| R51 | | 7 | 20 | 23 | 6 | 4 | | | 1 | 39 |
| R52 | | 6 | 20 | 23 | 4 | 1 | | | 1 | 45 |
| R53 | | 15 | 25 | 23 | 4 | 0 | | | 2 | 31 |
| R54 | | 5 | 20 | 24 | 7 | 5 | | | 1 | 38 |
| R55 | | 8 | 24 | 20 | 7 | 0 | | | 2 | 38 |
| R61 | | 6 | 18 | 13 | 21 | 1 | | | 2 | 38 |
| R62 | | 2 | 17 | 15 | 19 | 1 | | | 1 | 44 |
| R63 | | 5 | 17 | 13 | 13 | 1 | | | 1 | 50 |
| R64 | | 7 | 19 | 15 | 20 | 1 | | | 2 | 35 |
| R65 | | 4 | 14 | 23 | 14 | 3 | | | 1 | 40 |
| R66 | | 7 | 23 | 10 | 14 | 1 | | | 4 | 42 |
| R100 | | 19 | 25 | 18 | 2 | 0 | | | 4 | 32 |
| R101 | | 6 | 15 | 24 | 8 | 1 | | | 4 | 42 |
| R102 | | 8 | 14 | 29 | 1 | 1 | | | 4 | 43 |
| R103 | | 12 | 20 | 25 | 5 | 0 | | | 5 | 33 |
| R104 | | 5 | 24 | 21 | 6 | 2 | | | 4 | 38 |
| R105 | | 8 | 20 | 25 | 3 | 0 | | | 6 | 37 |
| R111 | | 6 | 15 | 18 | 17 | 1 | | | 4 | 39 |
| R112 | | 4 | 15 | 19 | 12 | 1 | | | 4 | 45 |
| R113 | | 4 | 21 | 12 | 13 | 0 | | | 4 | 46 |
| R114 | | 6 | 19 | 17 | 17 | 0 | | | 5 | 37 |
| R115 | | 5 | 11 | 17 | 21 | 1 | | | 4 | 42 |
| R116 | | 8 | 25 | 8 | 11 | 0 | | | 5 | 43 |
| R122 | | 0 | 6 | 31 | 15 | 12 | | | 2 | 33 |

| *Item Number* | *Response alternatives* *0* | *1* | *2* | *3* | *4* | *5* | *6* | *7* | *DK** | *NA*** |
|---|---|---|---|---|---|---|---|---|---|---|
| R123 | | 0 | 2 | 21 | 20 | 14 | | | 2 | 39 |
| R124 | | 0 | 12 | 21 | 14 | 9 | | | 4 | 39 |
| R125 | | 5 | 12 | 23 | 14 | 11 | | | 4 | 32 |
| R126 | | 2 | 5 | 12 | 21 | 23 | | | 2 | 35 |
| R127 | | 2 | 11 | 20 | 20 | 10 | | | 2 | 35 |
| R133 | | 1 | 15 | 13 | 29 | 2 | | | 2 | 37 |
| R134 | | 2 | 10 | 10 | 35 | 1 | | | 2 | 40 |
| R135 | | 2 | 15 | 10 | 23 | 2 | | | 4 | 43 |
| R136 | | 4 | 17 | 15 | 24 | 2 | | | 4 | 35 |
| R137 | | 1 | 10 | 8 | 39 | 2 | | | 2 | 37 |
| R138 | | 2 | 15 | 13 | 27 | 1 | | | 2 | 38 |
| R192 | | 1 | 18 | 32 | 10 | 5 | | | 10 | 25 |
| R214 | | 10 | 14 | 37 | 23 | 14 | | | 0 | 2 |
| R215 | | 17 | 23 | 39 | 14 | 2 | | | 1 | 4 |
| R218 | | 13 | 35 | 30 | 7 | 1 | | | 8 | 6 |
| R219 | | 7 | 18 | 33 | 24 | 4 | | | 10 | 5 |
| R220 | | 12 | 31 | 35 | 7 | 1 | | | 8 | 6 |
| R221 | | 5 | 20 | 21 | 18 | 24 | | | 7 | 5 |
| R226 | | 10 | 18 | 26 | 8 | 8 | | | 14 | 15 |
| R227 | | 7 | 20 | 42 | 14 | 5 | | | 5 | 7 |
| R229 | | 20 | 23 | 18 | 10 | 7 | | | 7 | 15 |
| R230 | | 4 | 14 | 29 | 19 | 17 | | | 6 | 12 |
| R231 | | 14 | 23 | 27 | 13 | 10 | | | 4 | 10 |
| R236 | | 2 | 13 | 29 | 17 | 13 | | | 8 | 18 |
| R237 | | 6 | 21 | 35 | 17 | 1 | | | 6 | 14 |
| R238 | | 19 | 32 | 29 | 10 | 1 | | | 2 | 6 |
| R239 | | 6 | 8 | 49 | 15 | 12 | | | 2 | 7 |
| R260 | | 21 | 33 | 12 | 6 | 13 | | | 8 | 6 |
| R263 | | 4 | 8 | 38 | 13 | 21 | | | 8 | 7 |
| R266 | | 19 | 30 | 23 | 6 | 6 | | | 10 | 7 |
| R269 | | 20 | 18 | 30 | 11 | 8 | | | 7 | 6 |
| R272 | | 20 | 27 | 29 | 4 | 7 | | | 7 | 6 |
| R275 | | 17 | 13 | 32 | 12 | 10 | | | 8 | 8 |
| R278 | | 5 | 14 | 32 | 19 | 17 | | | 7 | 6 |
| R281 | | 4 | 12 | 20 | 23 | 23 | | | 11 | 8 |
| R284 | | 11 | 25 | 20 | 15 | 13 | | | 10 | 6 |
| R287 | | 5 | 18 | 32 | 11 | 19 | | | 10 | 6 |
| R290 | | 20 | 42 | 12 | 5 | 0 | | | 15 | 6 |
| R291 | | 23 | 29 | 7 | 8 | 0 | | | 31 | 2 |
| R292 | | 12 | 25 | 12 | 7 | 0 | | | 40 | 4 |
| R293 | | 15 | 23 | 5 | 5 | 0 | | | 49 | 4 |
| R294 | | 15 | 43 | 11 | 4 | 0 | | | 21 | 6 |
| R295 | | 12 | 43 | 18 | 11 | 0 | | | 13 | 4 |
| R296 | | 2 | 25 | 29 | 21 | 0 | | | 18 | 5 |
| R297 | | 12 | 60 | 19 | 6 | 0 | | | 1 | 2 |
| R298 | | 12 | 27 | 29 | 18 | 0 | | | 8 | 6 |
| R299 | | 11 | 31 | 32 | 13 | 4 | | | 5 | 5 |
| R300 | | 5 | 15 | 24 | 37 | 7 | | | 7 | 5 |
| R301 | | 12 | 23 | 30 | 23 | 2 | | | 6 | 5 |
| R302 | | 7 | 21 | 27 | 24 | 4 | | | 11 | 6 |

| *Item Number* | *Response alternatives* 0 | *1* | *2* | *3* | *4* | *5* | *6* | *7* | *DK** | *NA*** |
|---|---|---|---|---|---|---|---|---|---|---|
| R303 | | 12 | 26 | 33 | 17 | 1 | | | 6 | 5 |
| R304 | | 15 | 39 | 27 | 8 | 0 | | | 5 | 5 |
| FF16*** | 33 | 25 | 11 | 8 | 14 | 1 | 4 | 3 | 0 | 0 |
| FF19 | 68 | 19 | 7 | 1 | 3 | 1 | 0 | 0 | 0 | 0 |
| FF37 | 28 | 28 | 24 | 8 | 7 | 3 | 1 | 0 | 0 | 0 |

* DK refers to 'don't know'. Some items had 'don't know' as a response or 'not done'. In other cases, respondents wrote 'don't know', 'can't guess', etc. All these responses are counted in the percentage figures given here.

** NA refers to 'not ascertained'. Responses included here are refusals, blank or incomplete items, or items with ambiguous responses (e.g. two numbers circled when one is required). First questionnaire item (indicated by 'F') percentages are based on a total of 72 respondents, those for the second questionnaire (indicated by 'R') on a total of 84 respondents.

*** As explained in Chapter 16, 'FF' variables are derived from records data.

## APPENDIX 14B

# *H.I.C. Outcomes – tension reduction*

Another possible H.I.C. Project outcome examined by the evaluation is the change or reduction in the tensions between top hospital staff. The organization of the hospital into three separate parts – the tripartite divisions (i.e. administrators, doctors, and nurses) – has often been cited as a source of difficulty for hospital functioning. It is possible that the H.I.C. Project has reduced some of the tensions, frictions, or conflicts between top members of the different divisions by sending them on courses together and by encouraging them to function as a team in carrying out projects in their respective hospitals.

First of all, the generally existing levels of tension between groups were established by a series of three questions (items F27, F28, and F29). *Figure 14B-i* shows that the relationships between 'top administrators and top nurses' seem to be characterized by less tension than those between 'top administrators and top doctors', or between 'top nurses and top doctors'. Next come the corresponding questions concerning the effects of H.I.C. in changing the level of tension (items F30, F31, and F32 in *Figure 14B-i*). The quite low responses here seem to indicate that relatively little decrease in tension has occurred in the H.I.C. hospitals (the mean values are either 2·2 or 2·3 for all three items).

Two further, rather more detailed, questions (not shown in the diagram) were asked about the level of tension within the respondent's own tripartite division and changes created by the H.I.C. Project in this level of tension (items F33 and F34). Using the same scale of responses as the items for tensions between 'top' members of the three divisions, respondents indicated that generally there was 'little tension' (mean of 2·1) 'between top people and lower echelons in the division'. This may mean that the respondents view the tensions between top members of different tripartite divisions as not serious, but greater than the tensions that are found between top people and lower echelons in the same tripartite divisions – where there is rather little tension.

In any event, the H.I.C. Project is again apparently seen as having little effect. The average rating for the item on changes in the degree of tension between top people and lower echelons within the tripartite division (item F34) is 2·2 on a scale in which 2 means 'H.I.C. has created no change'.

Thus, both between tripartite divisions and within tripartite divisions (specifically between the top and bottom), the H.I.C. Project is seen as having apparently little effect in reducing tensions. However, if the ratings of the levels of tension existing in H.I.C. hospitals can be taken to indicate that there is, in fact, relatively little tension at present in the system, then the failure of the H.I.C. Project to reduce tension is of little consequence.

FIGURE 14B-i *Tensions and Changes in Tensions between Top Tripartite Division Members*

(A diagram of mean responses superimposed on questionnaire items)

---

Here are some questions about the top people in this hospital—including the heads of the tripartite sections, their immediate deputies and associates.

One of the ideals of the Health Service is that the tripartite organization of the hospital functions in an integrative way. In this hospital, how much *tension* (strain or friction) is there at present between the *top people* in the following groups? (Circle one number on each line)

| | | *Very much* | *Much* | *Some* | *Little* | *None* |
|---|---|---|---|---|---|---|
| F27 | Between top administrators *and* top doctors (2.5)* | 5 | 4 | 3 | 2 | 1 |
| F28 | Between top nurses *and* top doctors (2.6) | 5 | 4 | 3 | 2 | 1 |
| F29 | Between top administrators *and* top nurses (2.1) | 5 | 4 | 3 | 2 | 1 |

---

What effect have the H.I.C. project activities had in changing the degree of tension between the top people in the hospital? (Circle one number on each line)

| | | *Much less tension* | *Less tension* | *No change* | *More tension* |
|---|---|---|---|---|---|
| F30 | Between top administrators *and* top doctors (2.2) | 4 | 3 | 2 | 1 |
| F31 | Between top nurses *and* top doctors (2.2) | 4 | 3 | 2 | 1 |
| F32 | Between top administrators *and* top nurses (2.3) | 4 | 3 | 2 | 1 |

---

* The mean response for all respondents ($N$=62 to 64) is given at the end of each item.

## APPENDIX 14C

# *Intercorrelations of H.I.C. outcome measures*

*Table 14C-i* shows the relationships among the criterion measures from the first survey. (The average responses are indicated in *Figures 14-1* and *14-2*.) These criterion measures deal with knowledge about problems, the solving of problems, information about functioning of others, and increases in the influence of respondents over others. The various measures are generally significantly correlated with one another, although there are some exceptions in the case of relationships between variables with referents of one kind and variables of another kind. Specifically, the influence measures are not always significantly related to knowledge about problems, and knowledge about problems is not always related to solving problems. But variables within areas are always significantly related to one another.

The next table (*Table 14C-ii*) shows the relationships among criterion measures from the second survey administered in December 1968 and January 1969. The first four measures (R214-R304) in the tables are based on (a) the respondent's perception of the outcomes of a project with which he had a high degree of contact (at least with the data or reports produced) or (b) the respondent's perception of improvements in his own work due to H.I.C. The pattern of correlations supports the view that the first pair of measures seem to reflect project-initiated actions, and the second pair of measures reflect improvements in work.

The remaining three measures in *Table 14C-ii* are based on ratings of changes in the behaviour of team members. It may be recalled that these changes were rated for each team member by all his colleagues on the hospital team. While these ratings of different kinds of communication changes in each team member are significantly intercorrelated among themselves, communication changes are not consistently related to improvements in the work of team members. The only possible exception seems to be changes in the knowledge and understanding of others' behaviour (item RC420).

*Table 14C-iii* shows the relationships between criteria from the first and from the second surveys. Any significant correlations in this table are rather more valid measures of relationships than those in the previous two tables,

TABLE 14C-i *Relationships among First Survey Criteria*

(*N*=62 to 69 individuals)

| | *F72* | *F76* | *F78* | *F87* | *F79* | *F82* | *F83* | *F85* | *F86* |
|---|---|---|---|---|---|---|---|---|---|
| F72 Team knowledge of problems | – | | | | | | | | |
| F76 Solve problems (hospital) | ·16 | – | | | | | | | |
| F78 Help set problems right | ·33** | ·66** | – | | | | | | |
| F87 Solve problems (own) | ·39** | ·45** | ·52** | – | | | | | |
| F79 Get respondents to solve | ·10 | ·44** | ·45** | ·26** | – | | | | |
| F82 Information about hospital | ·43** | ·26** | ·28** | ·18 | ·10 | – | | | |
| F83 Information about associates | ·27** | ·41** | ·41** | ·42** | ·20 | ·57** | – | | |
| F85 Increase influence generally | ·32** | ·33** | ·46** | ·21* | ·28** | ·42** | ·44** | – | |
| F86 Increase influence over associates | ·17 | ·34** | ·39** | ·39** | ·36** | ·25** | ·51** | ·61** | – |

* Significant at a probability less than 10 per cent, two-tailed test.
** Significant at a probability less than 5 per cent, two-tailed test.

TABLE 14C-ii *Relationships among Second Survey Criteria*

($N$=73 to 87 individuals)

| | | *R214* | *R215* | *R239* | *R304* | *RC100* | *RC260* | *RC420* |
|---|---|---|---|---|---|---|---|---|
| R214 | Administrative action | – | | | | | | |
| R215 | Worth of action | ·52** | – | | | | | |
| R239 | Improved work | ·36** | ·19* | – | | | | |
| R304 | Improved work | ·22* | ·12 | ·67** | – | | | |
| RC100 | Change – communication | ·19* | ·03 | ·14 | ·23** | – | | |
| RC260 | Change – listen | ·21* | ·19* | ·13 | ·19 | ·66** | – | |
| RC420 | Change – aware | ·30** | ·21* | ·33** | ·26** | ·57** | ·72** | – |

* Significant at a probability less than 10 per cent, two-tailed test.
** Significant at a probability less than 5 per cent, two-tailed test.

TABLE 14C-iii *Relationships between First and Second Survey Criteria*

($N$=55 to 68 individuals)

| | | Second survey criteria | | | | | | |
|---|---|---|---|---|---|---|---|---|
| | *First survey criteria* | *Admin action* R214 | *Worth of action* R215 | *Improved work* R239 | *Improved work* R304 | *Change-commun* RC100 | *Change-listen* RC260 | *Change-aware* RC420 |
| F72 | Team knowledge of problems | ·16 | −·14 | ·14 | ·38** | ·09 | ·05 | ·07 |
| F76 | Solve problems (hospital) | ·32** | ·42** | ·37** | ·36** | −0·4 | ·13 | ·29** |
| F78 | Help set problems right | ·34** | ·37** | ·22 | ·44** | ·00 | ·26** | ·17 |
| F87 | Solve problems (own) | ·49** | ·36** | ·41** | ·48** | −·02 | ·07 | ·14 |
| F79 | Get respondents to solve | ·14 | ·35** | ·28** | ·16 | −·21* | −·01 | −·02 |
| F82 | Information about hospital | −·08 | −·08 | ·27** | ·37** | ·07 | −·08 | ·08 |
| F83 | Information about associates | ·36** | ·15 | ·44** | ·37** | ·07 | ·06 | ·23* |
| F83 | Increase influence generally | ·17 | ·13 | ·24* | ·37** | ·07 | ·16 | ·21* |
| F86 | Increase influence over associates | ·38** | ·32** | ·42** | ·29** | −·03 | ·15 | ·33** |

* Significant at a probability less than 10 per cent, two-tailed test.
** Significant at a probability less than 5 per cent, two-tailed test.

since this table relates variables from two separate surveys. Any response-set covariance present must be minimal. By and large, the extent of knowledge acquired about problems is not related to any of the measures from the second survey.

However, problem-solving measures are quite consistently related to administrative actions and improvements in work behaviour. One might well expect the various problem-solving variables from the first survey to be related to the extent of administrative action, since the latter is one way in which problems are solved. For the most part, in our later analysis, we treat these variables as more or less different measures of the same thing – problem-solving – and we find that various determinants of H.I.C. outcomes are usually similarly related to the first survey measures of problem-solving and to 'administrative action' measured by the second survey.

Information about hospital functioning and increases in general influence tend not to show relationships with any of the second survey criteria, but information about associates and increased influence over the functioning of associates are related to, and perhaps determine and reflect, administrative actions and improvements in work behaviour, but not changes in communication behaviour.

With only a few exceptions, the colleague ratings of changes in a team member's communication behaviour are not related to his reports of problem-solving or acquiring knowledge of problems or information about others, or even increased influence over others. Apparently, these various direct outcomes of H.I.C. activity, plus administrative actions and work improvements mentioned above, are not associated with outcomes of communications behaviour in any clear, direct fashion.

An alternative explanation for this lack of correlation between the summed communication change items and other items is that the former are ratings obtained independently of the individual rated. This procedure prevents any response-set or 'halo' covariance occurring between these independent items and other items that are directly rated by the respondent himself. However, we shall see that, while this may partly explain the lack of correlations here, other similar variables are in fact correlated with colleague ratings, showing that the presence or absence of response-set covariance cannot wholly explain the presence or absence of correlations here.

## APPENDIX 16A

# *Analysis of feedback meeting transcripts*

In an exploratory analysis of feedback meeting transcripts we have attempted to determine what was discussed by whom, and whether these elements change over time.

This is basically a descriptive analysis. No control groups are used, and comparisons with other kinds of discussion groups, such as T-groups, are made in only a general way. However, comparisons or 'evaluations' can be made between activities, and their outcomes, and the ostensible or implied goals of various participants. Keeping in mind what participants seemed to want, did the discussion at meetings seem to be more facilitative of one goal than another?

We selected transcripts from four meetings – the first, fourth, sixth, and seventh – for this exploratory analysis. These meetings were chosen because the tapes were clear and audible and because the selection of early and late meetings provides some evidence of changes over the course of the meetings.

Contributions, or uninterrupted statements by participants, were categorized and counted in two ways. For 'process', a modified Bales (1950) system with the following main categories was used: giving, or asking for, (a) information, (b) opinions, and (c) suggestions for decisions or actions. For 'topic', the main categories were: (a) the hospital project scheduled for presentation and discussion, (b) other hospital projects, (c) the H.I.C. Project other than individual hospital projects, and (d) hospital problems or issues not part of a project.

In the data for each of the four meetings, the convener averages about one-sixth of all contributions, the remainder of the central team (including students), about one-tenth, and the hospital participants nearly three-quarters. Over the course of the four meetings analysed, the data show a trend towards fewer contributions by hospital participants, and more by the central team (excluding the convener), but this trend is rather slight. The overriding impression is the constancy in these proportions.

There would appear to be two important points evident from the differing proportions of contributions by various participants. The hospital participants did most of the talking, and this seems to conform to the planned nature of the meetings as a forum for hospital-team discussions.

The other point is the great preponderance of comments by the convener, in relation to the remainder of the central team. This suggests a central role by the convener in controlling, as well as organizing and creating, the meetings. The 'convener' was a 'leader' in this sense.

Taking the contributions of all participants together, we obtain a view of the feedback meetings as a forum for expressing opinions (two-fifths of all contributions) and reporting information (one-fifth). Requests for information or opinions totals another fifth of all contributions. Suggestions for action, or for a decision, are infrequent. Only one-twentieth of all contributions are suggestions about action or how to do something. Apparently, the meetings did not attend to the *solving* of problems nearly as much as to the expressing of views about the *state* of problems, whether general hospital problems or specific problems about doing projects (on problem-solving see Kelley and Thibaut, 1970). The meeting discussions were basically diagnostic (compare Bales and Strodtbeck, 1951; Cartwright and Zander, 1968, pp. 389-398).

In categorizing contributions giving or asking for information or opinions, we noted whether any dealt with the feelings or emotions of individuals either participating at the meeting or not present. If the meeting was to reflect a 'Tavy-type' group (see Rice, 1965) as the convener planned, then emotions, particularly of those present, would be an important topic. In fact, one-tenth of all contributions concern in some way the emotional states of individuals not present. These contributions include reports of survey information and items on feelings and attitudes, but also include giving, and asking for, opinions on these matters.

A further twentieth of all contributions concern some aspect of the emotions of those present at the meeting. This is not, strictly speaking, the 'here-and-now' that is discussed in T-groups (see Schein and Bennis, 1965; Rice, 1965), since our category includes recollections, or questions, by participants of emotional states at other times (e.g. 'How did you feel then?' would be categorized under emotions of meeting participants).

In conclusion, while the discussions of emotions would not seem to be a pervasive topic at these meetings, they certainly occurred at times, particularly if discussions about others not present at the meetings are included. These were by no means T-groups, but there was a perceptible element of similar activity.

The various overall figures given above do not, of course, hold for all of the different kinds of participants. For hospital participants, as one might expect since they contributed three-quarters of all contributions, the relative proportions of different kinds of contributions are very close to the proportions given for all participants. The only difference is that giving opinions totals one-half of all hospital contributions, while for all participants it is only two-fifths. Most of the deviations from the overall pattern of contributions are found for the convener and the remainder of the central team, including students.

Of contributions by all participants, the students provide only one-twenty-fifth. They probably had little impact on the meetings. This inference also conforms to our observations of the kinds of contributions made at the meetings. When students participated, it was to give information, or to give opinions (in the data, these aspects form over three-quarters of their contributions). Their behaviour, at least in these meetings, was to report on their project work, almost like another hospital-team member, although they did emphasize the giving of information rather more, and opinions rather less, than typical hospital-team members. It is our observation that students usually participated only if hospital-team members explicitly provided them with a role as presenters of a project report, or if the convener called upon them for a comment.

While the data show the students only infrequently asking questions, the other central-team members, and especially the convener, ask questions in one-third of their contributions. The convener differs from other central-team members in the extent to which she focuses on the feelings of those present at the meeting. One out of every ten of her contributions involves asking for the opinions of those present about various issues or comments dealing with the emotions or feelings of individuals. This confirms our general observation that the convener had in mind a T-group, or something similar, in running these meetings. A further difference in the data from the convener and other central-team members is that the latter tend to give rather more suggestions about decisions or action; this provides some evidence for our view that the central team, aside from the convener, had at least in part a problem-solving approach in the meetings.

Let us now turn to changes in the kinds of contributions over time, first of all changes within each meeting. Over the course of one day's meeting, giving information and also asking for information tend to decrease, and giving suggestions tends to increase. Giving and asking for opinions both remain more or less constant throughout the day. One might conclude from this that there were elements of a problem-solving group in the feedback meetings, since diagnosis decreases and suggestions for action increase. However, as we saw above, suggestions for action constitute a very small proportion of all activity. While there is movement towards problem-solution in the course of a day, the bulk of a meeting's discussion remains firmly centred on the expression of opinions.

As each meeting progresses, there is also usually an increase in the number of comments on the feelings of those present at the meeting, but the overall number of such contributions is small, so this generalization is quite tentative. Furthermore, any changes in the amount of discussion of emotions must be overshadowed by the very great preponderance of giving, and asking for, opinions on matters not concerning the emotions of those either present or absent.

While there are changes in emphasis on information and opinion over the course of a single day, the summary figures for each of the four meetings show no discernible changes over the course of the four meetings. As is the case with the figures for all participants together, taking different kinds of participants separately shows that different kinds of contributions retain their relative proportions when examined over time. There are fluctuations, in part probably because of the relatively small numbers involved for some kinds of contributions, but they display no discernible trend.

One factor that may have contributed to the apparent relative stability over time was the fixed format of presenting hospital project data for an hour or two, and then discussing the data reported. This probably ensured that at least a certain amount of information and opinion would be exchanged at each meeting (it should be noted that a presentation is counted as only a single contribution in the analysis of process). But why is there no increase over time in suggestions for action and the expression of opinion about emotional matters? A number of projects were presented at two separate meetings, and one would expect some movement towards problem-solving, and also an increase in exposure of the emotional aspects of the various problems, at the second presentation of a project.

However, despite pointed efforts by the convener and other central-team members in these (at times contradictory) directions, the hospital participants did not respond. Hospital-team members tended to present a new fund of data and new problems for discussion, rather than extensive reports on attempts at action or on the emotional aspects of attempting action, resistance to change, and so on. However, the relative stability of these factors over the series of meetings, despite increases during one meeting, may be due to the pattern of attendance at meetings, as well as the introduction of new projects.

A hypothesis for these phenomena must include the changing composition of those attending meetings. A large proportion of those at any one meeting were first- or second-time attenders, and as such they would no doubt have found it hard to discuss sensitive issues, such as the difficulties in getting others in their own hospital to change. Not only was the format of the meeting new to them, but the participants from other hospitals were relative strangers. For the more frequent attenders, the format probably presented no problems, but to ask for 'disclosures' about a person's own hospital, his own work, let alone his own emotions, in front of newcomers is asking a great deal. The data support the inference that hospital participants at any one meeting were able to move to some extent into these sensitive areas, but the altered composition at the next meeting would put the process of creating trust almost back to 'square one'.

The second way of examining the contributions in feedback meetings is in terms of the overt content or referents of questions and statements. In other words, what are the topics discussed?

In terms of topics, about three-quarters of all contributions are either about the hospital project presented or about hospital problems. Throughout the course of each meeting, discussion tends to move from the presented project to general hospital problems, and the same trend is apparent over the four meetings as a whole. That is, the last meeting has twice as much discussion of hospital problems compared to project discussion, while in the first meeting the proportions are reversed.

There are a number of possible explanations for this change in topics discussed. One might view projects as roundabout ways to get hospital participants talking about hospital problems. However, while hospital participants, and to some extent the convener, show this increasing emphasis over time on hospital problems, other central-team members, including students, do *not* do so. In fact, central-team contributions move from a strong emphasis on projects rather than general hospital problems, to an even stronger emphasis on projects. Thus, the roundabout approach does not seem to be a plan on the part of the central-team members other than the convener.

The increasing emphasis by hospital participants on hospital problems, as opposed to the projects themselves, is promising in terms of one set of desired outcomes from H.I.C. – namely problem-solving. Hospital problems are also desirable discussion topics since changes in the communications behaviour of these hospital participants must ultimately occur in the context of their hospital jobs. We noted, in our observations, that at times these kinds of discussion about hospital matters would elicit overt enthusiasm on the part of some hospital participants – as they found out how other tripartite division members did things, or how other hospitals did things. This was not always the case, for there could be quite a bit of defensiveness, and pointed remarks about the superiority of one's methods, in discussions of hospital problems – particularly those involving the activity of nurses. Nevertheless, the relatively large, and increasing, amount of discussion about hospital matters would appear to indicate that some awareness of 'other ways' and perhaps even some changes in patterns of openness and looking at other ways may have developed.

In any event, the constant central-team emphasis on projects leads us to conclude that discussion of hospital, or non-project, problems was not among their primary aims. We suggested above that the central team, excluding the convener, had a problem-solving orientation to the meetings. The 'problems' would appear, on this evidence, to be problems directly related to the hospital projects, and not non-project hospital problems. We would interpret the convener's behaviour, paralleling as it did that of the hospital participants in moving from project to hospital problems, as demonstrating an interest in getting hospital-team members to express themselves and to look at emotional behaviour, regardless of topic.

We conclude that the meetings displayed characteristics of both problem-solving groups and T-groups, but the number of contributions on these lines was relatively small. Suggestions for action, requests for such suggestions, and discussion about emotions or feelings played no major part in the discussions. Furthermore, since none of these elements showed an increase from meeting to meeting, the nature of the group did not move in the direction either of a problem-solving group or a T-group.

Our view is that the meetings were characterized essentially by diagnosis and evaluation of diagnosis. Hospital-team members exchanged information and opinions, thereby gaining, perhaps, more information about the matters discussed, or greater clarity about their own feelings and those of other people.

No major changes in sensitivity to emotional behaviour, or other outcomes typical of T-groups, seemed to have occurred; nor was there much evidence of problem-solving or commitments to a decided course of action – typical outcomes of problem-solving groups. While the convener and other central-team members appeared to be acting as if the groups were, respectively, T-groups or problem-solving groups, neither seemed to be achieving much success in terms of increases in the relevant processes over the series of observed meetings.

Of the topics under discussion, general hospital activities, rather than the hospital projects, seemed to receive increased emphasis by hospital-team members over the course of each meeting and over the course of the series of meetings. This is in contrast to an increased emphasis by central-team members on specific hospital project activities. The first trend may reflect the dissatisfaction of hospital-team members with discussions of projects, or it may indicate that they obtained some positive benefit from discussing general hospital activities. If the latter is true to any extent, it may be that hospital-team members have acquired a greater understanding of their respective hospital situations and hospital problems, although, as we suggest above, not necessarily moving closer to solving these problems.

# *References and Bibliography*


ABEL-SMITH, B. 1964. *The Hospitals 1800-1948.* London: Heinemann.

ADAMS, R. N. and PREISS, J. J. (Eds.) 1960. *Human Organization Research.* Homewood, Illinois: The Dorsey Press.

ADLINGTON, D. M. C. 1969. A Polemical Note on the National Training Scheme. *The Hospital,* **65**, (3).

ARGYRIS, C. 1956. Diagnosing Human Relations in Hospitals. A Case Study of a Hospital (multilith). New Haven: Yale University.

ARGYRIS, C. 1960. Creating Effective Relationships in Organizations. *Human Organization,* **17**, 34-40.

ARGYRIS, C. 1962. *Interpersonal Competence and Organizational Effectiveness.* Homewood, Ill.: Irwin-Dorsey.

ARGYRIS, C. 1964. *Integrating the Individual and the Organization.* London: Wiley.

ARGYRIS, C. 1967. On the Future of Laboratory Education. *Journal of Applied Behavioural Science,* **3**, 153-183.

ARIE, T. and FAIREY, M. J. 1969. Free Afternoon Visiting in a London Hospital. *British Journal of Hospital Medicine.* **2**. 4.

BALES, R. F. 1950. *Interaction Process Analysis: A Method for the Study of Small Groups.* Reading, Mass.: Addison-Wesley.

BALES, R. F. and STRODTBECK, F. C. 1951. Phases in Group Problem-solving. *Journal of Abnormal and Social Psychology,* **46**, 485-495. Also in D. Cartwright and A. Zander, 1968, 389-398.

BALINT, M., BALINT, E., GOSLING, R. and HILDEBRAND, P. 1966. *A Study of Doctors: Mutual Selection and the Evaluation of Results in a Training Programme for Family Doctors.* London: Tavistock; Philadelphia: Lippincott.

BARNES, E. (Ed.) 1961. *People in Hospital.* London: Macmillan.

BARNES, E. (Ed.) 1968. *Psychosocial Nursing, Studies from the Cassel Hospital.* London: Tavistock.

BARNES, L. B. 1967. Organizational Change and Field Experiment Methods. In V. H. Vroom (Ed.), *Methods of Organizational Research.* Pittsburgh: University of Pittsburgh Press.

BASS, B. M. and VAUGHAN, J. A. 1968. *Training in Industry: the Management of Learning.* Belmont, Calif.: Wadsworth; London: Tavistock.

BAVELAS, A. 1968. Communication Patterns in Task-oriented Groups. In D. Cartwright and A. Zander (Eds.), *Group Dynamics* (3rd edn.). New York: Harper & Row; London: Tavistock.

BEAHAN, P. H. 1966. Management Training and Career Development. *The Hospital,* **62**, (4).

BECKHARD, R. 1969. *Organization Development: Strategies and Models.* Reading, Mass.: Addison-Wesley.

BENDALL, E. R. D. 1965. Wastage, Sickness and Allocation. A Survey of Student Nurses. *Nursing Times,* **61**, 760-763.

BENNIS, W. G. 1961. A Typology of Change Process. In W. G. Bennis *et al.* (Eds.), *The Planning of Change: Readings in the Applied Behavioral Sciences.* New York: Holt, Rinehart, and Winston.

BENNIS, W. G. *et al.* (Eds.) 1961. *The Planning of Change.* New York: Holt, Rinehart, and Winston.

BENNIS, W. G. 1963. A New Role for the Behavioral Sciences: Effecting Organizational Change. *Administrative Science Quarterly*, **8**, 125-165.

BENNIS, W. G. 1965. Theory and Method in Applying Behavioral Science to Planned Organizational Change. *Journal of Applied Behavioral Science*, **1**, 337-339.

BENNIS, W. G. 1966. *Changing Organizations.* New York: McGraw-Hill.

BENNIS, W. G. 1969. *Organization Development: Its Nature, Origins, and Purposes.* Reading, Mass.: Addison-Wesley.

BENNIS, W. G., BENNE, K. D. and CHIN, R. (Eds.) 1969 (2nd edn.). *The Planning of Change.* New York: Holt, Rinehart, and Winston.

BION, W. R. 1959. *Experiences in Groups.* London: Tavistock; New York: Basic Books.

BLAKE, R. R., MOUTON, J. S., BARNES, L. B. and GREINER, L. E. 1964. Breakthrough in Organization Development. *Harvard Business Review*, **42**, 133-135.

BLAKE, R. R. and MOUTON, J. S. 1968. *Corporate Excellence Through Grid Organization Development: A Systems Approach.* Houston: Gulf.

BLALOCK, H. M. 1964. *Causal Inferences in Non-experimental Research.* Chapel Hill: University of North Carolina Press.

BRITISH MEDICAL JOURNAL, 1964. Internal Communications in Hospital. *British Medical Journal*, **ii**, 1456-1457.

BROWN, E. S. 1962. *Newer Dimensions of Patient Care: Part 2, Improving Staff Motivation and Competence in the General Hospital.* New York: Russell Sage Foundation.

BURNS, T. and STALKER, G. M. 1961. *The Management of Innovation.* London: Tavistock.

BUTTERFIELD, W. J. H. 1968. *Priorities in Medicine.* Oxford: Nuffield Provincial Hospitals Trust.

CAMPBELL, D. T. and STANLEY, J. C. 1963. Experimental and Quasi-experimental Designs for Research on Teaching. In N. L. Gage (Ed.) *Handbook of Research on Teaching.* Chicago: Rand McNally.

CARTWRIGHT, A. 1964. *Human Relations and Hospital Care.* London: Routledge and Kegan Paul.

CARTWRIGHT, D. and ZANDER, A. (Eds.) 1968. *Group Dynamics: Research and Theory* (3rd edn.). New York: Harper & Row; London: Tavistock.

CAUDILL, W. and ROBERTS, B. H. 1960. Pitfalls in the Organization of Interdisciplinary Research. In R. N. Adams and J. J. Preiss (Eds.), *Human Organization Research.* Homewood, Illinois: The Dorsey Press.

CENTRAL OFFICE OF INFORMATION, 1968. *Health Services in Britain.* London: HMSO.

CHAPPLE, E. O. and SAYLES, L. R. 1961. *The Measure of Management.* New York: Macmillan.

CHERNS, A. B. 1968. Social Research and its Diffusion. Loughborough University. (multilith)

CHESTLER, M. and FLANDERS, Mary 1967. Resistance to Research and Research Utilization: the Death and Life of a Feedback Attempt. *Journal of Applied Behavioral Science*, **3**, 469-487.

CHIN, R. 1961. The Utility of System Models and Developmental Models for Practitioners. In W. G. Bennis, *et al.* (Eds.), *The Planning of Change.* New York: Holt, Rinehart, and Winston.

CLARK, D. H. 1964. *Administrative Therapy.* London: Tavistock; Philadelphia: Lippincott.

COGHILL, N. F. 1969. Change and Growth in Hospitals. *Lancet*, **ii**, 1058-1061.

COLARELLI, N. J. and SIEGAL, S. M. 1966. *Ward H. An Adventure in Innovation.* New Jersey: Van Nostrand.

CRAIG, Janet. 1966. Hospital Internal Communications: Progress Report. *Nursing Times*, **62**, 681-683.

DALTON, W. 1970. Influence and Organizational Change. In A. R. Negandhi, *et al.* (Eds.), *Organization Behaviour Models.* Kent, Ohio: Bureau of Economic and Business Research, Kent State University.

DEAN, D. J., WATSON, J. P., WHITEHEAD, J. A. and CASSON, P. D. 1967. Patients' Views of a Psychiatric Hospital. *Nursing Times*, **63**, 887-889.

DEPARTMENT OF HEALTH AND SOCIAL SECURITY. 1970. *National Health Service.* The Future Structure of the National Health Service. London: HMSO.

DESSLER, G., KERRS, S., SCHIFFMAN, L. and TURNER, J. 1969. Review of 'Control in Organizations' by Arnold S. Tannenbaum. *Administrative Science Quarterly*, **14**, 318-321.

DUFF, R. S. and HOLLINGSHEAD, A. B. 1968. Sickness and Society. New York: Harper and Row.

DYER, W. G., MADDOCKS, R. F., MOFFITT, J. W., and UNDERWOOD, W. J. 1970. A Laboratory-consultation Model for Organizational Change. *Journal of Applied Behavioural Science*, **6**, 211-227.

DYKENS, J. W., HYDE, R. W., ORZACK, L. H. and YORK, R. H. 1964. *Strategies of Mental Hospital Change.* Boston: Mass. Department of Mental Health.

ECKSTEIN, H. 1959. *The English Health Service.* London: Oxford University Press.

EISENBERG, D. H. 1969. Automated Patient Questionnaire Program Measures Hospital's Effectiveness. *Hospitals*, **43**, (18), 66-68.

EMERSON, R. M. 1962. Power-dependence Relations. *American Sociological Review*, **27**, 31-41.

ENGLISH, H. B. and ENGLISH, A. G. 1958. *Comprehensive Dictionary of Psychological and Psychoanalytical Terms.* New York and London: Longmans, Green.

FAIREY, M., BARBER, B., WEBSTER, B., ARIE, T. and TOOLEY, P. 1970. A Study of Admission and Discharge Procedures 1966-1968. London: The London Hospital. (mimeo.)

FESTINGER, L. and KATZ, D. 1953. *Research Methods in the Behavioral Sciences.* New York: The Dryden Press.

FOUNDATION FOR RESEARCH ON HUMAN BEHAVIOR. 1960. *An Action Research Program for Organization Improvement* Ann Arbor, Michigan: Foundation for Research on Human Behavior.

FOUNDATION FOR RESEARCH ON HUMAN BEHAVIOR. 1960. *An Action Research Program for Organization Improvement.* Ann Arbor, Michigan: Foundation for Research on Human Behavior.

Further Communications, 1964. *The Hospital*, **60** (12).

GEORGOPOULOS, B. S. and MANN, F. C. 1962. *The Community General Hospital.* New York: Macmillan.

GEORGOPOULOS, B. S. and WIELAND, G. F. 1968. *Nationwide Study of Co-ordination and Patient Care in Voluntary Hospitals: Special*

*Report to Participating Hospitals.* Ann Arbor, Michigan: Institute for Social Research, University of Michigan.

GLASER, W. A. 1963. American and Foreign Hospitals. In E. Freidson (Ed.), *The Hospital in Modern Society.* New York: The Free Press.

GOLDSCHMIDT, P. G. 1968. *Project Paper Chase.* London: E.L.G. Marketing Ltd.

GOSS, M. E. W. 1961. Influence and Authority among Physicians. *American Sociological Review,* **26**, 39-50.

GREIG, F. W. 1966. How to Assess Your Training Needs. *Personnel Magazine,* August, 24-27.

GREINER, L. E. 1965. Organization Change and Development. Unpublished Ph.D. dissertation, Harvard University.

HAGE, J. and AIKEN, M. 1970. *Social Change in Complex Organizations.* New York: Random House.

HARRISON, R. 1970. Some Criteria for Choosing the Depth of Organisational Intervention Strategy. *Journal of Applied Behavioral Science,* **6**, 181-202.

HARRISON, R. and HOPKINS, R. L. 1967. The Design of Cross-cultural Training: an Alternative to the University Model. *Journal of Applied Behavioral Science,* **3**, 431-460.

HAVELOCK, R. G. and BENNE, K. D. 1966. An Exploratory Study of Knowledge Utilization. In G. Watson (Ed.), *Concepts for Social Change.* Washington, D.C.: National Training Laboratories.

HAWRYLYSHYN, B. 1969. Research on Effectiveness of Participative Teaching Methods. Genève: Centre d'Études Industrielles. (multilith).

HILLS, R. J. 1968. *Tdwards a Science of Organization.* Eugene, Oregon: Center for the Advanced Study of Educational Administration, University of Oregon.

HESSELING, P. 1966. *Strategy of Evaluation Research.* Assen: Van Gorcum.

HOLLOWAY, R. G., and LONERGAN, W. G. 1968. A Survey Program for Management and Organizational Development. *Hospitals,* **42**, 59-65.

Hospital Internal Communications. 1964. *British Hospital Journal and Social Service Review,* **74**, 1758-1760.

Hospital Internal Communications: A Three-day Course provided by King Edward's Hospital Fund, 1965. *British Hospital Journal and Social Service Review.*

Hospital Internal Communications, Conference at the Hospital Centre, 1964. *Nursing Times,* **60**, 1563-1564.

HOUGHTON, H. 1968. Problems of Hospital Communication: An Experimental Study. In G. McLachlan (Ed.), *Problems and Progress in Medical Care: Essays on Current Research, Third Series.* London: Oxford University Press.

HOUSE, R. J. 1967. T-Group Education and Leadership Effectiveness: a Review of the Empiric Literature and a Critical Evaluation. *Personnel Psychology,* **20**, 1-32.

HOUSE, R. J. 1969. T-Group Training: Good or Bad? *Business Horizons,* **12** (6), 69-78.

Human Relations in Hospitals. 1964. *Lancet,* **ii**, 1175.

HUNTER, T. D. 1967a. Hierarchy or Arena? The Administrative Implications of a Sociotherapeutic Regime. In H. Freeman and J. Farndale (Eds.), *New Aspects of the Mental Health Services.* Oxford: Pergamon.

HUNTER, T. D. 1967b. Self-run Hospitals. *New Society,* **10**, 356.

Internal Communications in Hospital. 1964. *British Medical Journal,* **ii**, 1456-1457.

JAHODA, M. 1963. *The Education of Technologists.* London: Tavistock.

JAQUES, E. 1951. *The Changing Culture of a Factory.* London: Tavistock/Routledge.

JOHNSON, K. 1968. People who 'Choose' to be Ill. *New Society*, **12**, 915-916.

JONES, M. 1962. *Social Psychiatry in the Community in Hospitals and in Prisons.* Springfield, Illinois: C. C. Thomas.

JONES, M. 1968. *Beyond the Therapeutic Community, Social Learning and Social Psychiatry.* New Haven: Yale University Press.

KAHN, R. L. 1960. Productivity and Job Satisfaction. *Personnel Psychiatry*, **13**, 275-287.

KAHN, R. L., WOLFE, D. M., QUINN, R. P., SNOEK, J. D. and ROSENTHAL, R. A. 1964. *Organizational Stress: Studies in Role Conflict and Ambiguity.* New York: Wiley.

KATZ, D. and KAHN, R. 1966. *The Social Psychology of Organizations.* New York: Wiley.

KELLEY, H. H. and THIBAUT, J. W. 1970. Group Problem Solving. In G. Lindzey and E. Aronson (Eds.), *The Handbook of Social Psychology*, **4** (2nd edn.). Reading, Mass.: Addison-Wesley.

KING, S. D. M. 1969. A New Look at Nursing Work Organization in a Psychiatric Hospital. *The Hospital*, **65** (3).

KLEIN, J. 1961. *Working with Groups.* London: Hutchinson.

KLEIN, L. 1969. Social Science: Customers Beware. *New Society*, **14**, 978-980.

KNAPP, L. and LARSON, C. E. n.d. Institutional Learning: a More Appropriate Definition of Roles. Milwaukee, Wisconsin: University of Wisconsin. (hectograph.)

KOONTZ, H. 1964. *Toward a Unified Theory of Management.* New York: McGraw-Hill.

LAKIN, M. 1969. Some Ethical Issues in Sensitivity Training. *American Psychologist*, **24**, 923-928.

LAWRENCE, P. R. and LORSCH, J. W. 1967. *Organization and Environment.* Boston: Harvard University.

LAWRENCE, P. R. and LORSCH, J. W. 1969. *Developing Organizations: Diagnosis and Action.* Reading, Mass.: Addison-Wesley.

LEVINE, J. and BUTLER, J. 1968. Lecture v. Group Discussion in Changing Behaviour. In A. Cartwright and D. Zander, 1968. *Group Dynamics: Research and Theory* (3rd edn.). New York: Harper & Row; London: Tavistock.

LEAVITT, H. 1965. Applied Organizational Change in Industry: Structural, Technological and Humanistic Approaches. In J. G. March (Ed.), *Handbook of Organizations.* Chicago: Rand McNally.

LEAVITT, H. J. and MUELLER, R. A. H. 1951. Some Effects of Feedback on Communication. *Human Relations*, **4**, 401-410.

LEWIN, K. 1968. Group Decision and Social Change. In G. E. Swanson *et al.* (Eds.), *Readings in Social Psychology.* New York: Holt.

LIKERT, R. 1961. *New Patterns of Management.* New York: McGraw-Hill.

LIKERT, R. 1967. *The Human Organization: Its Management and Value.* New York: McGraw-Hill.

LINDSAY, A. 1962. *Socialized Medicine in England and Wales: the National Health Service 1948-1961.* Chapel Hill: University of North Carolina Press.

LIPPITT, R., WATSON, J. and WESTLEY, B. 1958. *The Dynamics of Planned Change.* New York: Harcourt Brace.

LOOMIS, C. P. 1959. Tentative Types of Directed Social Change Involving Systemic Linkage. *Rural Sociology,* **24**, 383-390.

LORSCH, J. W. and LAWRENCE, P. 1969. The Diagnosis of Organizational

Problems. In W. G. Bennis *et al.* (Eds.), *The Planning of Change.* New York: Holt, Rinehart, and Winston.

LUSZKI, M. B. 1960. Team Research in Social Science: Major Consequences of a Growing Trend. In R. N. Adams and J. J. Preiss (Eds.), *Human Organization Research.* Homewood, Illinois: The Dorsey Press.

LYONS, T. F. 1966. Review of Attitudes and Turnover. Ann Arbor, Michigan. (hectograph).

MCGREGOR, D. 1960. *The Human Side of Enterprise.* New York: McGraw-Hill.

MCGREGOR, D. 1967. *The Professional Manager.* New York: McGraw-Hill.

MCQUITTY, L. L. 1964. Capabilities and Improvements of Linkage Analysis as a Clustering Method. *Educational and Psychological Measurement,* **24**, 441-456.

MAIER, N. R. F. 1950. The Quality of Group Discussion as Influenced by a Discussion Leader. *Human Relations,* **3**, 155-174.

MAIN, T. F. 1946. The Hospital as a Therapeutic Institution, *Bulletin of the Menninger Clinic,* **10**, 66-70. Also in E. Barnes (Ed.), 1968. *Psychosocial Nursing.* London: Tavistock.

MAIN, T. F. and RAPOPORT, R. N. 1962. Hospital Sociology. In A. T. Welford (Ed.), *Society, Problems and Methods of Study.* London: Routledge and Kegan Paul.

MANN, F. C. 1957. Studying and Creating Change: a Means to Understanding Social Organization. In C. M. Arensberg *et al.* (Eds.), *Research in Industrial Human Relations.* New York: Harper.

MANN, F. and LIKERT, R. 1952. The Need for Research on the Communication of Research Results. *Human Organization,* **11**, 15-19.

MANN, F. C. and WILLIAMS, L. K. 1960. Observations on the Dynamics of a Change to Electronic Data Processing Equipment. *Administrative Science Quarterly,* **5**, 217-256.

MANT, A. 1970. *The Experienced Manager.* London: British Institute of Management.

MARCH, J. G. and SIMON, A. 1958. *Organizations.* New York: Wiley.

MENZIES, I. E. P. 1960. A Case-study in the Functioning of Social Systems as a Defence against Anxiety. *Human Relations,* **13**, 95-121.

MERTON, R. K. 1957. *Social Theory and Social Structure.* Glencoe, Ill.: The Free Press.

MILBANK MEMORIAL FUND QUARTERLY. 1966. Discussion. *Milbank Memorial Fund Quarterly,* **44** (3), Part 2, 246-248.

MILES, M. B. 1959. *Learning to work in Groups.* New York: Bureau of Publications, Teachers College, Columbia University.

MILES, R. E. 1966. Human Relations or Human Resources? *Harvard Business Review,* **43** (4), 148-156.

MILLER, E. J. and RICE, A. K. 1967. *Systems of Organization: The Control of Task and Sentient Boundaries.* London: Tavistock.

MINISTRY OF HEALTH. 1966a. *Report of the Committee on Senior Nursing Staff Structure* (Chairman, Mr. B. Salmon). London: HMSO.

MINISTRY OF HEALTH. 1966b. *Report of a Sub-Committee of the Advisory Committee for Management Efficiency on the Management Functions of Hospital Doctors.* London: HMSO.

MINISTRY OF HEALTH. 1967. *First Report of the Joint Working Party on the Organization of Medical Work in Hospitals.* London: HMSO.

MOON, H. 1965. *The First Two Years. A Study of the Work Experience of Some Newly Qualified Medical Social Workers.* London: National Institute for Social Work Training.

MOUZELIS, N. P. 1967. *Organization and Bureaucracy: An Analysis of Modern Theories.* Chicago: Aldine.

PANTALL, J. and ELLIOTT, J. 1968. *Can Research Aid Hospital Management?* London: The Hospital Centre (Reprint 234).

PARSONS, T. 1951. *The Social System.* Glencoe, Ill.: The Free Press; London: Tavistock/Routledge.

PARSONS, T. *et al.* 1952. *Working Papers.* Glencoe, Ill.: The Free Press.

PARSONS, T. and BALES, R. F. 1955. *Family, Socialization and Interaction Process.* Glencoe, Ill.: The Free Press.

PEARSON, R. J. C., SMEDBY, B., BERFENSTAM, R., LOGAN, R. F. L., BURGESS, A. M. and PETERSON, O. L. 1968. Hospital Caseloads in Liverpool, New England, and Uppsala. *Lancet*, **ii**, 559-566.

PERKINS, M. E. and ROKER, E. G. 1967. Nursing Administration – Changing Patterns. *Nursing Times*, **63**, 890-894.

PERROW, C. 1965. Hospitals: Technology, Structure and Goals. In J. G. March (Ed.), *Handbook of Organizations.* Chicago: Rand McNally.

PERROW, C. 1969. Some Reflections on Technology and Organizational Analysis. In A. R. Negandhi *et al.* (Eds.), *Comparative Administration and Management: Conceptual Schemes and Research Findings.* Kent, Ohio: Bureau of Economic and Business Research, Kent State University.

RAPHAEL, W., 1969. *Patients and Their Hospitals.* London: King Edward's Hospital Fund.

RAPOPORT, R. N. 1957. Notes on the Disparagement of 'Sociologizing' in Collaborative Research. *Human Organization*, **16**, 14-15.

RAPOPORT, R. N. 1960. *Community as Doctor.* London: Tavistock.

REES, M. D. 1966. European School – American Style. *The Manager*, January/February, 45-47.

REVANS, R. W. 1964a. Conference on Hospital Internal Communication, Thursday, 19th November, 1964: Notes by Professor R. W. Revans. London: The Hospital Centre. (multilith, THC/64/428).

REVANS, R. W. 1964b. *Standards for Morale: Cause and Effect in Hospitals.* London: Oxford University Press.

REVANS, R. W. 1965a. Managers, Men and the Art of Listening. *New Society*, **5**, 13-15.

REVANS, R. W. 1965b. *Science and the Manager.* London: Macdonald.

REVANS, R. W. 1965c. Operation Babel. London: The Hospital Centre. (multilith, THC/65/73).

REVANS, R. W. 1966a. Hospital Internal Communication. Notes on the Project. London: The Hospital Centre. (multilith, THC/67/113).

REVANS, R. W. 1966b. *The Theory of Practice in Management.* London: Macdonald.

REVANS, R. W. 1967. Studies in Institutional Learning. Brussels: European Association of Management Training Centres. (mimeo).

REVANS, R. W. 1968. Hospital Internal Communications. *Nursing Times*, **64**, (11), 41-42.

REVANS, R. W. In press. *Hospitals: Communications, Choice, and Change.* London: Tavistock.

RICE, A. K. 1958. *Productivity and Social Organization.* London: Tavistock.

RICE, A. K. 1965. *Learning for Leadership.* London: Tavistock.

ROETHLISBERGER, F. J. and DICKSON, W. J. 1947. *Management and the Worker.* Cambridge, Mass.: Harvard University Press.

ROSNER, M. M. 1968. Economic Determinants of Organizational Innovation. *Administrative Science Quarterly*, **12**, 614-625.

ROSSI, P. 1967. Evaluating Social Action Programs. *Transaction*, **4** (7), 51-53.

SANFORD, N. 1969. Research with Students as Action and Education. *American Psychologist*, **24**, 544-546.

SCHEIN, E. H. 1958. The Chinese Indoctrination Program for Prisoners of War. *Psychiatry*, **19**, 149-172.

SCHEIN, E. H. 1969. *Process Consultation: Its Role in Organization Development.* Reading, Mass.: Addison-Wesley.

SCHEIN, E. H. and BENNIS, W. G. 1965. *Personal and Organizational Change via Group Methods.* New York: Wiley.

SCHMUCK, R. A. and RUNKEL, P. J. 1970. *Organizational Training for a School Faculty.* Eugene, Oregon: Center for Advanced Study of Educational Administration, University of Oregon.

SCHURR, M. C. 1969. A Comparative Study of Leadership in Industry and the Nursing Profession. *International Nursing Review*, **16**, 115-132.

SCOTTISH HOME AND HEALTH DEPARTMENT. 1967. *First Report of the Joint Working Party on the Organization of Medical Work in the Hospital Service in Scotland.* Edinburgh: HMSO.

SEASHORE, S. E. 1964. Field Experiments with Formal Organizations. *Human Organization*, **23**, 164-170.

SEASHORE, S. E. and BOWERS, D. G. 1970. Durability of Organizational Change. *American Psychologist*, **25**, 227-233.

SELLTIZ, C., JAHODA, M., DEUTSCH, M. and COOK, S. 1962. *Research Methods in Social Relations.* New York: Holt, Rinehart, and Winston; London: Methuen.

SIEGEL, S. 1956. *Nonparametric Statistics for the Behavioral Sciences.* New York: McGraw-Hill.

SKELLERN, E. 1953. Study of the Work of Ward Sisters. London: Royal College of Nursing. Also in E. Barnes, 1968. *Psychosocial Nursing.* London: Tavistock Publications.

SMITH, D. N. 1968. *The Ancillaries.* London: Guy's Hospital Medical School.

SMITH, P. B. 1968. Training and Developing Executives. In D. Pym (Ed.), *Industrial Society.* Harmondsworth: Penguin Books.

SOFER, C. 1955. Reactions to Administrative Change, Study of Staff Relations in Three British Hospitals. *Human Relations*, **8**, 291-316.

SOFER, C. 1961. *The Organization from Within.* London: Tavistock.

SOFER, C. 1964. The Assessment of Organizational Change. *Journal of Management Studies*, **1**, 128-142.

SOFER, C. and HUTTON, G. 1959. *New Ways in Management Training.* London: Tavistock.

STANTON, A. H. and SCHWARTZ, M. S. 1954. *The Mental Hospital.* New York: Basic Books.

STEVENS, R. 1966. *Medical Practice in Modern England.* Yale University Press.

STEWART, J. S. 1969. Cogwheel: A Physician's View of a Local Version. *British Medical Journal*, **iv**, 420-423.

STEWART, R. and SLEEMAN, J. 1967. *Continuously Under Review.* Occasional Papers in Social Administration, 20. London: G. Bell.

STRAUSS, G. 1963. Some Notes on Power-equalization. In H. J. Leavitt (Ed.), *The Social Science of Organizations: Four Perspectives.* Englewood Cliffs, N.J.: Prentice-Hall.

SUCHMAN, E. A. 1967. *Evaluative Research: Principles and Practice in Public Service and Social Action Programs.* New York: Russell Sage Foundation.

TANNENBAUM, A. S. 1962. Control in Organizations: Individual Adjustment and Organizational Performance. *Administrative Science Quarterly*, **7**, 236-237.

TANNENBAUM, A. S. 1966. *Social Psychology of the Work Organizations.* Belmont, Calif.: Wadsworth; London: Tavistock.

TANNENBAUM, A. S. (Ed.), 1968. *Control in Organizations.* New York: McGraw-Hill.

THE HOSPITAL CENTRE. 1966a. The Hospital Internal Communications Project. London: The Hospital Centre. (multilith, THC/66/97).

THE HOSPITAL CENTRE. 1966b. Note by Dr. R. W. Revans: The Intention of the Project. London: The Hospital Centre, Hospital Internal Communications Project. (multilith, THC/66/47).

THELEN, H. A. 1954. *Dynamics of Groups at Work.* New York: Chicago University Press.

THIBAUT, J. W. and KELLEY, H. H. 1959. *The Social Psychology of Groups.* New York: Wiley.

TRIST, E. L. and BAMFORTH, K. W. 1951. Some Social and Psychological Consequences of the Long-wall Method of Coal-getting. *Human Relations,* **4**, 3-38.

UNITED HOSPITAL FUND OF NEW YORK. 1968. *Analysing and Reducing Employee Turnover in Hospitals: A Special Study in Management Practices and Problems.* New York: United Hospital Fund.

URWICK, L. 1956. *The Pattern of Management.* Minneapolis: University of Minnesota Press.

VROOM, V. H. 1960. *Some Personality Determinants of the Effects of Participation.* Englewood Cliffs, N.J.: Prentice-Hall.

VROOM, V. H. 1964. *Work and Motivation.* New York: Wiley.

VROOM, V. H. (Ed.) 1967. *Methods of Organizational Research.* Pittsburgh: University of Pittsburgh Press.

WALTON, R. E. 1969. *Interpersonal Peacemaking: Confrontations and Third-Party Consultation.* Reading, Mass.: Addison-Wesley.

WARNER, W. K. and HAVENS, A. E. 1968. Goal Displacement and the Intangibility of Organizational Goals. *Administrative Science Quarterly,* **12**, 539-555.

WARRINER, C. K. 1965. The Problem of Organizational Purpose. *Sociological Quarterly,* **6**, 139-146.

WATSON, J. P. 1966. Hospital Internal Communications: An Account of the One Month Course. *British Hospital Journal and Social Service Review,* **74**, 116-117.

WEBSTER, B. 1967. Problems of the Admission of Patients. *Nursing Times,* **63**, 885-886.

WEDDELL, D. 1955. Human Relations in Nursing Administration. *Nursing Times,* **55**, 1474-1477. Also in E. Barnes (Ed.), 1968, *Psychosocial Nursing.* London: Tavistock.

WEICK, K. E. 1968. Systematic Observational Methods. In G. Lindzey and E. Aronson (Eds.), *The Handbook of Social Psychology,* **2** (2nd Edition). Reading, Mass.: Addison-Wesley.

WHITTAKER, G. 1965. *T-Group Training: Group Dynamics in Management Education.* Oxford: Blackwell.

WIELAND, G. F. 1965. Organizational Complexity and Coordination. University of Michigan: Doctoral Dissertation.

WIELAND, G. F. 1968a. Evaluating Action-research: Some Psychological Problems. *Revue Internationale de Sociologie,* Série II, **4**, 3-17.

WIELAND, G. F. 1968b. Hospitals and Social Research: a Review of Research Relevant to Management. *World Hospitals,* **4**, 201-205.

WIELAND, G. F. 1969a. The Determinants of Clarity in Organizational Goals. *Human Relations,* **22**, 161-172.

WIELAND, G. F. 1969b. Evaluating the Hospital Internal Communications

Project: the Use of Survey Methods in Evaluation. *International Nursing Review*, **16**, 106-114.

WIELAND, G. F. 1969c. Studying and Measuring Nursing Turnover. *International Journal of Nursing Studies*, **6**, 61-70.

YUCHTMAN, E. and SEASHORE, S. 1967. A System Approach to Organizational Effectiveness. *American Sociological Review*, **32**, 891-903.

ZOLLSCHAN, G. K. and HIRSCH, W. (Eds.), 1964. *Explorations in Social Change*. London: Routledge & Kegan Paul.

ZUCKER, E. and SMITH, D. 1967. Rethinking Medical Social Work. *New Society*, **9**, 462-463.

# *Indexes*

# Author index

# *Subject index*